Virtual Medical Office

for

Proctor: Kinn's The Medical Assistant,
12th Edition

D0534390

Virtual Medical Office

for

Proctor: Kinn's The Medical Assistant, 12th Edition

Study Guide prepared by

Tracie Fuqua, BS, CMA (AAMA)
Program Director
Medical Assistant Program
Wallace State Community College
Hanceville, Alabama

Textbook by

Deborah B. Proctor, EdD, RN
Professor and
Medical Assistant Program Director
Butler County Community College
Butler, Pennsylvania

Alexandra Patricia Adams, MA, BA, RMA, CMA (AAMA)
Former Health Information Specialist
Program Director and
Administrative Medical Assisting Instructor
Ultrasound Diagnostic School
(now Sanford-Brown College)
Professional Writer
Grand Prairie, Texas

Software developed by

Wolfsong Informatics, LLC
Tucson, Arizona

ELSEVIER
SAUNDERS

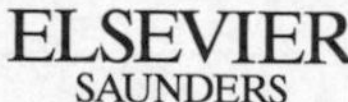

3251 Riverport Lane
Maryland Heights, Missouri 63043

ISBN: 978-0-323-22097-2

VIRTUAL MEDICAL OFFICE FOR
PROCTOR: KINN'S THE MEDICAL ASSISTANT
TWELFTH EDITION
Copyright © 2014, 2011, 2007 by Saunders, an imprint of Elsevier Inc.

All rights reserved. No part of this publication may be reproduced or transmitted in any form or by any means, electronic or mechanical, including photocopying, recording, or any information storage and retrieval system, without permission in writing from the publisher. Permissions may be sought directly from Elsevier's Rights Department: phone: (+1) 215 239 3804 (US) or (+44) 1865 843830 (UK); fax: (+44) 1865 853333; e-mail: healthpermissions@elsevier.com. You may also complete your request on-line via the Elsevier website at http://www.elsevier.com/permissions.

Although for mechanical reasons all pages of this publication are perforated, only those pages imprinted with an Elsevier Inc. copyright notice are intended for removal.

Notice

Knowledge and best practice in this field are constantly changing. As new research and experience broaden our knowledge, changes in practice, treatment and drug therapy may become necessary or appropriate. Readers are advised to check the most current information provided (i) on procedures featured or (ii) by the manufacturer of each product to be administered, to verify the recommended dose or formula, the method and duration of administration, and contraindications. It is the responsibility of the practitioner, relying on their own experience and knowledge of the patient, to make diagnoses, to determine dosages and the best treatment for each individual patient, and to take all appropriate safety precautions. To the fullest extent of the law, neither the Publisher nor the Authors assumes any liability for any injury and/or damage to persons or property arising out or related to any use of the material contained in this book.

ISBN: 978-0-323-22097-2

Executive Content Strategist: Jennifer Janson
Content Development Strategist: Karen Baer
Publishing Services Manager: Debbie Vogel
Project Manager: Pat Costigan

Printed in the United States of America

Last digit is the print number: 9 8 7 6 5 4 3 2 1

Working together to grow
libraries in developing countries

www.elsevier.com | www.bookaid.org | www.sabre.org

ELSEVIER BOOK AID International Sabre Foundation

Table of Contents

GETTING STARTED

The product you have purchased is part of the Evolve Learning System. Please read the following information thoroughly to get started.

HOW TO ACCESS YOUR VMO RESOURCES ON EVOLVE

There are two ways to access your VMO Resources on Evolve:

1. If your instructor has enrolled you in your VMO Evolve Resources, you will receive an email with your registration details.

2. If your instructor has asked you to self-enroll in your VMO Evolve Resources, he or she will provide you with your Course ID (for example, 1479_jdoe73_0001). You will then need to follow the instructions at https://evolve.elsevier.com/cs/studentEnroll.html.

HOW TO ACCESS THE ONLINE VIRTUAL MEDICAL OFFICE

The Virtual Medical Office simulation is available through the Evolve VMO Resources. There is no software to download or install: the Virtual Medical Office simulation runs within your Internet browser, directly linked from the Evolve site.

HOW TO ACCESS THE WORKBOOK

There are two ways to access the workbook portion of *Virtual Medical Office:*

1. Print workbook
2. An electronic version of the workbook, available within the VMO Evolve Resources

TECHNICAL SUPPORT

Technical support for *Virtual Medical Office* is available by visiting the Technical Support Center at http://evolvesupport.elsevier.com or by calling 1-800-222-9570 inside the United States and Canada.

Copyright © 2014, 2011, 2007 by Saunders, an imprint of Elsevier Inc. All rights reserved.

GETTING SET UP

TECHNICAL REQUIREMENTS

To use an Evolve Online Product, you will need access to a computer that is connected to the Internet and equipped with web browser software that supports frames. For optimal performance, it is recommended that you have speakers and use a high-speed Internet connection. Dial-up modems are not recommended for *Virtual Medical Office*.

Windows®

Windows PC
Windows XP, Windows Vista™
Pentium® processor (or equivalent) @ 1 GHz (Recommend 2 GHz or better)
800 x 600 screen size
Thousands of colors
Soundblaster 16 soundcard compatibility
Stereo speakers or headphones
Internet Explorer (IE) version 6.0 or higher
Mozilla Firefox version 2.0 or higher

Macintosh®

Mozilla Firefox version 2.0 or higher

WEB BROWSERS

Supported web browsers include Microsoft Internet Explorer (IE) version 6.0 or higher and Mozilla Firefox version 2.0 or higher.

Copyright © 2014, 2011, 2007 by Saunders, an imprint of Elsevier Inc. All rights reserved.

SCREEN SETTINGS

For best results, your computer monitor resolution should be set at a minimum of 800 x 600. The number of colors displayed should be set to "thousands or higher" (High Color or 16 bit) or "millions of colors" (True Color or 24 bit).

WINDOWS

1. From the **Start** menu, select **Settings**, then **Control Panel**.
2. Double-click on the **Display** icon.
3. Click on the **Settings** tab.
4. Under **Screen resolution** use the slider bar to select **800 x 600 pixels**.
5. Access the **Colors** drop-down menu by clicking on the down arrow.
6. Select **High Color (16 bit)** or **True Color (24 bit)**.
7. Click on **Apply**, then **OK**.
8. You may be asked to verify the setting changes. Click **Yes**.
9. You may be asked to restart your computer to accept the changes. Click **Yes**.

MACINTOSH

1. Select the **Monitors** control panel.
2. Select **800 x 600** (or greater) from the **Resolution** area.
3. Select **Thousands** or **Millions** from the **Color Depth** area.

Copyright © 2014, 2011, 2007 by Saunders, an imprint of Elsevier Inc. All rights reserved.

Enable Cookies

Browser	Steps
Internet Explorer (IE) 6.0 or higher	**1.** Select **Tools → Internet Options**. **2.** Select **Privacy** tab. **3.** Use the slider (slide down) to **Accept All Cookies**. **4.** Click **OK**. **-OR-** **3.** Click the **Advanced** button. **4.** Click the check box next to **Override Automatic Cookie Handling**. **5.** Click the **Accept** radio buttons under **First-party Cookies** and **Third-party Cookies**. **6.** Click **OK**.
Mozilla Firefox 2.0 or higher	**1.** Select **Tools → Options**. **2.** Select the **Privacy** icon. **3.** Click to expand Cookies. **4.** Select **Allow sites to set cookies**. **5.** Click **OK**.

Set Cache to Always Reload a Page

Browser	Steps
Internet Explorer (IE) 6.0 or higher	**1.** Select **Tools → Internet Options**. **2.** Select **General** tab. **3.** Go to the **Temporary Internet Files** and click the **Settings** button. **4.** Select the radio button for **Every visit to the page** and click **OK** when complete.
Mozilla Firefox 2.0 or higher	**1.** Select **Tools → Options**. **2.** Select the **Privacy** icon. **3.** Click to expand Cache. **4.** Set the value to "**0**" in the **Use up to: __ MB of disk space for the cache** field. **5.** Click **OK**.

Copyright © 2014, 2011, 2007 by Saunders, an imprint of Elsevier Inc. All rights reserved.

Plug-Ins

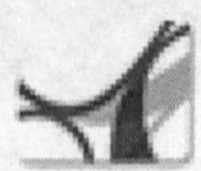

Adobe Acrobat Reader—With the free Acrobat Reader software, you can view and print Adobe PDF files. Many Evolve products offer student and instructor manuals, checklists, and more in this format!

Download at: http://www.adobe.com

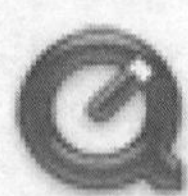

Apple QuickTime—Install this to hear word pronunciations, heart and lung sounds, and many other helpful audio clips within Evolve Online Courses!

Download at: http://www.apple.com

Adobe Flash Player—This player will enhance your viewing of many Evolve web pages, as well as educational short-form to long-form animation within the Evolve Learning System!

Download at: http://www.adobe.com

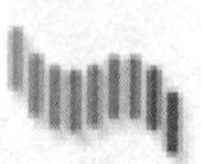

Adobe Shockwave Player—Shockwave is best for viewing the many interactive learning activities within Evolve Online Courses!

Download at: http://www.adobe.com

Microsoft Word Viewer—With this viewer Microsoft Word users can share documents with those who don't have Word, and users without Word can open and view Word documents. Many Evolve products have testbank, student and instructor manuals, and other documents available for downloading and viewing on your own computer!

Download at: http://www.microsoft.com

Copyright © 2014, 2011, 2007 by Saunders, an imprint of Elsevier Inc. All rights reserved.

Quick Office Tour

Welcome to *Virtual Medical Office*, a virtual office setting in which you can work with multiple patient simulations and also learn to access and evaluate the information resources that are essential for providing high-quality medical assistance.

In the virtual medical office, Mountain View Clinic, you can access the Reception area, Exam Room, Laboratory, Office Manager, and Check Out area, plus a separate room for Billing and Coding.

■ BEFORE YOU START

Make sure you have your textbook nearby when you use *Virtual Medical Office* online. You will want to consult topic areas in your textbook frequently while working online and using this study guide.

■ HOW TO SIGN IN

- After entering the access code included inside this study guide, enter your name on the Medical Assistant identification badge.
- Click on **Start Simulation**.

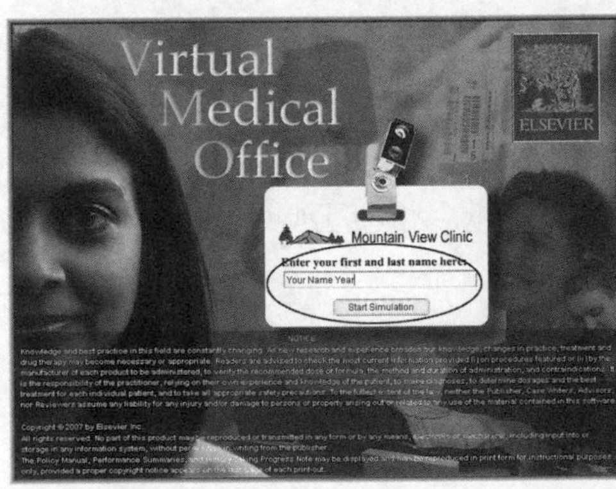

Copyright © 2014, 2011, 2007 by Saunders, an imprint of Elsevier Inc. All rights reserved.

- This takes you to the office map screen. Across the top of this screen is the list of patients available for you to follow throughout their office visit.

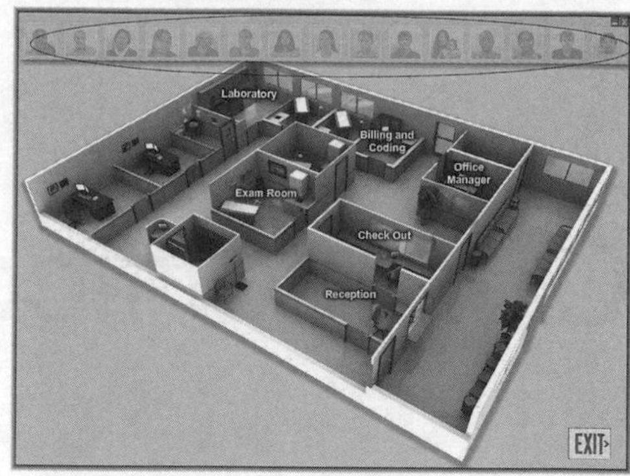

PATIENT LIST

1. **Janet Jones (age 50)**—Ms. Jones has sustained an on-the-job injury. She is in pain and impatient. By working with Ms. Jones, students will learn about managing difficult patients, as well as the requirements involved in workers' compensation cases.

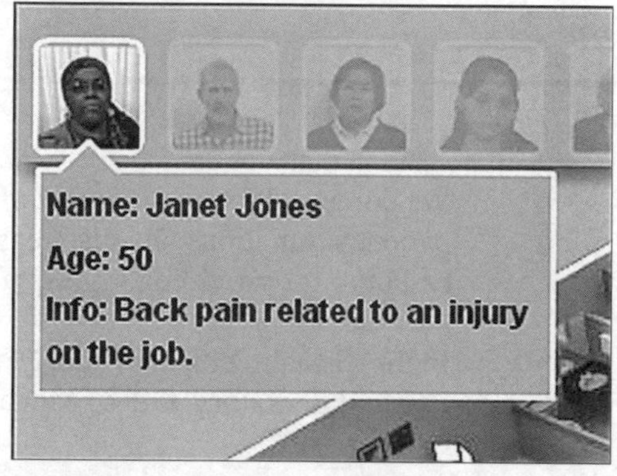

2. **Wilson Metcalf (age 65)**—A Medicare patient, Mr. Metcalf is being seen for multiple symptoms of abdominal pain, nausea, vomiting, and fever. He is seriously ill and might need more specialized care in a hospital setting.

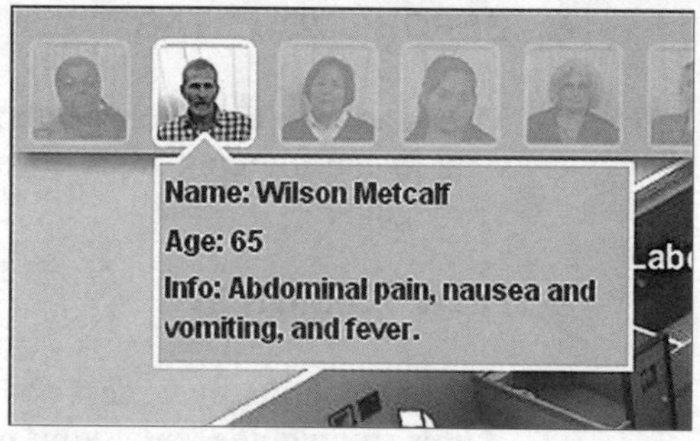

3. **Rhea Davison (age 53)**—An established patient with chronic and multiple symptoms, Ms. Davison does not have medical insurance.

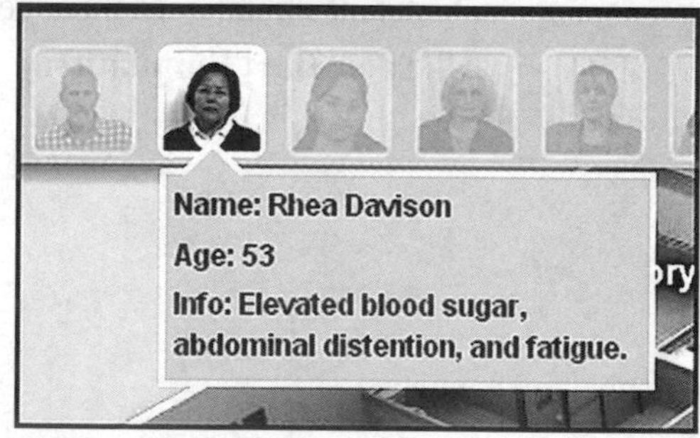

Copyright © 2014, 2011, 2007 by Saunders, an imprint of Elsevier Inc. All rights reserved.

4. **Shaunti Begay (age 15)**—A new patient, Shaunti Begay is a minor who has an appointment for a sports physical. Upon arrival, Shaunti and her family learn that Mountain View Clinic does not participate in their health insurance.

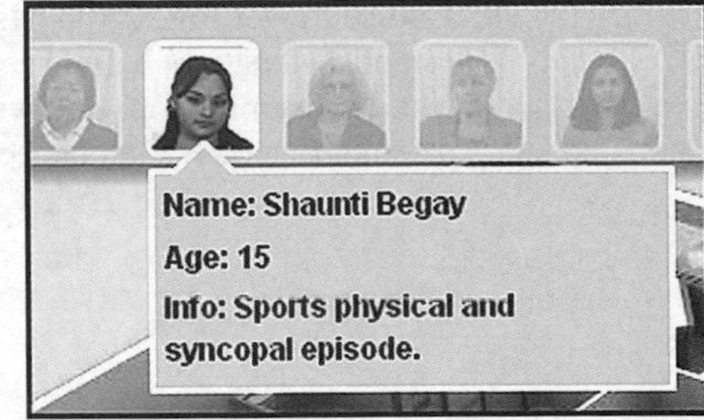

5. **Jean Deere (age 83)**—Accompanied by her son, Ms. Deere is an established Medicare patient being evaluated for memory loss and hearing loss.

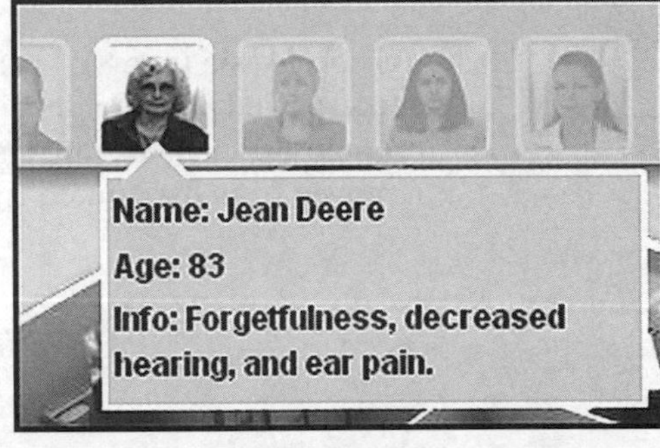

6. **Renee Anderson (age 43)**—Ms. Anderson scheduled her appointment for a routine gynecological examination but exhibits symptoms that suggest she is a victim of domestic violence.

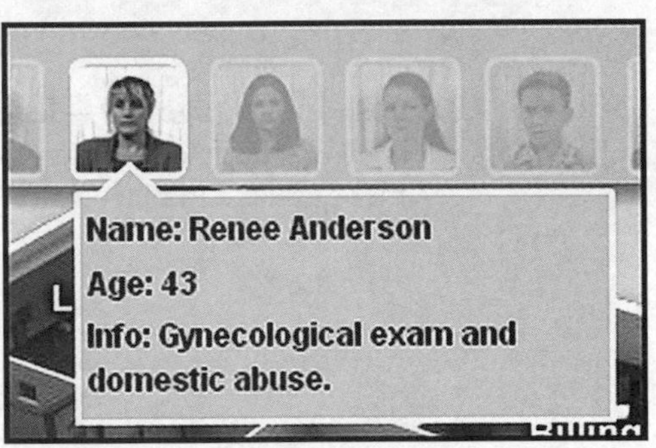

7. **Teresa Hernandez (age 16)**—Teresa is a minor patient who is unaccompanied by a parent for her appointment. She is seeking contraceptive counseling and STD testing.

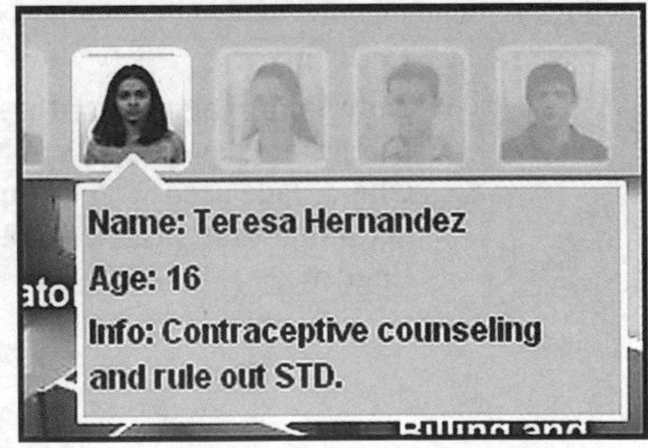

Copyright © 2014, 2011, 2007 by Saunders, an imprint of Elsevier Inc. All rights reserved.

8. **Louise Parlet (age 24)**—Ms. Parlet is an established patient being seen for a pregnancy test and examination. She will also need to be referred to an OB/GYN specialist.

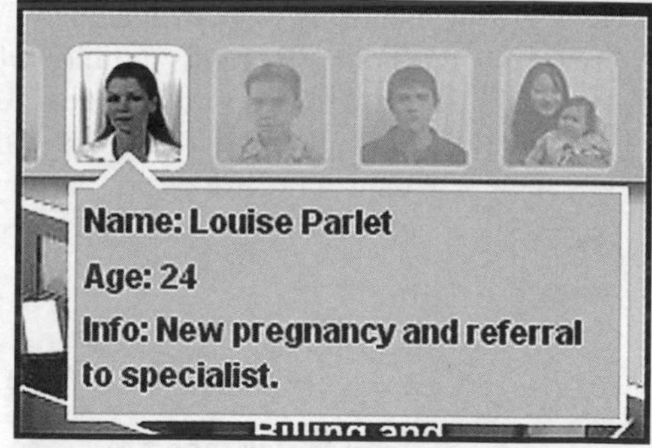

9. **Tristan Tsosie (age 8)**—A minor patient accompanied by his older sister and younger brother, Tristan is having a splint and sutures removed from his injured right arm.

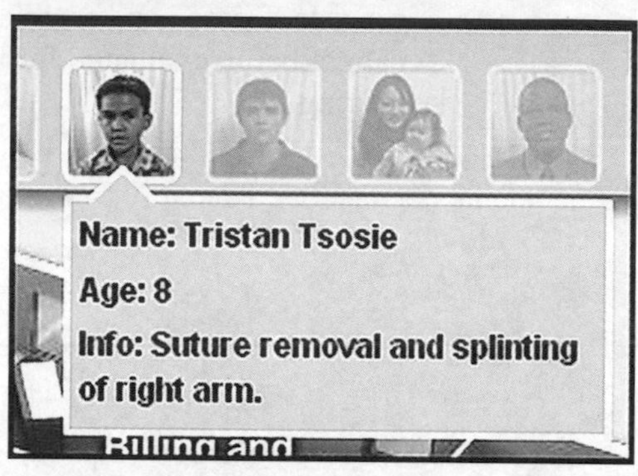

10. **Jose Imero (age 16)**—Jose is a minor patient who is scheduled for an emergency appointment to have the laceration on his foot sutured.

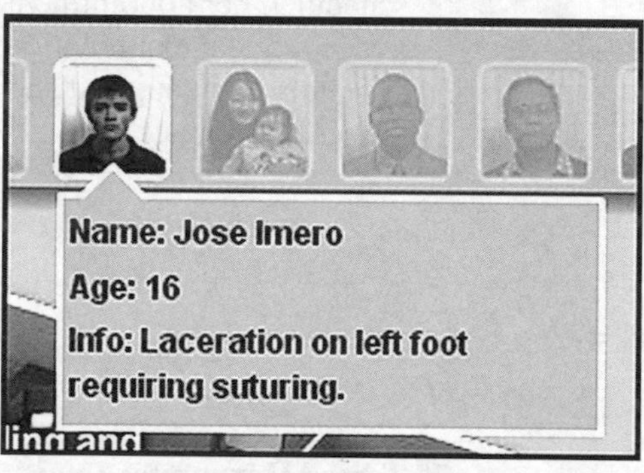

11. **Jade Wong (age 7 months)**—Jade and her parents are new patients to Mountain View Clinic. Jade needs a checkup and updates to her immunizations. Her mother does not speak English.

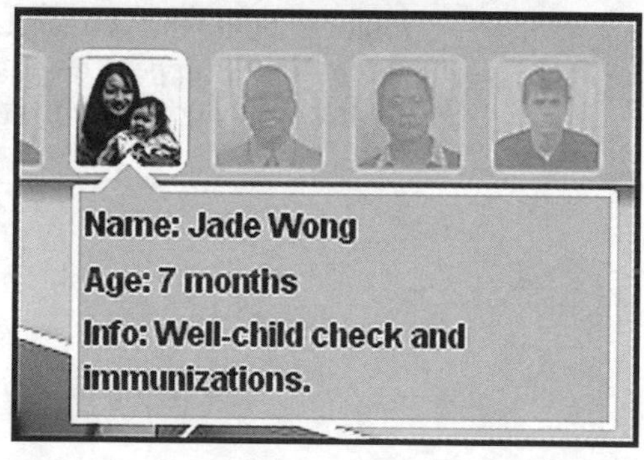

Copyright © 2014, 2011, 2007 by Saunders, an imprint of Elsevier Inc. All rights reserved.

12. **John R. Simmons (age 43)**—Dr. Simmons is a new patient with a history of high blood pressure and recent episodes of blood in his urine.

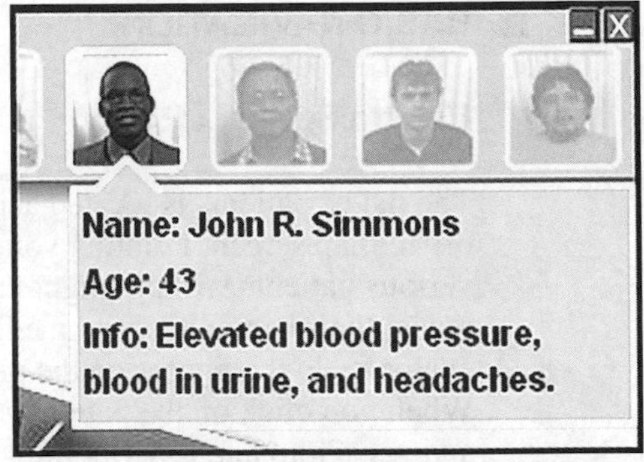

13. **Hu Huang (age 67)**—Mr. Huang developed a severe cough and fever after returning from a recent trip to Asia.

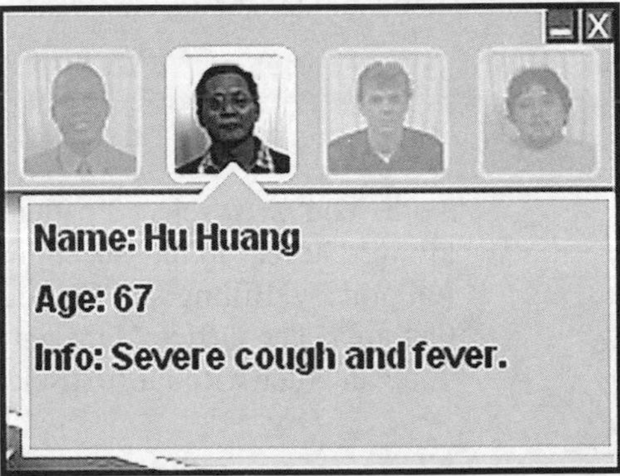

14. **Kevin McKinzie (age 18)**—Mr. McKinzie has made an appointment because of his nausea and vomiting. He is insured through the restaurant where he works.

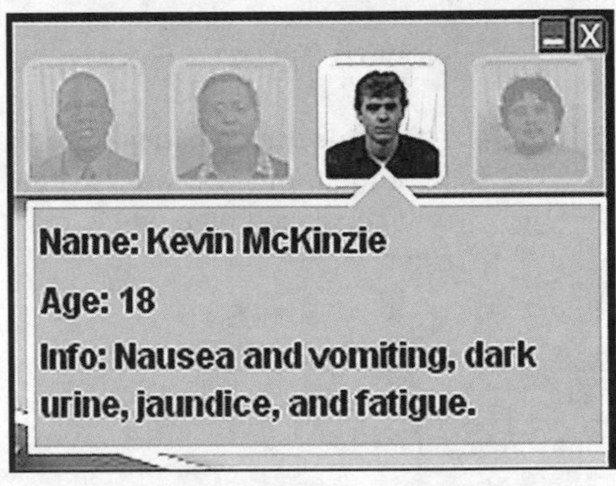

15. **Jesus Santo (age 32)**—Mr. Santo has been brought to the office as a walk-in appointment by his employer for leg pain and a fever. He has no insurance or identification, but his employer has offered to pay for the visit.

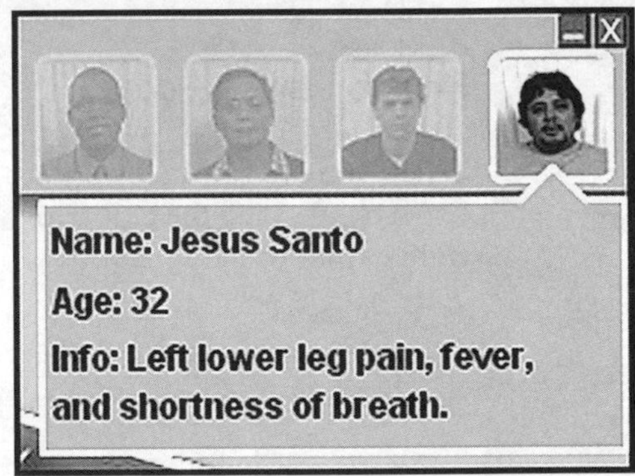

Copyright © 2014, 2011, 2007 by Saunders, an imprint of Elsevier Inc. All rights reserved.

BASIC NAVIGATION

How to Select a Patient

The list of patients is located across the top of the office map screen. Pointing your cursor at the various patients will highlight their photo and reveal their name, age, and medical problem (see examples in the photos on the previous pages). When you click on the patient you wish to review, a larger photo and description will appear in the lower left corner of the screen.

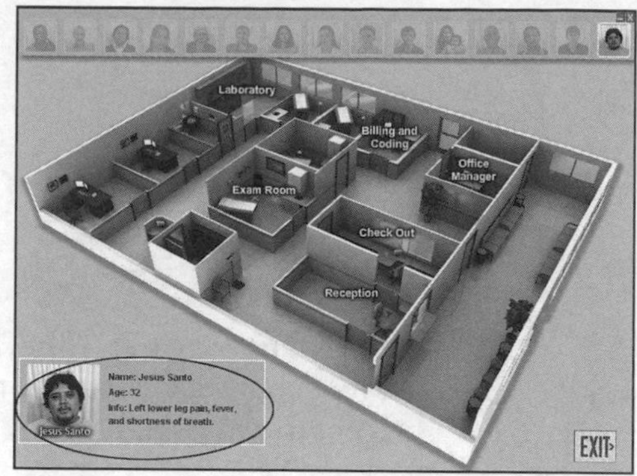

Note: You ***must*** select a patient before you are allowed access to the Reception area, Exam Room, Laboratory, Billing and Coding office, or Check Out area. The Office Manager area is the only room you can enter without first selecting a patient.

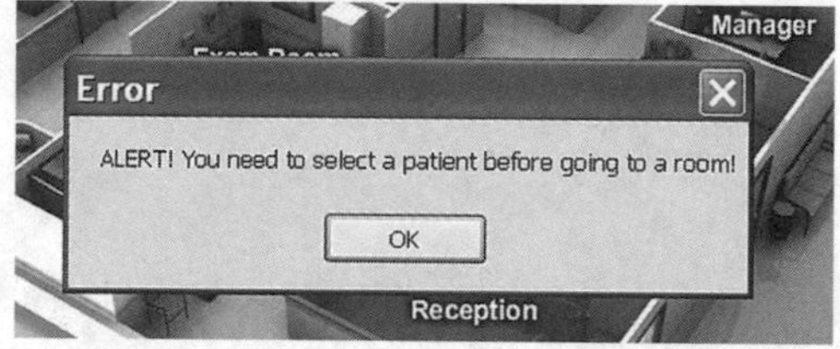

How to Select a Room

After selecting a patient, use your cursor to highlight the room you want to enter. The active room will be shaded blue on the map. Click to enter the room.

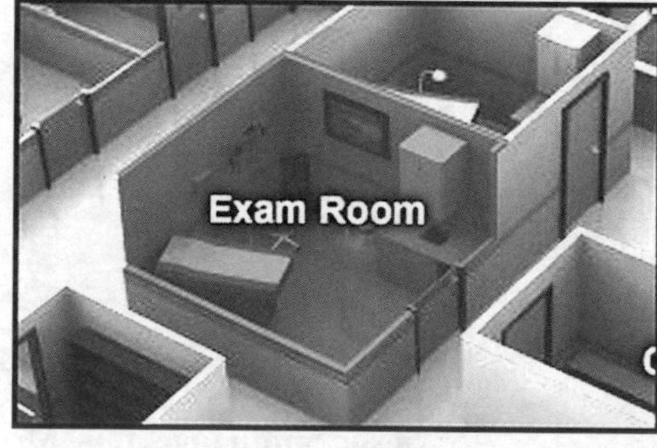

How to Leave a Room

When you are finished working in a room, you can leave by clicking the exit arrow found at the bottom right corner of the screen.

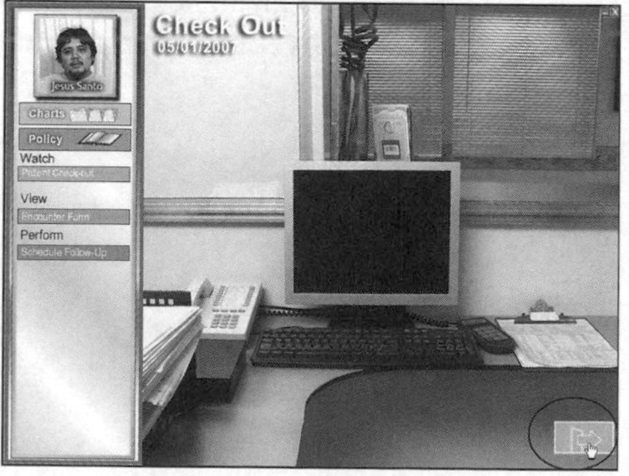

Copyright © 2014, 2011, 2007 by Saunders, an imprint of Elsevier Inc. All rights reserved.

Leaving a room will automatically take you to the Summary Menu.

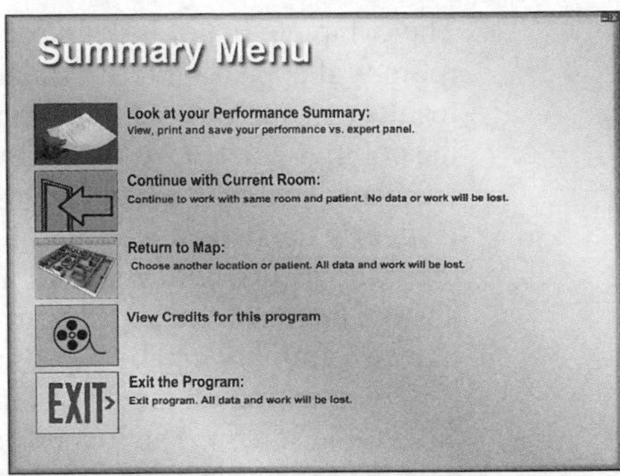

From the Summary Menu, you can choose to:

- **Look at Your Performance Summary**
  In each room there are interactive wizards or tasks that can be completed. The Performance Summary lets you compare your answers with those of the experts.
- **Continue with Current Room**
  This takes you back to the last room in which you worked. This option is not available if you have already reviewed your Performance Summary.
- **Return to Map**
  This reopens the office map for you to select another room and/or another patient.
- **View Credits for This Program**
  This provides a complete listing of software developers, publisher, and authors.
- **Exit the Program**
  This closes the *Virtual Medical Office* software. You will need to sign in again before you can use the program.

How to Use the Performance Summary

If you completed any of the interactive wizards in a room, you can compare your answers with those of the experts by accessing your Performance Summary. The Performance Summary is not a grading tool, although it is valuable for self-assessment and review.

From the Summary Menu, click on **Look at Your Performance Summary**.

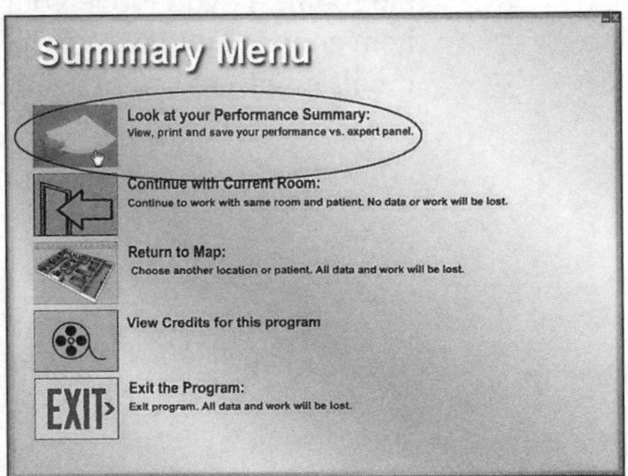

Copyright © 2014, 2011, 2007 by Saunders, an imprint of Elsevier Inc. All rights reserved.

The complete list of tasks associated with the active room will appear with two columns showing the results of your choices. Your answers will appear in the column labeled **Your Performance**, and the answers chosen by the expert will appear in the **Expert's Performance** column. A check mark in the same box in both columns indicates that your answer matched the expert's answer. The Performance Summary can be saved to your computer or disk by clicking on the disk icon at the upper right side of the screen. The saved file can be printed or emailed to your instructor. A hard copy can also be printed without saving by clicking on the printer icon at the upper right corner of the screen.

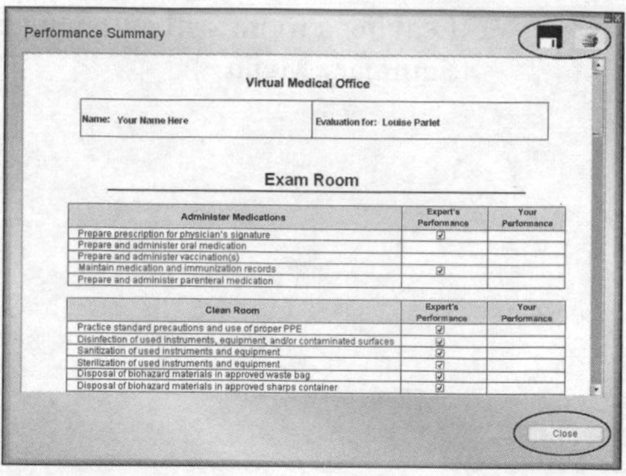

Administer Medications	Expert's Performance	Your Performance
Prepare prescription for physician's signature	☑	
Prepare and administer oral medication		
Prepare and administer vaccination(s)		
Maintain medication and immunization records	☑	
Prepare and administer parenteral medication		

Clean Room	Expert's Performance	Your Performance
Practice standard precautions and use of proper PPE	☑	
Disinfection of used instruments, equipment, and/or contaminated surfaces	☑	
Sanitization of used instruments and equipment	☑	
Sterilization of used instruments and equipment	☑	
Disposal of biohazard materials in approved waste bag	☑	
Disposal of biohazard materials in approved sharps container	☑	

■ ROOM DESCRIPTIONS

Each room can be entered at any time in any order. You can follow a patient's visit from Reception to Check Out, or you can choose to observe each patient at any point in their care. Below is a description of the information and activities that can be found in various rooms.

ALL ROOMS

- In all rooms you can access the patient's medical record and the office Policy Manual.
- In all rooms in which there are interactive tasks to be completed, you can select tasks or features from the menu on the left of the screen, as shown on this sample of the menu in the Reception area.

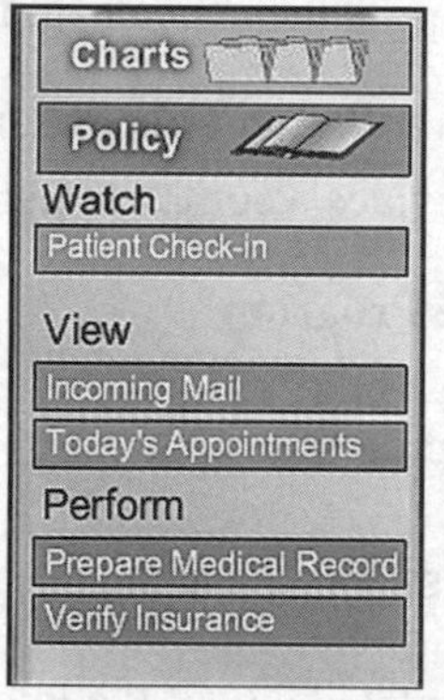

- As an alternative to using the menu, you can click on the corresponding items in the photo of the room. As you move your cursor over each item connected to one of the tasks on the menu, it will highlight and become active.

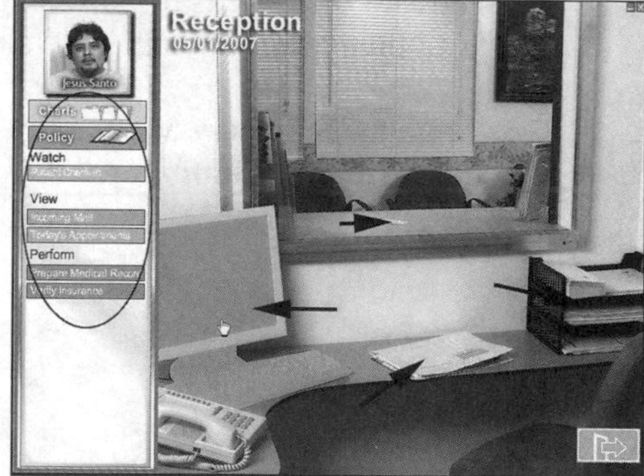

Copyright © 2014, 2011, 2007 by Saunders, an imprint of Elsevier Inc. All rights reserved.

RECEPTION

In the Reception area, you can choose:

- **Charts**—Look at the patient's chart. *Note:* For new patients, there will be no information available in the chart at this time, although you do have the option of assembling a new medical record.
- **Policy**—Open the office Policy Manual and review the established administrative, clinical, and laboratory policies for Mountain View Clinic. Within the Policy Manual you will also find the Coding and Billing Manual.
- **Watch**—Watch a video of the patient's arrival. Each patient is shown checking in at the front desk so that you can observe the procedures typically performed by the receptionist and consider some of the various problems that might arise.
- **Incoming Mail**—Look at the incoming mail for the day. Mountain View Clinic has received a wide range of correspondence that must be read and responded to accordingly.
- **Today's Appointments**—Review the appointment schedule for the day. You can check the schedule to find out what time patients are supposed to arrive, the reason for their visit, and how much time the physician will need for the examination.
- **Prepare Medical Record**—Practice preparing the medical record. This interactive feature allows you to build a medical record for a new patient or update information for an established patient.
- **Verify Insurance**—Verify a patient's insurance. Also interactive, this feature allows you to ask patients about the status of their insurance and to view their insurance cards.

EXAM ROOM

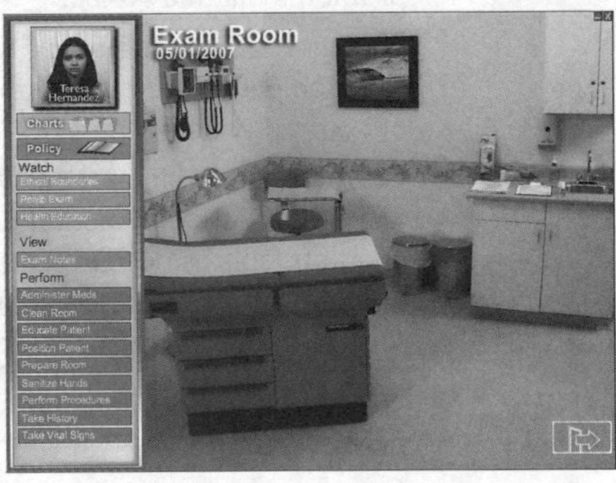

- **Charts** and **Policy**—Access the patient's chart and the office Policy Manual.
- **Watch**—View video clips of different parts of the patient's examination. Observe the actions of the medical assistants in the videos and critique the competencies demonstrated.
- **Exam Notes**—Review the physician's documented findings for the current visit. These notes are added to the full Progress Notes in the patient's chart as the patient continues on to Check Out.
- **Perform**—Perform multiple tasks that are required of a clinical medical assistant, such as preparing the room for the examination, taking vital signs and patient history, and properly positioning the patient for an examination.

Copyright © 2014, 2011, 2007 by Saunders, an imprint of Elsevier Inc. All rights reserved.

Laboratory

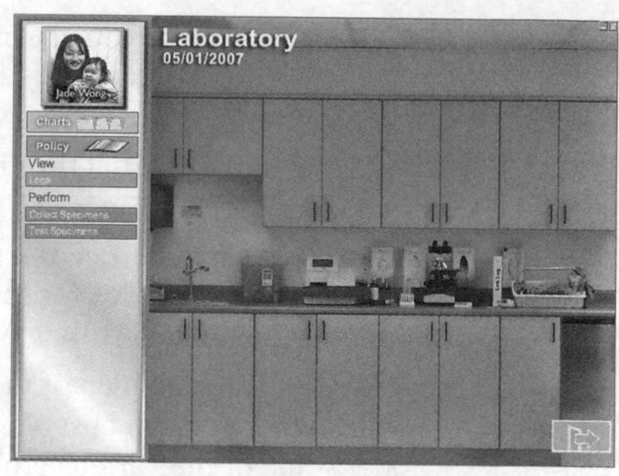

- **Charts** and **Policy**—Access the patient's chart and the office Policy Manual.
- **View: Logs**—View the laboratory's log of specimens sent out for testing. Opportunities to practice filling out laboratory logs are included in the workbook exercises.
- **Perform**—Perform specific tasks as needed in the laboratory, such as collecting and testing specimens. These interactive wizards walk you through the steps for collecting and testing specimens ordered by the physician as part of the patient's examination. The Progress Notes are available throughout so that you can review the physician's directions.

Check Out

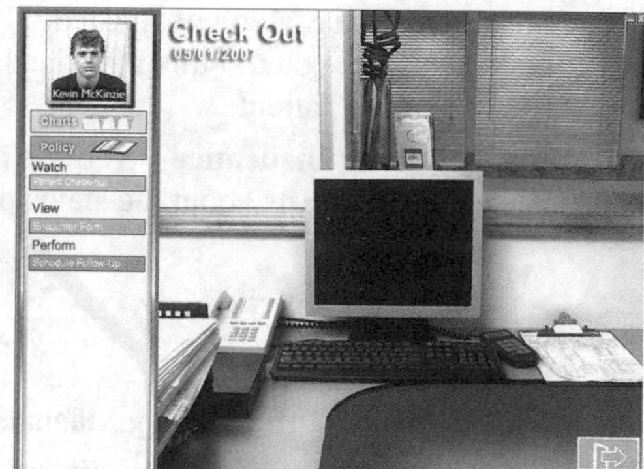

- **Charts** and **Policy**—Access the patient's chart and the office Policy Manual.
- **Watch**—Watch a video clip of the patient checking out of the office at the end of the visit. Observe the administrative medical assistants as they schedule follow-up appointments, accept payments, and manage the various duties and problems that may arise.
- **View**—Look at the Encounter Form completed for each patient and verify that the form is filled out correctly and completely.
- **Perform**—Certain patients will require a return visit to the office. Schedule their follow-up appointments as needed. Opportunities to work with the appointment book and additional scheduling tasks are included in the study guide.

Billing and Coding

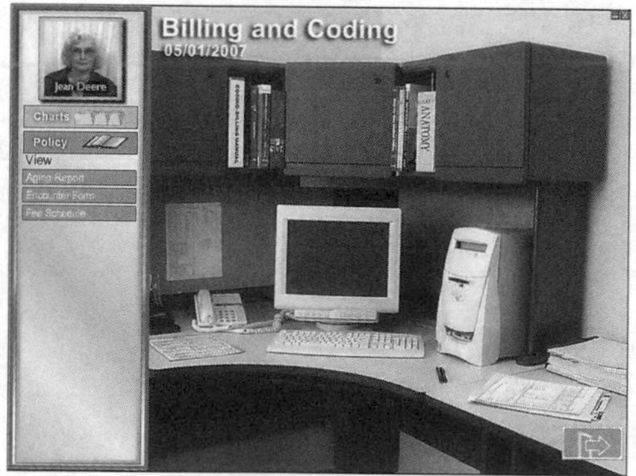

- **View: Aging Report**—Review the outstanding balances on various patient accounts and assess when to implement different collection techniques.
- **View: Encounter Form**—Review the patient's Encounter Form and determine whether the proper procedures were followed to ensure accurate billing and coding.
- **View: Fee Schedule**—Review the office's fee schedule to calculate the proper charges for the patient's visit.

Copyright © 2014, 2011, 2007 by Saunders, an imprint of Elsevier Inc. All rights reserved.

OFFICE MANAGER

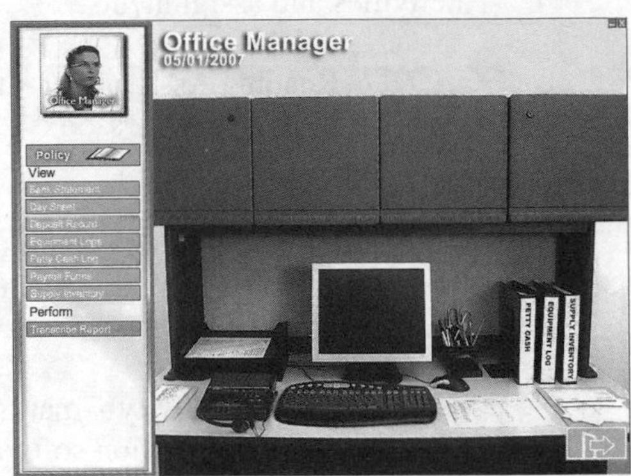

- **Policy**—View the office Policy Manual. Note that patient charts are not available from the manager's office, and there is no need to select a patient to enter the Office Manager area.
- **View**—A variety of financial and administrative documents are available for viewing in the manager's office. Banking deposits and payments can be tracked through these documents, and opportunities to practice managing office finances are included in the study guide.
- **Perform: Transcribe Report**—A recorded medical report is included for transcription practice with full player controls.

EMBEDDED ERRORS

The individual lessons and patient scenarios associated with the *Virtual Medical Office* program were designed to stimulate critical thinking and analytical skills and to help develop the competencies on which you will be tested on as part of your course work. Thus deliberate errors have been embedded into each of the 15 patient scenarios and in the Billing and Coding and Office Manager activities. Many of the exercises in the study guide draw attention to these errors so that you can work through how and why a correction needs to be made. Other errors have not been specifically addressed, and you may discover them as you work through the various rooms and tasks. Instructors and students alike are encouraged to use any errors they find to further develop the essential critical thinking and decision-making skills needed for the clinical office.

Copyright © 2014, 2011, 2007 by Saunders, an imprint of Elsevier Inc. All rights reserved.

The following icons are used throughout the study guide to help you quickly identify particular activities and assignments:

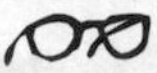 Reading Assignment—tells you which textbook chapter(s) you should read before starting each lesson

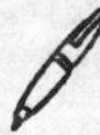 Writing Activity—certain activities focus on written responses such as filling out forms or completing documentation

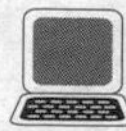 Online Activity—marks the beginning of an activity that uses the *Virtual Medical Office* simulation software

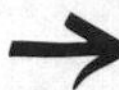 Online Instructions—indicates the steps to follow as you navigate through the software

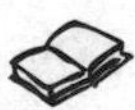 Reference—indicates questions and activities that require you to consult your textbook

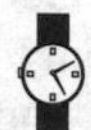 Time—indicates the approximate amount of time needed to complete the exercise

Copyright © 2014, 2011, 2007 by Saunders, an imprint of Elsevier Inc. All rights reserved.

LESSON 1

Performing Professional Duties

Reading Assignment: Chapter 3—The Medical Assisting Profession
Chapter 4—Professional Behavior in the Workplace
Chapter 5—Interpersonal Skills and Human Behavior

Patient: Rhea Davison

Note: The first exercise does not involve Rhea Davison, but you must choose a patient to access the clinic rooms. We have selected Rhea Davison because she will be your patient later in this lesson.

Learning Objectives:

- Describe the necessary documentation of licensure and accreditation.
- Recognize the need for confidentiality and HIPAA regulations.
- Prepare a travel itinerary for a physician who will be speaking at the national American Association of Medical Assistants (AAMA) conference.
- Locate resources and information for the employer.
- Understand different credentials medical assistants may obtain.

Overview:

In this lesson you will prepare documentation needed for assisting the physician in various areas related to office policies and the physician's professional needs. The ethical and legal aspects of confidentiality are addressed. The Internet will be used to research travel arrangements for a conference one of the physicians needs to attend.

Copyright © 2014, 2011, 2007 by Saunders, an imprint of Elsevier Inc. All rights reserved.

Exercise 1

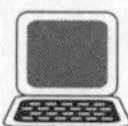

Online Activity—Maintaining Licensure and Credentials

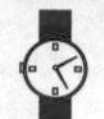

15 minutes

- Sign in to Mountain View Clinic.
- Select **Rhea Davison** from the patient list.
- Click on **Reception**.
- Under the Watch heading, click on **Patient Check-In** and watch the video.

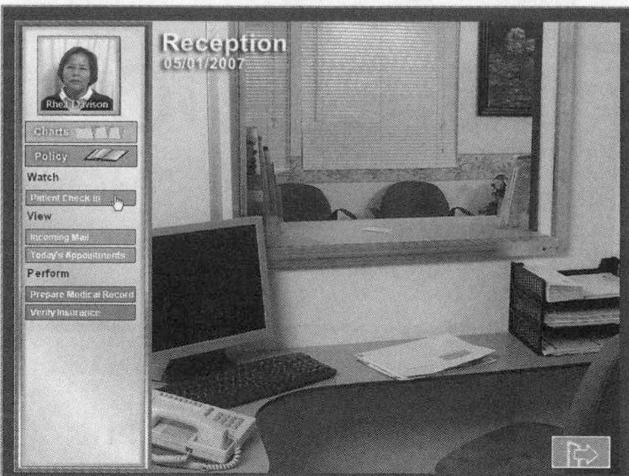

In the video, the medical assistant discusses the CMA (AAMA) credential. However, the RMA is another credential that is recognized on a national level. (*Note:* The CMA credential must now be written as CMA (AAMA) to be distinguished from other CMA credentials that are not Certified Medical Assisting Credentials.)

1. Look up the CMA (AAMA) and RMA credentials and name the organizations that award these credentials. What did you find?

2. Research your state to see if there are any state or regional examinations or credentials awarded by area or region.

Copyright © 2014, 2011, 2007 by Saunders, an imprint of Elsevier Inc. All rights reserved.

3. On arrival this morning, Dr. Meyer states that you need to check on the status of her renewed medical license because it has not arrived. She reminds you that her current license expires on June 1. Go to the Internet and find the name and address of the medical examining board for the state in which you live. Also find the time limit for medical licensure and any necessary components for renewal of the license. Print your findings for your instructor.

4. What are some other credentials medical assistants may obtain?

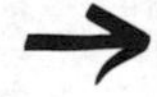

- Click the **X** on the video screen to close the video.
- Remain in the Reception area with Rhea Davison as your patient to continue to the next exercise.

Exercise 2

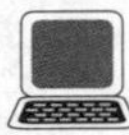

Online Activity—Maintaining Confidentiality and Explaining Office Policy to the Patient

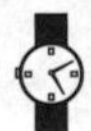

40 minutes

1. Ms. Davison is an established patient. Did Kristin handle Ms. Davison's late arrival in a professional manner? Explain your answer.

Copyright © 2014, 2011, 2007 by Saunders, an imprint of Elsevier Inc. All rights reserved.

2. Would you have expected Ms. Davison to be upset if her appointment had to be rescheduled?

3. What was your feeling about Kristin and the issue of confidentiality just before the arrival of the office manager?

4. The office manager appeared to be upset with Ms. Davison. However, do you think she was more upset with Ms. Davison or with her employee Kristin? Explain your answer.

5. The office manager explained the need to follow HIPAA policy and the need for confidentiality of medical records. How do you feel about the attitude of the office manager while discussing the matter of confidentiality?

Copyright © 2014, 2011, 2007 by Saunders, an imprint of Elsevier Inc. All rights reserved.

6. Why does the office manager need to explain the HIPAA policy in such a specific manner?

- Click the exit arrow.
- Click **Return to Map**, then click **Yes** at the pop-up menu to return to the office map or click **Exit the Program**.

Exercise 3

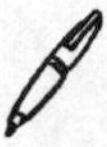

Writing Activity—Obtaining Travel Itineraries and Locating Information for the Physician

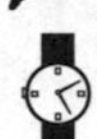

90 minutes

1. Prepare and provide a travel itinerary for one of the physicians at Mountain View Clinic, following these steps:
   a. Using the Internet as your tool, make travel arrangements for Dr. Meyer to attend the next American Association of Medical Assistants (AAMA) Conference. Dr. Meyer is scheduled to speak on Saturday afternoon at 4 p.m. and would like to arrive at the airport by noon that day. She plans to spend one night and would like a return flight on Sunday arriving no later than 7 p.m.
   b. Decide on the best flight to meet Dr. Meyer's needs from your site (your geographic location) of practice. Record the fare, times of departure and arrival, and any special identification or security requirements.
   c. Make arrangements for Dr. Meyer at the hotel where the conference is being held, showing the room fee including taxes. Make a notation of the check-in time and the check-out time at the hotel.
   d. Finally, arrange for land transportation for Dr. Meyer from the airport to the hotel and back to the airport. Some hotels have a complimentary shuttle or can recommend a shuttle company. You can also check the price of renting a car or the approximate cost for taxi service.

Copyright © 2014, 2011, 2007 by Saunders, an imprint of Elsevier Inc. All rights reserved.

2. Travel restrictions and requirements change frequently, particularly for travel outside of the United States. Using the Internet as a resource, locate websites that provide updated information on security, restrictions, and requirements for travelers.

3. Dr. Meyer is scheduled to present a speech on sleep apnea at the conference. She asks you to consult the Internet and find five links she can use as information resources as she prepares her speech. What did you find?

(1)

(2)

(3)

(4)

(5)

Copyright © 2014, 2011, 2007 by Saunders, an imprint of Elsevier Inc. All rights reserved.

LESSON **2**

Telephone Techniques

Reading Assignment: Chapter 5—Interpersonal Skills and Human Behavior
• The Process of Communication
Chapter 9—Telephone Techniques

Patients: Louise Parlet, Wilson Metcalf

Learning Objectives:

- Describe how nonverbal and verbal communication are apparent when using the telephone.
- Understand the need for ethical and legal behavior on the telephone.
- Identify ways to ensure confidentiality when using the telephone in the medical office.
- Manage telephone calls professionally while handling other administrative duties.

Overview:

In this lesson the legal and ethical issues related to the use of the telephone will be discussed. Issues of confidentiality when using the phone to make arrangements for transfer of a patient to an inpatient facility will also be covered. Proper telephone techniques are important in setting the mood for the entire office. This lesson is designed to provide basic understanding of these techniques.

Copyright © 2014, 2011, 2007 by Saunders, an imprint of Elsevier Inc. All rights reserved.

Exercise 1

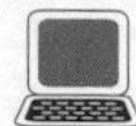

Online Activity—Proper Use of the Telephone in the Medical Office

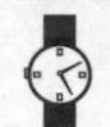

40 minutes

- Sign in to Mountain View Clinic.
- Select **Louise Parlet** from the patient list.
- Click on **Reception**.
- Under the Watch heading, click on **Patient Check-In** and watch the video.

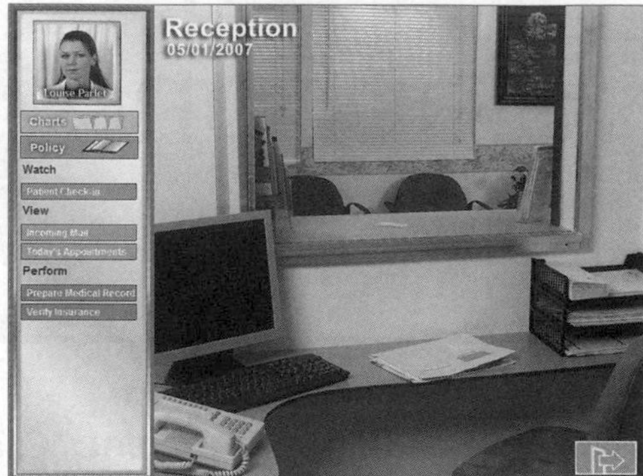

1. As Kristin answers the phone, how does she identify herself? Was her identification a correct procedure? Why or why not?

2. What nonverbal communication does Kristin convey when she answers the phone?

3. Kristin did not close the privacy window while talking on the telephone. Was this a break in confidentiality? Why or why not?

4. When should the privacy window be closed when the medical assistant is on the telephone?

Copyright © 2014, 2011, 2007 by Saunders, an imprint of Elsevier Inc. All rights reserved.

5. Kristin said "Please excuse me" so that she could answer the telephone. When she completed the phone call, she apologized for the interruption. Was this a proper telephone technique? Give a reason for your answer.

6. What was your opinion about the way the sales representative behaved while Ms. Parlet was at the counter?

7. Could Kristin have handled the sales representative's intrusion into their conversation in a more sensitive way from Ms. Parlet's perspective?

8. Assume that Kristin is engaged in a phone call that involves personal information about the medical condition of a patient. How can she determine whether she is communicating with a person to whom she can legally and ethically release the information?

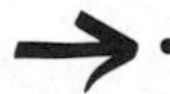

- Click the **X** on the video screen to close the video.
- Click the exit arrow.
- Click **Return to Map** and select **Yes** at the pop-up menu to return to the office map.
- Select **Wilson Metcalf** from the patient list.
- Click on **Check Out**.
- Under the Watch heading, click on **Patient Check-Out** and watch the video.

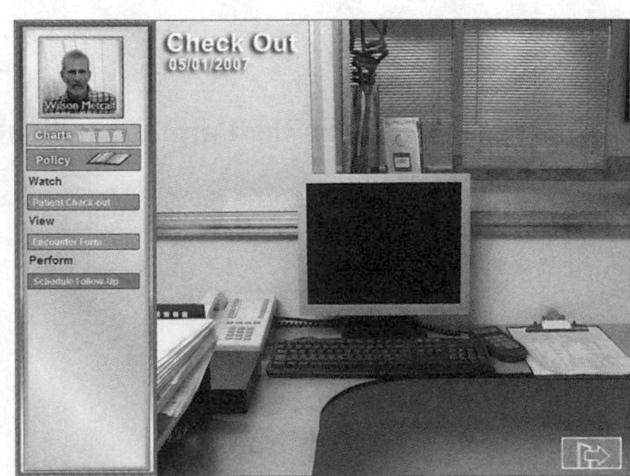

Copyright © 2014, 2011, 2007 by Saunders, an imprint of Elsevier Inc. All rights reserved.

9. How is Mr. Metcalf's confidentiality safeguarded while the medical assistant is on the telephone?

10. How did the medical assistant verify the exact location of the patient transfer so that the orders could be sent as needed?

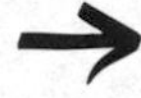

- Click the **X** on the video screen to close the video.
- Click on **Charts**.
- Click on the **Patient Medical Information** tab and select **7-Release of Information Authorization**.

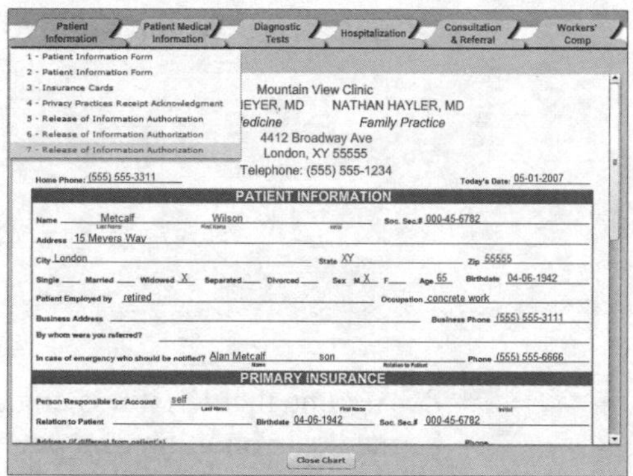

11. Was it permissible for Leah to call Mr. Metcalf's son concerning his transfer to the hospital? Why or why not?

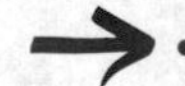

- Click on the **Patient Medical Information** tab and select **1-Patient Information Form**.

Copyright © 2014, 2011, 2007 by Saunders, an imprint of Elsevier Inc. All rights reserved.

12. What telephone number was given for Mr. Metcalf's son Alan?

13. Would it have been better, in your opinion, to have Mr. Metcalf's son's phone number on the Release of Information Authorization? Why?

- Click **Close Chart** to return to the Check Out area.
- Click **Return to Map**, then click **Yes** at the pop-up menu to return to the office map or click **Exit the Program**.

Exercise 2

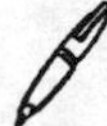

Writing Activity

15 minutes

1. List different acceptable ways to introduce yourself if you were working at Mountain View Clinic, keeping in mind the rules for answering the phone that are discussed in your textbook. Practice each way out loud while holding the telephone. Choose which introduction seems most comfortable to you and be prepared to share your personal preference with your classmates.

Copyright © 2014, 2011, 2007 by Saunders, an imprint of Elsevier Inc. All rights reserved.

2. What do most incoming calls pertain to in the medical office?

3. How far should the medical assistant hold the telephone receiver from his or her mouth when speaking into the handset?

4. List seven vital pieces of information to include on a telephone message.

5. Which types of calls require operator assistance?

6. When possible, why should operator-assisted calls be avoided?

Copyright © 2014, 2011, 2007 by Saunders, an imprint of Elsevier Inc. All rights reserved.

LESSON 3

Scheduling and Managing Appointments

Reading Assignment: Chapter 10—Scheduling Appointments

Patient: Janet Jones

Learning Objectives:

- Discuss the rationale for providing space in a day's appointment schedule for emergency appointments.
- Explain the need for a matrix on the appointment schedule.
- Describe the role of the Policy Manual in appointment scheduling.
- Explain the importance of verbal communication concerning appointment delays.
- Apply the skills of scheduling appointments in person and by telephone.
- Apply the skills of maintaining the appointment book.
- Identify office policies concerning rescheduling appointments.
- Apply the skills of rescheduling appointments.

Overview:

In this lesson you will schedule and manage appointments using the policies established for this office. The patient, Janet Jones, is upset because she has not been seen immediately. You will discuss the proper way to deal with such a situation. After today's appointment, Janet Jones will need to come back for a follow-up appointment. You will schedule this appointment for her at the appropriate time and schedule other appointments for established and new patients.

Copyright © 2014, 2011, 2007 by Saunders, an imprint of Elsevier Inc. All rights reserved.

Exercise 1

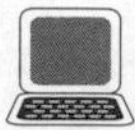

Online Activity—Using a Specific Daily Appointment Schedule

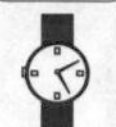

25 minutes

- Sign in to Mountain View Clinic
- Select **Janet Jones** from the patient list.
- Click on **Reception**.
- Click on the **Computer**.
- Scroll down the appointment book to see both the morning and afternoon schedules.

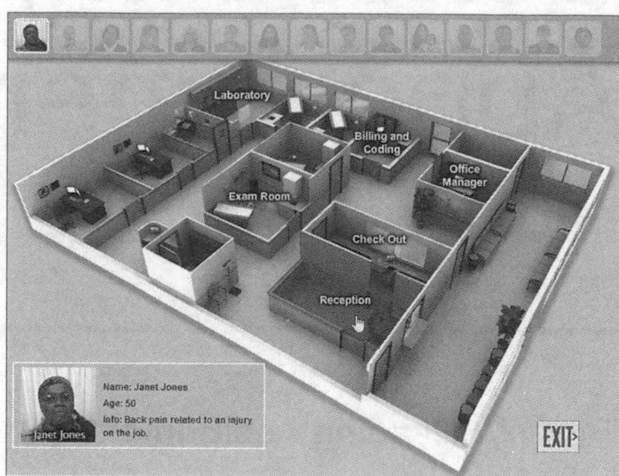

1. According to the appointment schedule, what time is Janet Jones' appointment?

2. If Janet Jones signed in at 1:30 p.m., would she have been on time for her appointment? Explain your answer.

- Click **Finish** to return to the Reception area.
- Under the Watch heading, click on **Patient Check-In** and watch the video.

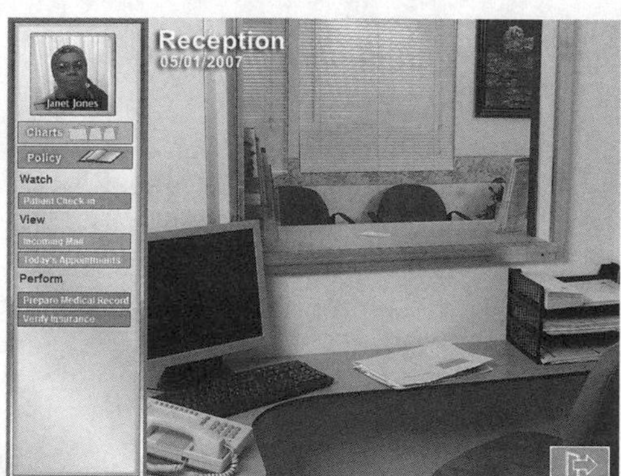

3. Janet Jones is upset when she arrives at the counter. How does Kristin handle the patient in a professional way through verbal and nonverbal communication?

Copyright © 2014, 2011, 2007 by Saunders, an imprint of Elsevier Inc. All rights reserved.

4. Assuming that Ms. Jones checked in at 1:30 p.m., what would have been an appropriate statement for the receptionist to make to the patient as she checked in to prevent her from becoming so upset?

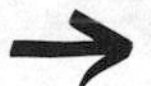

- Click the **X** on the video screen to close the video.
- Click on **Policy** to open the office Policy Manual.
- Type "appointment scheduling" in the search bar and click on the magnifying glass.
- Read the section of the Policy Manual on scheduling appointments.
- Keep the Policy Manual open to answer the following questions.

5. What is the length of time needed for an appointment during which a history and physical examination must be completed for a new patient?

6. Why is it necessary to set up a matrix before making appointments?

7. What buffer times are available for emergency appointments, and why is it important to have this time available?

Copyright © 2014, 2011, 2007 by Saunders, an imprint of Elsevier Inc. All rights reserved.

8. According to the office Policy Manual, what would have been appropriate concerning rescheduling Janet Jones' appointment?

9. Why is it important to identify workers' compensation appointments at the time of scheduling rather than at the time of the appointment?

10. Is the patient's time just as valuable as the physician's time? Explain your answer.

→ • Click **Close Manual** to return to the Reception area.
- Click the exit arrow.
- Click **Return to Map** and select **Yes** at the pop-up menu to return to the office map.

Copyright © 2014, 2011, 2007 by Saunders, an imprint of Elsevier Inc. All rights reserved.

Exercise 2

Writing Activity—Adding Appointments to a Schedule

20 minutes

At the end of the day on April 31, a list of patients needing appointments on May 1 was shown to Dr. Hayler and Dr. Meyer. Both physicians stated that because few patients were currently in the hospital, they would be able to see patients in the clinic earlier than usual the next morning. Dr. Hayler and Dr. Meyer will begin seeing patients at 8:15 a.m. The staff has been informed of the early start. The white areas of the appointment book indicate buffer times for adding patients who need to see the doctor today or for those patients with emergent needs. You may choose a patient, go to the Reception desk, open the Policy Manual, and type "appointment scheduling" in the search bar to review the length of time you will need to block off for each appointment.

1. a. Insert the following appointments for Dr. Hayler into the morning schedule on the next page.

    (1) Robert Leuker is a patient who has not been to the clinic in 5 years and wants to be seen for a lump in his arm. He has a past history of cancer and needs to be seen ASAP. He should be seen first in the morning so that he can be referred as necessary. He is insured through BlueCross/BlueShield (BC/BS). His phone number is (555) 555-8890.

    (2) Lindsey Repp needs a follow-up appointment for an earache and recurrent fever. She is insured through Central Health HMO and can be double-booked at the end of the appointment for Louise Parlet. Her telephone number is (555) 555-9004.

    (3) John Price, who needs a follow-up appointment for his blood pressure, has Medicare. His blood pressure was low when he took it yesterday, and he feels dizzy. He simply wants Dr. Hayler to reevaluate his medication. After discussing this with Dr. Hayler, he can be seen just before lunch and will be "worked in" with the other scheduled patients. Mr. Price's phone number is (555) 555-1998.

   b. After completing Dr. Hayler's appointments, add the following appointments for Dr. Meyer in the morning, using the same schedule on the next page.

    (1) Catherine Lake needs a follow-up appointment for pyelonephritis. She forgot to make her follow-up appointment when she was last seen. Ms. Lake is going out of town for 2 weeks and needs to see Dr. Meyer before leaving. Her insurance coverage is through BC/BS. Dr. Meyer will see her at the earliest appointment time. Catherine Lake's phone number is (555) 555-1865.

    (2) Lucille Meryl needs to be seen for a follow-up to a thyroid test. Dr. Meyer wants to see her as a double-booking at the end of the appointment for Rhea Davison. Her insurance is through Drake. Her phone number is (555) 555-3219.

    (3) An established patient, Simon Reed, calls at 11:30 a.m. to tell you that he has some chest pain, and even though he has an appointment for tomorrow, he does not think he should wait. Mr. Reed has experienced a heart attack in the past. When you discuss this with Dr. Meyer, she tells you to phone 911 while keeping the patient on the line. She also says that she will go to the hospital to see Mr. Reed once he is in the emergency room. What notation should you make on the schedule?

Copyright © 2014, 2011, 2007 by Saunders, an imprint of Elsevier Inc. All rights reserved.

	Dr. Hayler Name	Insurance	Dr. Meyer Name	Insurance
8:00 AM	(Hospital rounds) Joe Smitty- Chem 12, CBC Marsha Brady-fasting BS		(Hospital rounds)	
8:15 AM	(Hospital rounds)		(Hospital rounds) Joanne Crosby-PT, PTT	
8:30 AM	Louise Parlet - Est. Pt. New pregnancy/pelvic (555) 555-3214	Teachers'	Rhea Davison - Est. Pt. Elevated blood sugar, abdominal distention, pelvic- (555) 555-5656	None
8:45 AM				
9:00 AM				
9:15 AM				
9:30 AM			Hu Huang - Est. Pt. Severe cough, fever (555) 555-1454	Medicare
9:45 AM	Jade Wong - NP 7 mos. well child checkup/ immunization- (555) 555-3345	Central Health HMO		
10:00 AM			~~Chris O'Neil - back pain~~ (pt. cancelled- resched 5/7) Jesus Santo - NP Leg pain, SOB (walk-in)	None
10:15 AM				
10:30 AM			Jean Deere - Est. Pt. Memory loss, ear pain (555) 555-6361	Medicare
10:45 AM	Tristan Tsosie - Est. Pt. Suture removal (555) 555-1515	BC/BS		
11:00 AM				
11:15 AM			Wilson Metcalf - Est. Pt. N/V, abdominal pain, difficulty urinating- (555) 555-3311	Medicare
11:30 AM	LUNCH			
11:45 AM				
12:00 PM				

Copyright © 2014, 2011, 2007 by Saunders, an imprint of Elsevier Inc. All rights reserved.

2. You must now call John Price to inform him that Dr. Hayler will see him just before lunch. Below, write the information that Mr. Price will need to be told. Why did Dr. Hayler need to be contacted before making the appointment for Mr. Price?

3. You must also call Lucille Meryl to inform her that Dr. Meyer wants to see her about her test results. What information do you need to provide, and how would you answer her if she questions why she needs to be seen so quickly?

Exercise 3

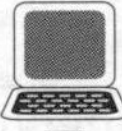

Online Activity—Preparing an Appointment Schedule

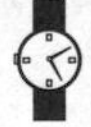

30 minutes

- Select **Janet Jones** from the patient list.
- Click on **Check Out**.
- Click on the **Encounter Form** clipboard.

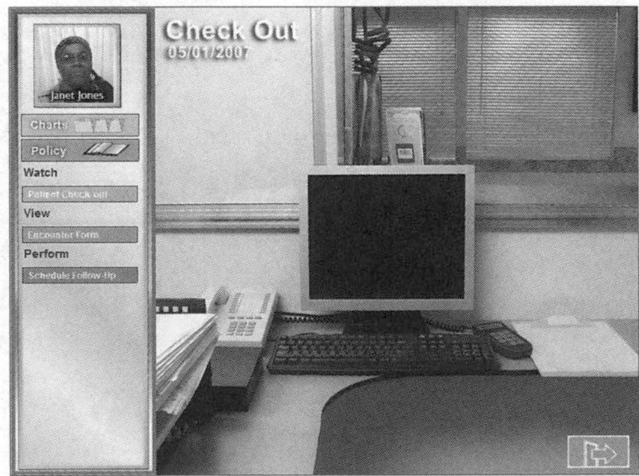

Copyright © 2014, 2011, 2007 by Saunders, an imprint of Elsevier Inc. All rights reserved.

1. What is the date that Janet Jones should return to the clinic for a follow-up appointment?

2. How much time should be allotted to the follow-up appointment for Ms. Jones?

- Click **Finish** to return to the Check Out area.
- Under the Watch heading, click on **Patient Check-Out** and watch the video.

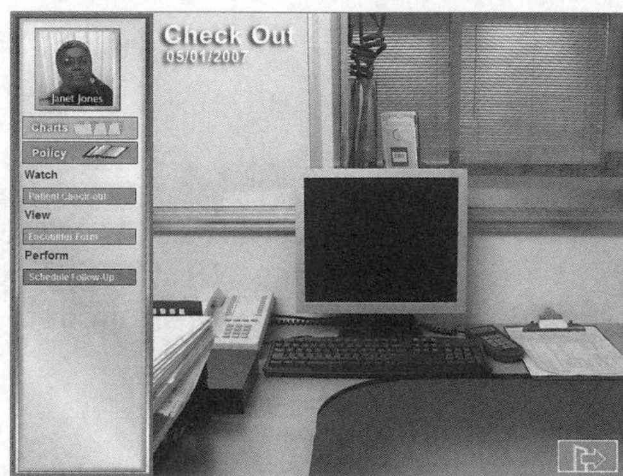

3. At what time of day was Ms. Jones' follow-up appointment made?

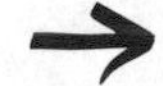

- Click the **X** on the video screen to close the video.
- Click the exit arrow.
- Click **Return to Map** and select **Yes** at the pop-up menu to return to the office map or click **Exit the Program**.

Copyright © 2014, 2011, 2007 by Saunders, an imprint of Elsevier Inc. All rights reserved.

Complete the following activities using the appointment sheets in questions 4 and 5 on the next two pages.

(1) Set up the appointment sheet for the date that Janet Jones is to return for her follow-up visit at the same time the medical assistant in the video scheduled her appointment.

(2) Using the information in the Policy Manual, set up the matrix for that day. (*Note:* If you need to review this, return to the Policy Manual, type "hours of operation" in the search bar, and click once on the magnifying glass.

(3) Add an appointment at 11:00 a.m. for Kay Soto (an established patient) with Dr. Meyer. Ms. Soto has been prescribed a weight loss program and is coming in for a weight check. Her insurance is through Metro HMO. Ms. Soto's phone number is (555) 555-0054.

(4) George Smith, age 15, is to be seen by Dr. Hayler for a football injury the night before. He has State Agricultural Insurance and is an existing patient. George needs to be seen as early as possible so that he can go to school. Mr. Smith's phone number is (555) 555-8778.

(5) Callie Agree, a new patient, is to be seen for a possible sinus infection. She has Medicare and will be accompanied by her daughter. The daughter prefers to see Dr. Meyer in the midmorning so that her mother will have time to dress. Ms. Agree's phone number is (555) 555-3452.

(6) Sophie Coats, age 6 months, is an established patient who will be seen by Dr. Hayler for a well-baby visit. She is due to have immunizations at this visit. Her mother prefers to have an appointment as early in the morning as possible. Sophie is covered by her father's insurance with Banker's Health. Ms. Coats' phone number is (555) 554-0090.

(7) Mamie Mack, age 18, is an established patient who needs a physical examination for college. She prefers to be seen by Dr. Hayler. Either late morning or early afternoon is better for her since she is still in school. She is covered through George Allen Insurance at her mother's place of employment. Ms. Mack's phone number is (555) 554-8745.

(8) Kay Soto calls to cancel her appointment for the day because she has to leave town to take care of her ill mother. She does not want to reschedule at this time.

(9) Dr. Hayler will need to leave at 11:15 a.m. for a dental appointment but will be back in the afternoon by 1:00 p.m. Mark this on the appointment sheet.

(10) Dr. Meyer is scheduled to be off the afternoon of this day. Mark this on the appointment sheet.

Copyright © 2014, 2011, 2007 by Saunders, an imprint of Elsevier Inc. All rights reserved.

4.

/ /2007	Dr. Hayler		Dr. Meyer	
Time	Patient Name	Insurance	Patient Name	Insurance
8:00 AM				
8:15 AM				
8:30 AM				
8:45 AM				
9:00 AM				
9:15 AM				
9:30 AM				
9:45 AM				
10:00 AM				
10:15 AM				
10:30 AM				
10:45 AM				
11:00 AM				
11:15 AM				
11:30 AM				
11:45 AM				
12:00 PM				
12:15 PM				

Copyright © 2014, 2011, 2007 by Saunders, an imprint of Elsevier Inc. All rights reserved.

5.

__/__/2007	Dr. Hayler		Dr. Meyer	
Time	Patient Name	Insurance	Patient Name	Insurance
12:30 PM				
12:45 PM				
1:00 PM				
1:15 PM				
1:30 PM				
1:45 PM				
2:00 PM				
2:15 PM				
2:30 PM				
2:45 PM				
3:00 PM				
3:15 PM				
3:30 PM				
3:45 PM				
4:00 PM				
4:15 PM				
4:30 PM				
4:45 PM				
5:00 PM				

Copyright © 2014, 2011, 2007 by Saunders, an imprint of Elsevier Inc. All rights reserved.

6. What is the necessary procedure for canceling Kay Soto's appointment?
   a. Erase the canceled appointment and tell Ms. Soto that there will be a charge because she did not give 24 hours notice.
   b. Cross out the appointment (using the office-preferred writing implement) and record the cancellation in the patient medical record or in the database if using electronic records.
   c. Report the cancellation to Dr. Meyer.
   d. Tell her that she must reschedule this appointment today for continued medical care.

7. Why is it important to document a canceled appointment in the patient's medical record?

8. When is it appropriate to report a canceled appointment to the physician?

Copyright © 2014, 2011, 2007 by Saunders, an imprint of Elsevier Inc. All rights reserved.

LESSON 4

Scheduling Admissions and Procedures

Reading Assignment: Chapter 10—Scheduling Appointments
- Scheduling Other Types of Appointments

Chapter 14—The Paper Medical Record
- Releasing Medical Record Information

Patients: Wilson Metcalf, Shaunti Begay

Learning Objectives:

- Recognize the patient information that needs to be sent to a medical facility if your office is making a referral.
- Check the patient's records to verify who is authorized by the patient to receive information regarding the patient.
- Use the Policy Manual to determine the responsibility of the medical assistant in making arrangements for inpatient admissions and referrals to other physicians.
- Explain why it is important to arrange outpatient appointments at a time convenient for the patient.
- Recognize confidentiality issues that must be followed when making arrangements to transfer a patient to a hospital.

Overview:

In this lesson you will make the necessary arrangements for moving Wilson Metcalf from the office to the hospital. You will ensure that his family has been notified of the move. With Shaunti Begay, you will make arrangements for outpatient testing and schedule an office appointment for providing her test results. This patient will also need to see a specialist, so any questions concerning the insurance for these appointments will need to be answered.

Copyright © 2014, 2011, 2007 by Saunders, an imprint of Elsevier Inc. All rights reserved.

Exercise 1

Online Activity—Scheduling Inpatient Admissions and Procedures

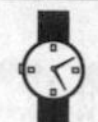

30 minutes

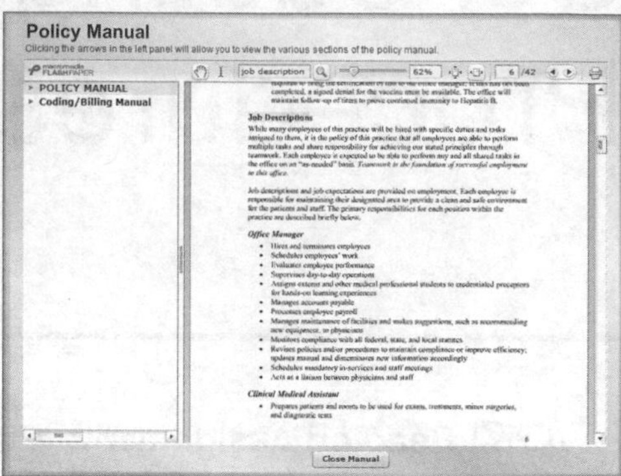

- Sign in to Mountain View Clinic.
- Select **Wilson Metcalf** from the patient list.
- Click on **Check Out**.
- Click on **Policy** to open the office Policy Manual.
- Type "job description" in the search bar and click once on the magnifying glass.
- Read the section of the Policy Manual on the job descriptions for the medical assistants.

1. According to office policy, which medical assistant has the primary duty of making the arrangements for inpatient admissions and for making referrals to other physicians?

- Click **Close Manual** to return to the Check Out area.
- Under the Watch heading, click on **Patient Check-Out** and watch the video. (*Note:* You may have already watched this video in Lesson 2. Review to answer the following question.)

2. Which documents are being copied and sent to the hospital with Mr. Metcalf? Select all that apply.

_____ Medicare card

_____ Private insurance card

_____ Authorization form

_____ Office registration

_____ Physician's orders

Copyright © 2014, 2011, 2007 by Saunders, an imprint of Elsevier Inc. All rights reserved.

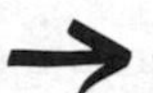

- Click on **Charts**.
- Click on the **Patient Information** tab and select **3-Insurance Cards**. Click on **next card** to view the second card.
- Click on the **Patient Information** tab and select **1-Patient Information Form**.
- Click on the **Patient Information** tab and select **6-Release of Information Authorization Form**.
- Note that both the Patient Information Form and the Release of Information Authorization Form are dated 5-1-2007.

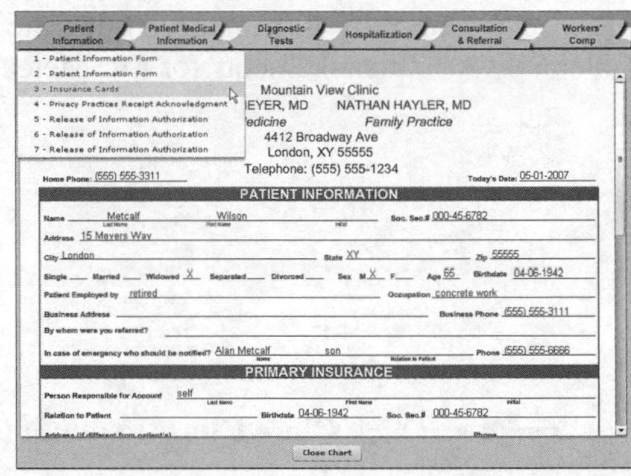

3. Why would it be appropriate to send the office registration and authorization form to the hospital for Wilson Metcalf's admission?

4. Who may receive information concerning Mr. Metcalf's medical condition? Can the entire medical record be released?

5. Did Leah act within the ethical and legal boundaries to release the information she gave to the hospital for Mr. Metcalf? Explain your answer.

Copyright © 2014, 2011, 2007 by Saunders, an imprint of Elsevier Inc. All rights reserved.

6. Why is it important that the window to the waiting room be closed while Leah is making arrangements for Mr. Metcalf to be transferred to the hospital?

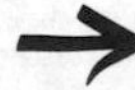

- Click **Close Chart** to return to the Check Out area.
- Click the exit arrow.
- Click **Return to Map** and select **Yes** at the pop-up menu to return to the office map.

Exercise 2

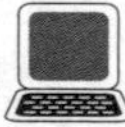

Online Activity—Scheduling Outpatient Admissions and Procedures

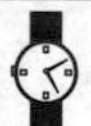

20 minutes

- Select **Shaunti Begay** from the patient list.
- Click on **Check Out**.
- Click on **Charts**.
- Click on the **Patient Medical Information** tab and select **2-Progress Notes**.

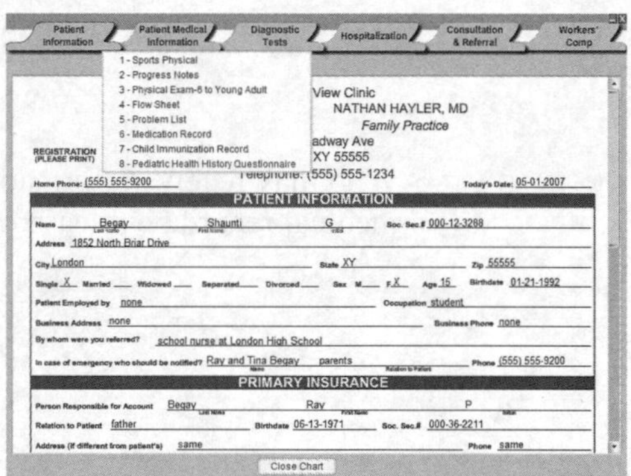

1. What appointments does the check-out medical assistant need to make?

2. Why is it important for Leah to obtain a referral preauthorization, or precertification for the tests to be performed?

Copyright © 2014, 2011, 2007 by Saunders, an imprint of Elsevier Inc. All rights reserved.

3. From the Progress Notes, what patient diagnosis is the physician interested in "ruling out" by this referral?

- Click **Close Chart** to return to the Check Out area.
- Under the Watch heading, click on **Patient Check-Out** and watch the video.

4. Did Leah make sure the referral for outpatient admission and procedures was scheduled at a time convenient for the patient and her family?

Critical Thinking Question

5. Why is it important to check that referrals and appointments to specialists are made at a time that is convenient for the patient?

6. Why is it important to document a canceled appointment in the patient's medical record?

7. Shaunti's father, Mr. Begay, is concerned with the financial aspects of the visit since his insurance is not a provider for this medical office. Leah provided the information about his insurance carrier and the referral. However, she did not provide information that was needed to assist Shaunti in the referral. Can you name two items that were not discussed with or given to Mr. Begay?

Copyright © 2014, 2011, 2007 by Saunders, an imprint of Elsevier Inc. All rights reserved.

8. Refer to the Progress Notes and then look at the referral authorization in Shaunti's chart; compare it with the Progress Notes. Did Leah gain approval for all the tests the doctor wants the patient to have?

9. Mr. Begay was concerned about the amount of the bill for Shaunti. Do you think that Leah was professional in her handling of verbal and nonverbal communication in this interaction? In what way, if any, would you have changed what was said or done? Did Leah act in an ethical manner?

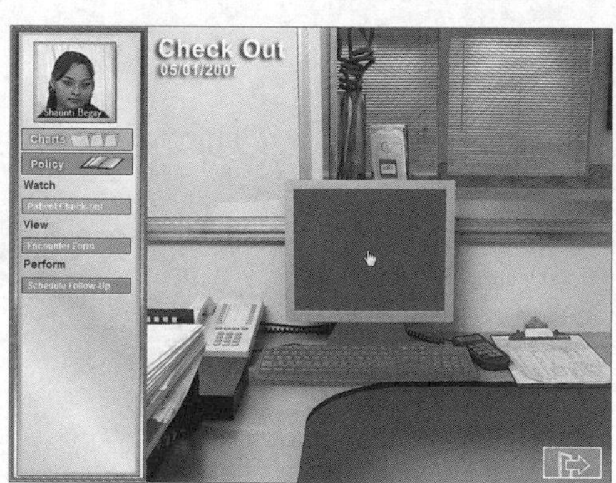

- Click the **X** on the video screen to close the video.
- Click on the **Encounter Form** clipboard.
- Review the information necessary to schedule a follow-up visit.
- Click **Finish** to return to the Check Out area.
- Click on the **Computer**.
- Use the checkboxes to select the actions required to schedule the patient's next visit.
- Click **Finish** to return to the Check Out area.
- Click the exit arrow.
- On the Summary Menu, click on **Look at Your Performance Summary**.
- Scroll down the Performance Summary and compare your answers with those chosen by the experts. The summary can be printed or saved for your instructor.
- Click **Close** to return to the Summary Menu.
- Click **Return to Map**, then click **Yes** at the pop-up menu to return to the office map or click **Exit the Program**.

Copyright © 2014, 2011, 2007 by Saunders, an imprint of Elsevier Inc. All rights reserved.

LESSON 5

Maintaining a Proper Inventory

Reading Assignment: Chapter 12—The Office Environment and Daily Operations
- Supplies and Equipment in the Physician's Office

Patients: None

Learning Objectives:

- Describe the steps necessary for replenishing supplies.
- Discuss how having too many or too few supplies can affect the efficiency of the office.
- Decide which items to reorder and the amount to reorder.
- Explain the necessity of checking equipment for maintenance on a regular basis.
- Discuss the role of the medical assistant in suggesting new equipment for the medical office.
- Describe the proper disposal of controlled substances that are found to be out of date.

Overview:

Ensuring the availability of supplies and equipment when needed is essential to the efficiency of the medical office practice. The proper inventory of supplies and equipment helps to ensure their availability. In some cases, it is more efficient to order supplies in larger quantities. The medical assistant also has the responsibility of making sure that the equipment ordered is the most currently used in the field. Finally, when medications are found to be out of date, proper disposal is necessary. This lesson will focus on supplies and equipment and their importance to office efficiency.

Copyright © 2014, 2011, 2007 by Saunders, an imprint of Elsevier Inc. All rights reserved.

Exercise 1

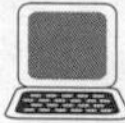

Online Activity—Deciding When to Replenish Supplies

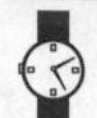

30 minutes

- Sign in to Mountain View Clinic.
- Click on **Office Manager**.
- Click on the **Supply Inventory** binder.
- To view the record for each item in the inventory, click on the corresponding tab headings.

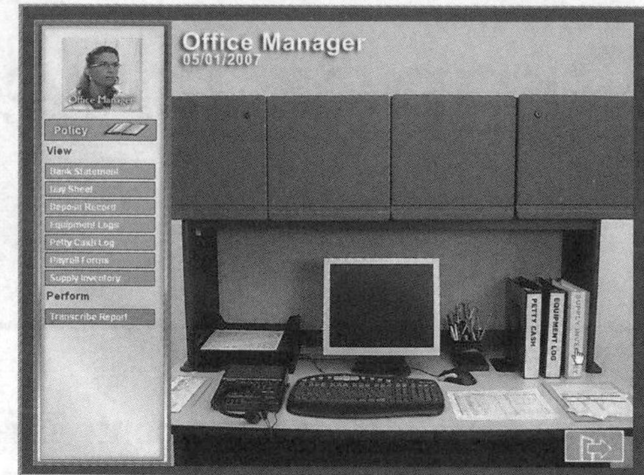

1. What is the reorder point for sutures?

2. Looking at the record from 2006, how many packages of sutures were previously used in May?

→ • Click on **Gauze** to view the inventory record.

3. What is the reorder point for gauze?

4. Looking at the record from 2006, how many bags of gauze were previously used in May?

5. The inventory for gauze is recorded as bags, but gauze can also be ordered by the case. How many bags are in one case?

Copyright © 2014, 2011, 2007 by Saunders, an imprint of Elsevier Inc. All rights reserved.

6. What is the unit price? Does this represent the price per bag or the price per case?

7. What is the discount offered for ordering four or more cases of gauze?

8. After looking at the inventory supply sheet for gauze, should gauze be reordered? If so, why and how much? If not, why not? If you reorder, what will be the net amount of the purchase?

→ • Click on the tab heading for **EKG Paper** to view the inventory record.

9. When was the last order placed for EKG paper? How much was ordered?

10. When was this order received?

11. What is the reorder point for EKG paper?

12. How many packs of EKG paper are currently in inventory?

Copyright © 2014, 2011, 2007 by Saunders, an imprint of Elsevier Inc. All rights reserved.

13. Should EKG paper be reordered now? If so, why? If not, why not? If you reorder, what quantity should be reordered?

14. The order for EKG paper is prepaid. What are some possible reasons for setting up a prepaid order for this item? *Use your critical thinking skills while answering this question.*

→ • Click on **Envelopes** to view the inventory record.

15. How often does the office normally order envelopes?

16. On February 28, 2007, the office ordered four more boxes of envelopes. When did this order arrive?

17. Why is there so much time between when the order is placed and when the order is received?

Copyright © 2014, 2011, 2007 by Saunders, an imprint of Elsevier Inc. All rights reserved.

18. From what you see on the inventory form, do the envelopes need to be reordered? How could the office lower the price of the envelopes? Do you see a problem with the reorder point, and does this need to be changed? If the envelopes should be reordered in bulk, what would be the price?

→ • Click on **Paper** to view the inventory record for copier paper.

19. After examining the inventory supply card for copier paper, what is the cost for three cases?

20. What is the cost for ordering five cases?

Copyright © 2014, 2011, 2007 by Saunders, an imprint of Elsevier Inc. All rights reserved.

21. Below, fill out the purchase order for three cases of copier paper. The shipping fee is $6.00 and the sales tax is 6%.

Office Station

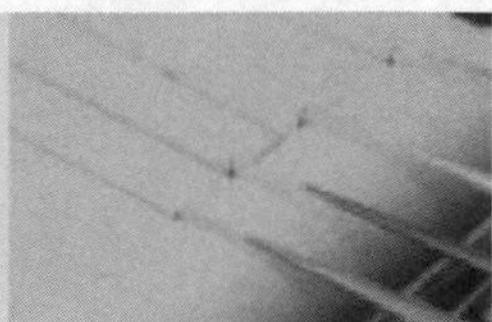

Purchase Order

Bill To:
Mountain View Clinic
4412 Broadway
London, XY 55555

Ship To:
Mountain View Clinic
4412 Broadway
London, XY 55555

Order #:
Date:

Delivery Required By:

Sales Contact	Terms	Tax ID

Item	Quantity	Description	Unit Price	Disc %	Total

Shipping	
Subtotal	
Tax %	
Balance Due	

145 Oceanus Way, St. Pinot, XY 53559
Phone: (123) 456 7890 Fax: (123) 456 7899 CSR@officestation.com

Copyright © 2014, 2011, 2007 by Saunders, an imprint of Elsevier Inc. All rights reserved.

Here is a copy of the supplier's invoice for the copier paper you ordered. Use the information on this invoice to complete question 22 on the next page.

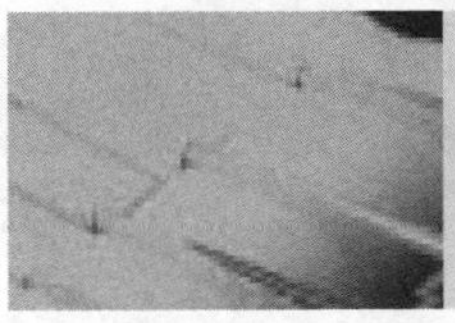

Office Station

INVOICE #2297

Bill To:
Mountain View Clinic
4412 Broadway
London, XY 55555

Ship To:
Mountain View Clinic
4412 Broadway
London, XY 55555

Order #: 105699

Delivery Required By:

Date:

Sales Contact	Terms	Tax ID

Item	Quantity	Description	Unit Price	Disc %	Total
CPO-117	3 cases	Copier Paper	$71.27 / 3 cases		$71.27

Shipping	$6.00
Subtotal	$77.27
Tax %	$4.64
Balance Due	$81.91

145 Oceanus Way, St. Pinot, XY 53559
Phone: (123) 456 7890 Fax: (123) 456 7899 CSR@officestation.com

Copyright © 2014, 2011, 2007 by Saunders, an imprint of Elsevier Inc. All rights reserved.

22. Using the information on invoice 2297 from the Office Station (previous page), complete the check below to pay for the delivered supplies.

173980

DATE: ____________

TO: ____________

FOR: ____________

ACCOUNT NO. ____________

AMOUNT PAID $ ____________

MOUNTAIN VIEW CLINIC
4412 Broadway
London, XY 55555

173980
94-72/1224

Date: ____________

Pay to the order of: ____________

____________ Dollars $ ____________

Clarion National Bank
Member FDIC
90 Grape Vine Road
London, XY 55555-0001

____
Authorized Signature

⑈005503⑈ ⑆446782011⑆ 678800470

23. How should the ordered supplies be handled when they arrive at the office?

- Click **Finish** to return to the manager's office.
- Click the exit arrow.
- Click **Return to Map** and select **Yes** at the pop-up menu to return to the office map.

Exercise 2

Writing Activity—Properly Disposing Medications

10 minutes

- Sign in to Mountain View Clinic and select any patient from the patient list.
- Click on **Reception**.
- Click on **Policy** to open the office Policy Manual.
- Type "**22**" into the search box to navigate to page 22.
- Read the section of the Policy Manual on the disposal of medications.

1. While checking supplies, Cathy noticed that some of the nonscheduled medications are out of date. These medications are oral tablets and capsules. What means of disposal is correct for these medications?

Copyright © 2014, 2011, 2007 by Saunders, an imprint of Elsevier Inc. All rights reserved.

2. If part of a schedule II medication ampule has to be disposed of, how many clinical medical assistants need to witness the disposal?

- Click on the exit arrow.
- Click **Return to Map** and select **Yes** at the pop-up menu to return to the office map or click **Exit the Program**.

Exercise 3

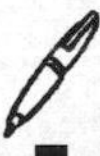

Writing Activity—Maintaining Administrative Equipment

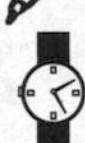

10 minutes

1. When filling the copier with paper, Cathy notices that it is time for regular maintenance of the machine and the representative has not been to the office. What should be Cathy's next step?

2. The toner cartridges are low, and Cathy sees a need for replenishing these. What should she do?

Copyright © 2014, 2011, 2007 by Saunders, an imprint of Elsevier Inc. All rights reserved.

Exercise 4

Writing Activity—Suggestions for Equipment and Supplies

10 minutes

1. Ameeta has observed that not all patients with diabetes are using the same glucose meters at home. The physicians are asking that quality control be checked with patients more often. However, if the office does not have the same glucometers and supplies that some of the patients use at home, it is difficult to provide accurate patient teaching. What steps should Ameeta take to ensure that patient teaching is accurate and helpful to each patient?

2. Leah, as an administrative assistant, has found that the phone line for the fax machine is often busy when a fax needs to be received. Often the person attempting to send the fax has called to complain of the difficulty of getting important information to the physicians. What steps should Leah take to show the need for another fax line for the hospital? *Use your critical thinking skills while answering this question.*

Copyright © 2014, 2011, 2007 by Saunders, an imprint of Elsevier Inc. All rights reserved.

LESSON 6

Written Communications

Reading Assignment: Chapter 13—Written Communication and Document Processing
Chapter 25—Medical Practice Management and Human Resources
- Problem Patients

Patient: Wilson Metcalf

Note: The exercises in this lesson do not specifically involve Wilson Metcalf, but a patient must be selected in order to access the required records.

Learning Objectives:

- Prepare letters in response to the mail received.
- Use correct grammar, spelling, and formatting techniques in letter writing.
- Read mail correspondence correctly.

Overview:

In this lesson you will be asked to respond to incoming mail that includes an NSF check and a letter from a collection agency.

Copyright © 2014, 2011, 2007 by Saunders, an imprint of Elsevier Inc. All rights reserved.

Exercise 1

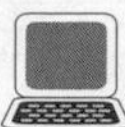

Online Activity—Composing a Letter for an NSF Check

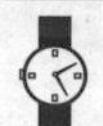

40 minutes

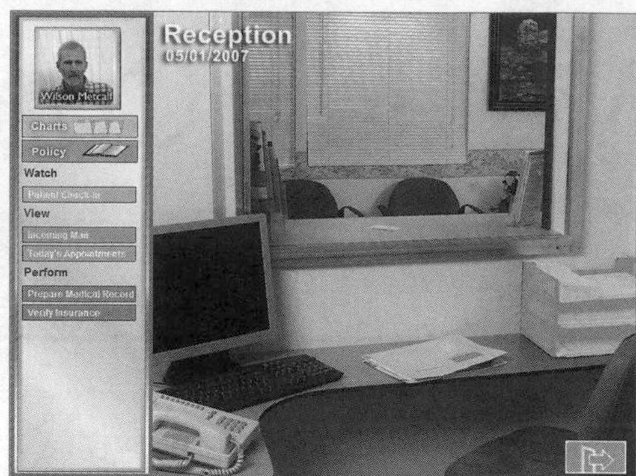

- Sign in to Mountain View Clinic.
- Select **Wilson Metcalf** from the patient list.
- Click on **Reception**.
- Click on the **Stackable Trays**.
- Click the numbers or arrows at the top of the page to examine and read each piece of mail.

1. Were any payments received in the mail today?

2. List the people from whom payments were received.

3. What is the name of the physician who sent a consultation letter to Dr. Meyer?

4. Who was the letter in reference to?

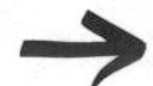

- Click the number **7** and read that piece of mail.

5. On the next page, write your letter to the patient about the NSF check, using an acceptable format. Be sure your message conveys the need to handle this matter within a certain number of days and include the charges from the bank in addition to the amount owed the office. Also, include that no further checks will be accepted for this patient's medical care at Mountain View Clinic. This should be prepared for a signature by the office manager.

Copyright © 2014, 2011, 2007 by Saunders, an imprint of Elsevier Inc. All rights reserved.

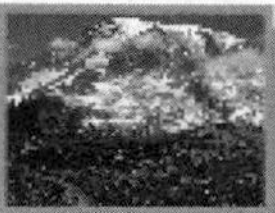

Mountain View Clinic

4412 Broadway / London, XY 55555 / Phone: (555) 555-1234 / Fax: (555) 555-1239

Nathan Hayler, MD - Family Practice / Katarina Meyer, MD - Internal Medicine

Copyright © 2014, 2011, 2007 by Saunders, an imprint of Elsevier Inc. All rights reserved.

Exercise 2

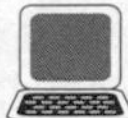

Online Activity—Composing a Letter in Response to an Inaccurate Accounts Payable

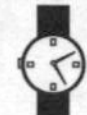

30 minutes

- Click the number **10** and read that piece of mail.
- From the list of mail at the top of the screen, click on **10** to read the letter from Summer Oxygen Company.
- Click **Finish** to return to the Reception area.
- Click the exit arrow.
- Click **Return to Map** and select **Yes** at the pop-up menu to return to the office map.
- Click on **Office Manager**.
- Click on **Bank Statement** file folder.
- Click on the **Check Ledger** tab.

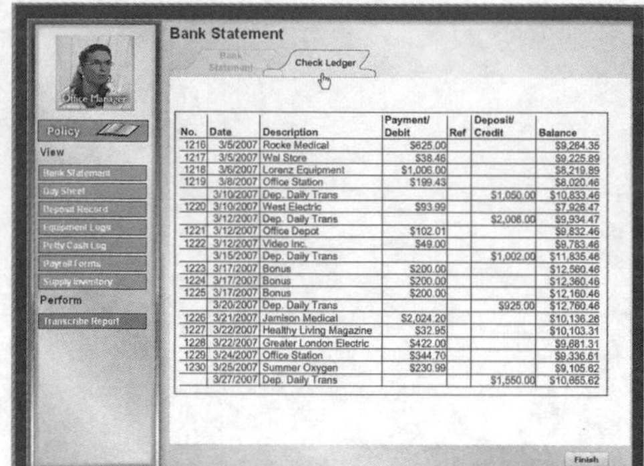

No.	Date	Description	Payment/ Debit	Ref	Deposit/ Credit	Balance
1216	3/5/2007	Rocke Medical	$625.00			$9,264.35
1217	3/5/2007	Wal Store	$38.46			$9,225.89
1218	3/6/2007	Lorenz Equipment	$1,006.00			$8,219.89
1219	3/8/2007	Office Station	$199.43			$8,020.46
	3/10/2007	Dep. Daily Trans			$1,050.00	$10,833.46
1220	3/10/2007	West Electric	$93.99			$7,926.47
	3/12/2007	Dep. Daily Trans			$2,008.00	$9,934.47
1221	3/12/2007	Office Depot	$102.01			$9,832.46
1222	3/12/2007	Video Inc.	$49.00			$9,783.46
	3/15/2007	Dep. Daily Trans			$1,002.00	$11,835.46
1223	3/17/2007	Bonus	$200.00			$12,560.46
1224	3/17/2007	Bonus	$200.00			$12,360.46
1225	3/17/2007	Bonus	$200.00			$12,160.46
	3/20/2007	Dep. Daily Trans			$925.00	$12,760.46
1226	3/21/2007	Jamison Medical	$2,024.20			$10,136.26
1227	3/22/2007	Healthy Living Magazine	$32.95			$10,103.31
1228	3/22/2007	Greater London Electric	$422.00			$9,681.31
1229	3/24/2007	Office Station	$344.70			$9,336.61
1230	3/25/2007	Summer Oxygen	$230.99			$9,105.62
	3/27/2007	Dep. Daily Trans			$1,550.00	$10,655.62

1. There was a payment made to Summer Oxygen Company for $230.99.

   a. According to the check ledger, what was the date the payment was made?

   b. What was the check number?

→ • Click on the **Bank Statement** tab to review the account activity for April 2007.

2. Did check #1230 for $230.99 clear the account, according to the bank statement?

Copyright © 2014, 2011, 2007 by Saunders, an imprint of Elsevier Inc. All rights reserved.

3. Below, compose a rough draft for a letter to the Oxygen Supply Company in response to the claim that the invoice has not been paid. Write your letter to the oxygen company using an acceptable format. Be sure your message includes all information needed to clear the accounts payable, and that a copy of the canceled check is enclosed with the letter. This should be prepared for signature by the office manager.

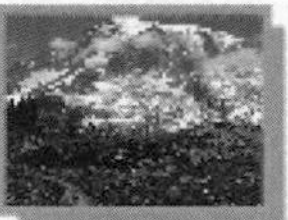

Mountain View Clinic

4412 Broadway / London, XY 55555 / Phone: (555) 555-1234 / Fax: (555) 555-1239

Nathan Hayler, MD - Family Practice / Katarina Meyer, MD - Internal Medicine

Copyright © 2014, 2011, 2007 by Saunders, an imprint of Elsevier Inc. All rights reserved.

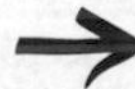

- Click **Finish** to return to the manager's office.
- Click the exit arrow.
- Click **Return to Map** and select **Yes** at the pop-up menu to return to the office map.

Exercise 3

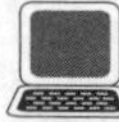

Online Activity—Writing a Termination Letter

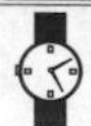

15 minutes

- Select **Wilson Metcalf** from the patient list.
- Click on **Reception**.
- Click on the **Computer**.
- Scroll down the appointment book to see both the morning and afternoon schedules.

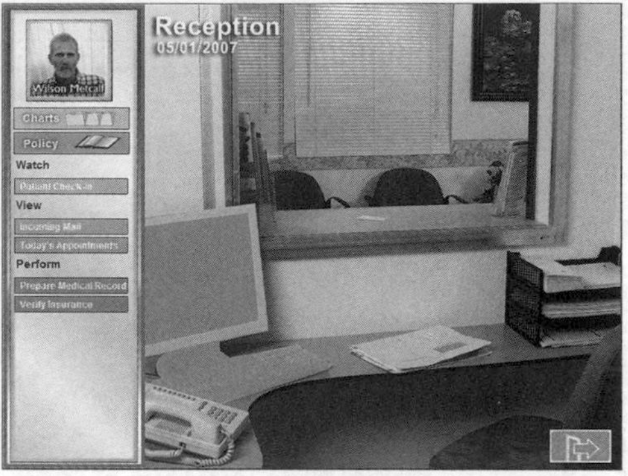

1. What is the name of the patient who has canceled the appointment, and what is the chief complaint?

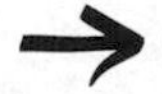

- Click **Finish** to return to the Reception area.
- Click on **Policy** to open the office Policy Manual.
- Type "cancel" in the search bar and click on the magnifying glass.
- Read the section of the Policy Manual on canceled appointments.

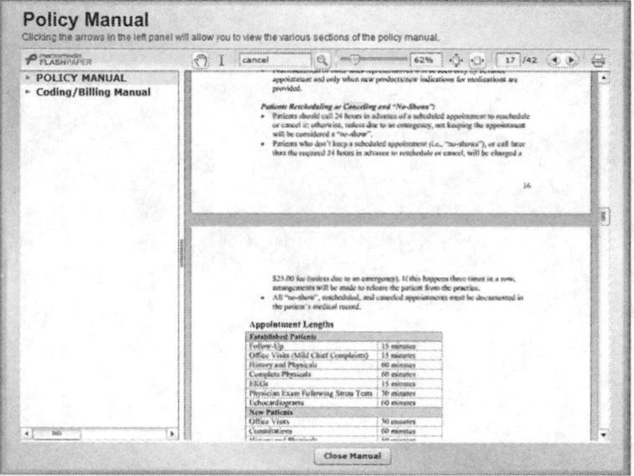

Copyright © 2014, 2011, 2007 by Saunders, an imprint of Elsevier Inc. All rights reserved.

2. Below, compose a letter to the patient you identified in question 1. In the letter, describe the reason for possible termination and the necessary steps needed to remain a patient of Dr. Meyer. The letter should include all of the reasons for possible termination and the need for the patient to keep appointments as made. The letter can also state that Dr. Meyer is concerned about continuity of care and the need for patient safety through this continuity of care.

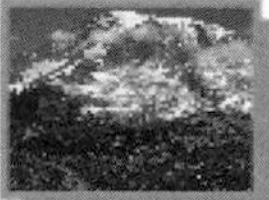

Mountain View Clinic

4412 Broadway / London, XY 55555 / Phone: (555) 555-1234 / Fax (555) 555-1239

Nathan Hayler, MD - Family Practice / Katarina Meyer, MD - Internal Medicine

Copyright © 2014, 2011, 2007 by Saunders, an imprint of Elsevier Inc. All rights reserved.

3. Why does the letter need to be sent by certified mail?

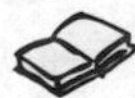

4. If a decision is made to terminate a patient, how much time must be allowed between notification and the termination? (*Hint:* Refer to the Problem Patients section in Chapter 25 to answer this question.)

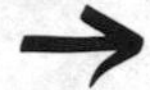

- Click **Close Manual** to return to the Reception area.
- Click the exit arrow.
- Click **Return to Map**, then click **Yes** at the pop-up menu to return to the office map or click **Exit the Program**.

Copyright © 2014, 2011, 2007 by Saunders, an imprint of Elsevier Inc. All rights reserved.

LESSON 7

Organizing a Patient's Medical Record

Reading Assignment: Chapter 11—Patient Reception and Processing

- Registration Procedures

Chapter 14—The Paper Medical Record

- Creating an Efficient Medical Records Management System
- Organization of the Medical Record
- Contents of the Complete Case History
- Making Additions to the Patient Record
- Keeping Records Current
- Filing Procedures (Conditioning)

Chapter 15—The Electronic Medical Record

- Executive Order to Promote Interoperability of EMR Systems
- Technological Terms in Health Information
- American Recovery and Reinvestment Act (ARRA)
- HITECH ACT and Meaningful Use

Patients: Renee Anderson, Tristan Tsosie

Learning Objectives:

- Discuss why proper organization of the medical record is essential.
- Identify and describe the forms found in a medical record.
- Apply principles of medical record organization to choose forms that would be needed when preparing a new patient's medical record.
- Determine whether forms need to be added to the medical record for an established patient.
- Describe the appropriate care of a damaged medical record.
- Determine the appropriate division of medical records when a new record must be established.
- Understand the difference between the terms electronic health record (EHR), electronic medical record (EMR), and personal health record (PHR).
- Identify the goal of EMR interoperability.

Copyright © 2014, 2011, 2007 by Saunders, an imprint of Elsevier Inc. All rights reserved.

Overview:

In this lesson we will explore the importance of preparing a patient's medical record correctly. Because the medical record is a legal document that shows the chronological care of the patient, this document must be correctly organized to ensure that information can be located as needed. Incorrectly organized charts not only cause frustration, but also decrease the efficiency of the medical practice. In this lesson you will organize a medical record for a new patient. For an established patient, you will ensure that information received from other sources has been properly organized and that the information is readily available when the patient arrives for an appointment. You will also be asked to distinguish between the terms *electronic medical record* and *electronic health record*.

Exercise 1

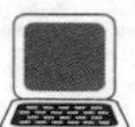

Online Activity—Organizing a Medical Record for a New Patient

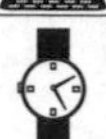

30 minutes

- Sign in to Mountain View Clinic.
- Select **Renee Anderson** from the patient list.
- Click on **Reception**.
- Click on **Policy** to open the Policy Manual.
- Type "medical record" in the search bar and click on the magnifying glass.
- Read the section of the Policy Manual on the duties assigned to the various types of medical assistants in the office.

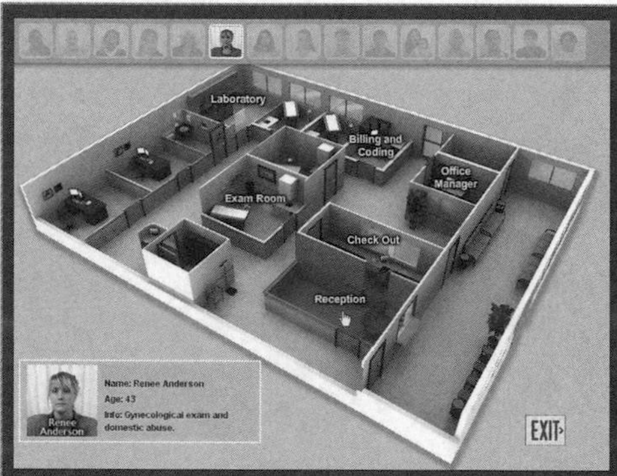

1. At Mountain View Clinic, the Policy Manual states that the ________________________ medical assistant is responsible for preparing and organizing the medical record.

Critical Thinking Question

2. Why do you think it is important for the administrative medical assistant to provide the necessary forms in a medical record for a new patient after the patient is "checked" in at the registration desk?

Copyright © 2014, 2011, 2007 by Saunders, an imprint of Elsevier Inc. All rights reserved.

- Click on **Close Manual** to return to the Reception area.
- Click on the **Medical Record**.
- Click on the **Perform** button next to Assemble Medical Record.
- Add forms needed in the Patient Information tab by clicking on the forms from the Forms Available list and clicking **Add** to confirm your choice.
- Make note of all the forms you add into the table below.
- Continue adding forms to the appropriate tabs in the patient's medical record. To select a new tab, either click on the tab on the medical record or use the drop-down menu on the right.
- If you wish to remove a chosen form, highlight the form and click **Remove** at the bottom of the screen.

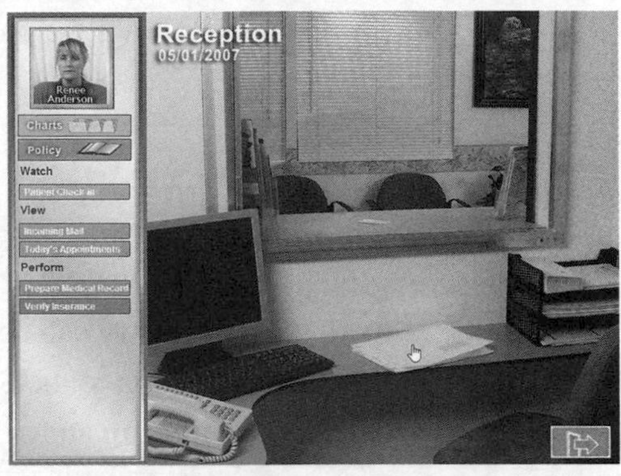

3. Below, list the forms you added to Renee Anderson's medical record.

- Click **Finish** to close the chart and return to the Reception area.
- Click on the **Insurance Card**.
- Identify the appropriate question to ask the patient regarding her insurance and click on **Ask**.
- Use the checkboxes to select which procedures are needed to verify the patient's insurance.
- Click **Finish** to return to the Reception area.

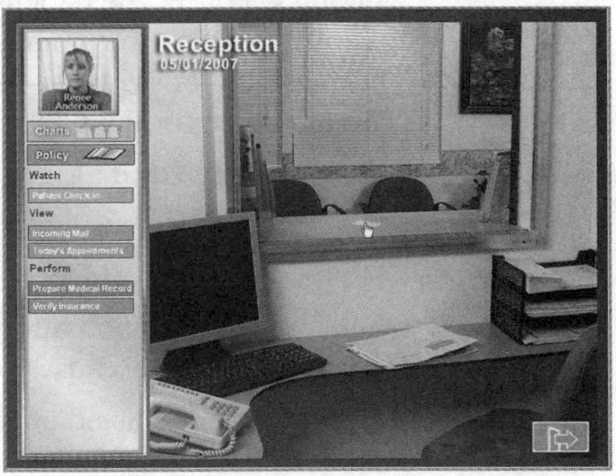

4. The form that contains the patient's demographic information is the

____.

5. The form in the medical record that contains subjective information about the patient's illnesses in the past is the ____.

6. The legal document that must be signed to allow information to be used to file insurance is the ____.

Copyright © 2014, 2011, 2007 by Saunders, an imprint of Elsevier Inc. All rights reserved.

7. The form that allows the physician to record findings in the medical record is the

____.

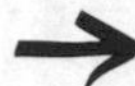

- Click the exit arrow.
- On the Summary Menu, click on **Look at Your Performance Summary**.
- Scroll down the Performance Summary and compare your answers with those chosen by the experts. The summary can be printed or saved for your instructor.
- Click **Close** to return to the Summary Menu.
- Click **Return to Map** and select **Yes** at the pop-up menu to return to the Office Map.

Exercise 2

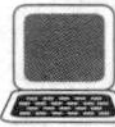

Online Activity—Determining Whether to Add Forms to the Medical Record of an Established Patient

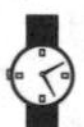

30 minutes

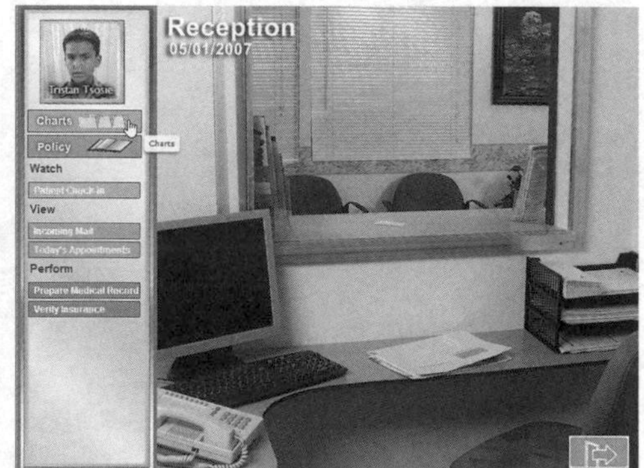

- Select **Tristan Tsosie** from the patient list.
- Click on **Reception**.
- Click on **Charts**.
- Click on the **Hospitalization** tab and select **1-ED Record**.
- Read the ED Record to decide what other forms should be available for the physician for this office visit and to determine whether Tristan is following the orders of the physician who saw him in the Emergency Department. Think about which procedures the patient had while at the Emergency Department and which procedure should have a report to be filed in his chart. Then look under the tabs to see whether you can find the report that you would also need to have available for the physician.
- Click on **Close Chart** to return to the Reception area.

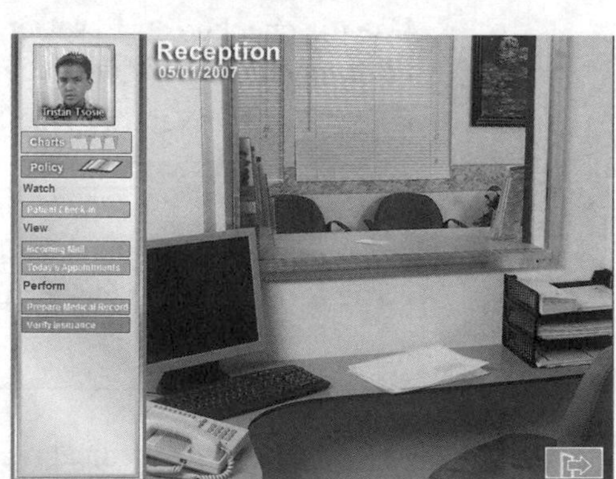

- Click on the **Medical Record**.
- Click on the **Perform** button next to Review and Update Medical Records.
- Review the forms listed under the Patient Information tab. Add any forms that are missing from the Patient Information tab by clicking on the forms from the Forms Available list and clicking **Add** to confirm your choice. The forms you select will appear under the tabs at the bottom of the screen.
- When you have completed the Patient Information section, continue reviewing and adding forms to the appropriate tabs in Tristan Tsosie's medical record. To select a new tab, either click on the tab on the medical record itself or use the drop-down menu on the right.

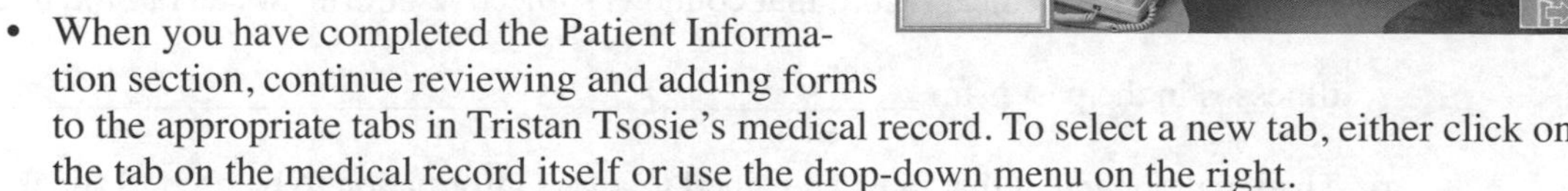

- If you wish to remove a chosen form, highlight the form in the tab and click **Remove** at the bottom of the screen.

Copyright © 2014, 2011, 2007 by Saunders, an imprint of Elsevier Inc. All rights reserved.

1. According to the ED Record, with what department was Tristan supposed to follow-up?

2. According to the Consultation Notes, when was Tristan supposed to follow up with the physician? (*Note:* Specify in number of days.)

3. Explain the difference between the terms electronic medical record (EMR) and electronic health records (EHR).

4. If the medical office were sharing information with the hospital, would the record be called EMR or EHR?

5. Did the Emergency Department report advise the patient of when (number of days) to follow up with the doctor? Could this omission of information lead to problems with the patients follow-up care?

Copyright © 2014, 2011, 2007 by Saunders, an imprint of Elsevier Inc. All rights reserved.

6. Other than the ED Record, do any reports related to the ED visit appear in the record? If so, identify the report(s).

7. When adding an abnormal report to the paper medical record, the medical assistant should:
   a. be sure the physician has seen the report before filing it.
   b. place the forms in the medical record in chronological order, with the earliest record on top.
   c. always be sure the date of arrival has been stamped on the report.
   d. wait to file the form just before the patient's arrival for an appointment.
   e. do both a and d.

8. When the medical assistant files materials in the medical record of an established patient, the materials should be filed in what order?

9. When accessing Tristan's medical record on arrival, you notice that the forms from the hospital have been torn during transmittal. What steps do you need to take to maintain the record from further damage?

10. If a patient folder is old, torn, or simply worn, what should the medical assistant do?

11. If a chart is overcrowded and a second chart needs to be established, how far back should the records go that are moved to the new chart? How should the record be marked to show that more than one medical record is available?

Copyright © 2014, 2011, 2007 by Saunders, an imprint of Elsevier Inc. All rights reserved.

12. If the medical office is using an EMR that is interoperable with the hospitals EMR, would the physician have been able to access Tristan's records without having a paper copy in the medical record?

13. What is the goal of EMR interoperability?

14. Who manages, shares, and controls the information in the Personal Health Record (PHR)?

15. What component of the American Recovery and Reimbursement Act (ARRA) awards financial incentives for physicians for using electronic health records.

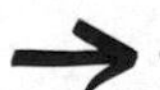

- Click **Finish** to close the chart and return to the Reception area.
- Click the exit arrow.
- On the Summary Menu, click **Look at Your Performance Summary**.
- Scroll down the Performance Summary to the Patient Records section and compare your answers with those chosen by the experts. The summary can be saved or printed for your instructor.
- Click **Close** to return to the Summary Menu.
- On the Summary Menu, click **Return to Map** and select **Yes** at the pop-up menu to return to the Office Map or click **Exit the Program**.

Copyright © 2014, 2011, 2007 by Saunders, an imprint of Elsevier Inc. All rights reserved.

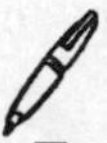

Exercise 3

Writing Activity—Medical Record Matching Exercise

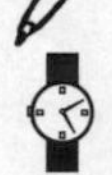

20 minutes

1. Read the following records and then identify which of the following sections of the medical record each item would be filed in. Write your answer in the lettered blank above each item.

   Consent documents
   Diagnostic procedure documents
   Hospital documents
   Medical office administrative documents
   Medical office clinical documents
   Problem-oriented record
   Therapeutic service documents

Copyright © 2014, 2011, 2007 by Saunders, an imprint of Elsevier Inc. All rights reserved.

a. ______________________________

HISTORY AND PHYSICAL
ST. MERCY HOSPITAL

Patient Name: Carol Jacobs Room #: 215
Physician: Charles Thomas, MD Hospital #: 5422
Admission Date: 12/14/12

CHIEF COMPLAINT: Chest pain

HISTORY OF PRESENT ILLNESS: Patient is an 85-year-old female complaining of chest pain. Patient was found to have abnormal cardiac enzymes in the Emergency Room consistent with acute myocardial infarction. Patient denied any pain radiating; however, she did complain of left-sided chest pain and lower back pain. Patient did not admit to any shortness of breath, nausea, or diaphoresis.

MEDICATIONS: Lasix, Darvocet-N 100, Lisinopril, Lopressor, Glynase, Relafen, Cytotec, and Micro K.

ALLERGIES: No drug allergies known.

PAST MEDICAL HISTORY: Significant for congestive heart failure, chronic obstructive pulmonary disease, diabetes mellitus type 2, coronary atherosclerosis, hypertension, and osteoporosis.

SOCIAL HISTORY: Not a drinker and not a smoker. Patient resides in a nursing home.

PHYSICAL EXAMINATION:

General: Patient is in acute distress. She is obese.
HEENT: She has 2 centimeters jugular venous distention. Pupils are equal and reactive to light and accommodation. No evidence of scleral or conjunctival icterus.
Chest: +2 bibasilar rales.
Heart: Regular rate and rhythm. +2/6 systolic ejection murmur in the left sternal border.
Abdomen: Soft, nontender, no splenomegaly and no hepatomegaly and positive bowel sounds.
Extremities: No evidence of edema or deep venous thrombosis.
Neurological: Cranial nerves II through XII grossly intact.

IMPRESSIONS: Congestive heart failure
Rule out myocardial infarction

Charles Thomas, MD

Charles Thomas, MD

Copyright © 2014, 2011, 2007 by Saunders, an imprint of Elsevier Inc. All rights reserved.

b. ______________________________

COLLEGE HOSPITAL
4567 BROAD AVENUE
WOODLAND HILLS, MD 21532

RADIOLOGY REPORT

Examination Date:	June 14, 2012	**Patient:**	Rose Baker
Date Reported:	June 14, 2012	**X-ray No.:**	43200
Physician:	Harold B. Cooper, M.D.	**Age:**	19
Examination:	PA Chest, Abdomen	**Hospital No.:**	80-32-11

FINDINGS

PA CHEST: Upright PA view of chest shows the lung fields are clear, without evidence of an active process. Heart size is normal. There is no evidence of pneumoperitoneum.

IMPRESSION: NEGATIVE CHEST

ABDOMEN: Flat and upright views of the abdomen show a normal gas pattern without evidence of obstruction or ileus. There are no calcifications or abnormal masses noted.

IMPRESSION: NEGATIVE STUDY

RADIOLOGIST: *Marian B. Skinner*
Marian B. Skinner, MD

Copyright © 2014, 2011, 2007 by Saunders, an imprint of Elsevier Inc. All rights reserved.

c. ________________________________

DISCHARGE SUMMARY

Brennan, Susan
97-32-11
June 18, 2012

ADMISSION DATE: June 14, 2012 **DISCHARGE DATE:** June 16, 2012

HISTORY OF PRESENT ILLNESS:
This 19-year-old female, nulligravida, was admitted to the hospital on June 14, 2012, with fever of 102°, left lower quadrant pain, vaginal discharge, constipation, and a tender left adnexal mass. Her past history and family history were unremarkable. Present pain had started two to three weeks prior to admission. Her periods were irregular, with latest period starting on May 30, 2012, and lasting for six days. She had taken contraceptive pills in the past but had stopped because she was not sexually active.

PHYSICAL EXAMINATION:
She appeared well developed and well nourished, and in mild distress. The only positive physical findings were limited to the abdomen and pelvis. Her abdomen was mildly distended, and it was tender, especially in the left lower quadrant. At pelvic examination, her cervix was tender on motion, and the uterus was of normal size, retroverted, and somewhat fixed. There was a tender cystic mass about 4-5 cm in the left adnexa. Rectal examination was negative.

PROVISIONAL DIAGNOSIS:
1. Probable pelvic inflammatory disease (PID).
2. Rule out ectopic pregnancy.

LABORATORY DATA ON ADMISSION:
Hgb 10.8, Hct 36.5, WBC 8,100 with 80 segs and 18 lymphs. Sedimentation rate 100 mm in one hour. Sickle cell prep+ (turned out to be a trait). Urinalysis normal. Electrolytes normal. SMA-12 normal. Chest x-ray negative, 2-hour UCG negative.

HOSPITAL COURSE AND TREATMENT:
Initially, she was given cephalothin 2 gm IV q6h, and kanamycin 0.5 gm IM bid. Over the next two days the patient's condition improved. Her pain decreased and her temperature came down to normal in the morning and spiked to 101° in the evening. Repeat CBC showed Hgb 9.8, Hct 33.5. The pregnancy test was negative. She was discharged on June 16, 2012 in good condition. She will be seen in the office in one week.

DISCHARGE DIAGNOSIS:
Pelvic inflammatory disease.

Harold B. Cooper, MD
Harold B. Cooper, MD

Copyright © 2014, 2011, 2007 by Saunders, an imprint of Elsevier Inc. All rights reserved.

d. ______________________________

EMERGENCY DEPARTMENT REPORT
CAMDEN CLARK HOSPITAL

Name: John Larimer
DOB: 2/2/72
ER Physician: John Parsons, MD
Date: 7/7/12
ER Number: 07398
Physician: James Woods, MD

NATURE OF ILLNESS/INJURY: This 40-year-old male presents to the Emergency Department complaining of a laceration of the sole of his right foot. Patient cut his foot on a rock 2 days ago and thinks he might have an infection now. Patient also complains of coughing over the past several days.

PHYSICAL EXAMINATION: Temperature 97.4, Pulse 76, Respirations 20, Blood Pressure 120/70. Patient is alert and oriented and is in no acute distress. ENT is normal. Lungs show diffuse rhonchi without crackles or wheezing. Heart has a regular rate and rhythm. Right great toe with marked tenderness with edema and erythema and heat.

DIAGNOSIS: Asthmatic Bronchitis
Cellulitis, right foot first MTP

TREATMENT: PCMX scrub to right foot. Bacitracin dressing. Tetanus Diphtheria 0.5 cc IM. Biaxin 500 mg bid x 10 days. Guaifenesin with codeine 2 tsp q4h prn. Entex LA,1 bid prn. Debridement of skin flap.

PATIENT INSTRUCTIONS: Patient to follow up with family doctor in 7 days. Discussed bronchospasms with the patient.

James Woods, MD
James Woods, MD

Copyright © 2014, 2011, 2007 by Saunders, an imprint of Elsevier Inc. All rights reserved.

e. ______________________________

(Attach label or complete blanks.)

First name: ______________ Last name: ______________

Date of Birth: ______ Month ______ Day ______ Year

Account Number: ______________________________

Procedure Consent Form

I, ____, hereby consent to have Dr. ______________ perform ____.

I have been fully informed of the following by my physician:

1. The nature of my condition
2. The nature and purpose of the procedure
3. An explanation of risks involved with the procedure
4. Alternative treatments or procedures available
5. The likely results of the procedure
6. The risks involved with declining or delaying the procedure

My physician has offered to answer all questions concerning the proposed procedure.

I am aware that the practice of medicine and surgery is not an exact science, and I acknowledge that no guarantees have been made to me about the results of the procedure.

Patient ______________________________ Date ______________
(or guardian and relationship)

Witnessed ______________________________ Date ______________

Copyright © 2014, 2011, 2007 by Saunders, an imprint of Elsevier Inc. All rights reserved.

f. ______________________________

PROBLEM ORIENTED - PROGRESS NOTES

Date	Time	Problem Number	FORMAT: Problem Number and TITLE: S = Subjective O = Objective A = Assessment P = Plan
11/15/12	9:30 AM	1	S: Mother states that her child has had a runny nose and her throat has been
			sore for 2 days.
			O: Vital signs: T 98.8 P 96 R 24
			Weight: 42 lb
			General: alert and active. HEENT: sclera clear. TMs negative. Positive clear
			rhinorrhea. Pharynx benign. Heart: regular without murmur.
			Lungs: clear to auscultation and percussion. Abdomen: negative tenderness.
			Positive bowel x 4. GU: negative. Neuro: good tone.
			A: Upper respiratory tract infection.
			P: 1. A prescription for Rondec DM, 1/2 tsp q6h prn cough and congestion.
			2. Instructed mother to contact office if child does not improve.

NAME-Last	First	Middle	Attending Physician	Record No.	Room/Bed
Michaels	Jessica	L	Frank Edwards, MD	1	24

PROBLEM ORIENTED - PROGRESS NOTES

Copyright © 2014, 2011, 2007 by Saunders, an imprint of Elsevier Inc. All rights reserved.

g. ______________________________

OPERATIVE REPORT
ST. MARY'S HOSPITAL

Name: Natalie Boyer

Hospital #: 291734 Room #: OP

Surgeon: Paul Cain, M.D. Date of Surgery: 1/6/12

Assistants: N/A Anesthesia: General

Anesthesiologist: John Adams, M.D.

PRE-OP DIAGNOSIS: Abnormal Pap test with history of cervical carcinoma.

POST-OP DIAGNOSIS: Same and awaiting path report.

PROCEDURE: D&C, laser cone of the cervix.

The patient to the operating room, lithotomy position, perineum and vagina were prepped, and moist sterile drape was used. Laser precautions all in place. Bimanual examination revealed a uterus enlarged with a second-degree uterine prolapse. The cervix was dilated. Uterus sounded to around 9 cm. The endocervical canal was dilated and D&C was performed with tissue recovered and submitted to Pathology. The cervix was stained with iodine, and the nonstaining area was identified. The laser was brought in, 50 watts of current were used to remove laser cone, and we submitted that to Pathology. We then vaporized beyond the margins of the cone, 3-4 mm to a depth of 4-5 mm. Hemostasis was adequate. We placed O Vicryl figure-of-eight sutures at the 3 and the 9 o'clock positions in the cervix, and then we put Monsel solution on the cervix. Hemostasis adequate. Sponge and needle counts correct times two. The patient tolerated the procedure well, and she returned to the recovery room in stable condition. She will be discharged home when awake and stable on Cipro 250 mg twice a day for a week, Darvocet-N 100, #20 as needed for pain. If she continues to have abnormal Pap tests, we will probably want to do a vaginal hysterectomy.

SURGEON: Paul Cain, MD
Paul Cain, MD

Copyright © 2014, 2011, 2007 by Saunders, an imprint of Elsevier Inc. All rights reserved.

h. ______________________________

HAROLD B. COOPER, M.D.
6000 MAIN STREET
VENTURA, CA 93003

June 15, 2012

John F. Millstone, M.D.
5302 Main Street
Ventura, CA 93003

Dear Dr. Millstone:

RE: Elaine J. Silverman

This 69-year-old woman was seen at your request. The patient was admitted to the hospital yesterday because of chills, fever, and abdominal and back pain.

REVIEW OF HEALTH HISTORY: The history has been reviewed. A prominent feature of the history is the presence of intermittent, severe, shaking chills for four days with associated left lower back pain, left lower quadrant abdominal pain, and fever to as high as 103 or 104 degrees. The patient has had hypertension for a number of years and has been managed quite well with Aldomet 250 mg twice a day.

PHYSICAL EXAMINATION: On examination her temperature at this time is 100.6 degrees. The pulse is 110 and regular. Blood pressure is 190/100. The patient has partial bilateral iridectomies, the result of previous cataract surgery. Otherwise, the head and neck are not remarkable. Lung fields are clear throughout. The heart reveals a regular tachycardia, and heart sounds are of good quality. No murmurs are heard, and there is no gallop rhythm present. The abdomen is soft. There is no spasm or guarding. A well-healed surgical scar is present in the right flank area. There is considerable tenderness in the left lower quadrant of the left mid abdomen, but as noted, there is no spasm or guarding present. Bowel sounds are present. Peristaltic rushes are noted, and the bowel sounds are slightly high pitched. The extremities are unremarkable.

IMPRESSIONS: I believe the patient has acute diverticulitis. She may have some irritation of the left ureter in view of the findings on the urinalysis. She appears to be responding to therapy at this time in that her temperature is coming down and there has been a slight reduction in the leukocytosis from yesterday.

RECOMMENDATIONS: I agree with the present program of therapy, and the only suggestion would be to possibly increase the dose of gentamicin to 60 mg q8h, rather than the 40 mg q8h that she is now receiving.

Thank you for asking me to see this patient in consultation.

Sincerely,

Harold B. Cooper

Harold B. Cooper, M.D.

mtf

Copyright © 2014, 2011, 2007 by Saunders, an imprint of Elsevier Inc. All rights reserved.

i. ________________________________

PHYSICAL THERAPY EVALUATION

OBJECTIVE DATA TESTS AND SCALES PRINTED ON REVERSE.

DATE OF SERVICE 9 / 23 / 12

HOMEBOUND REASON: ☐ Needs assistance for all activities ☐ Residual weakness
☐ Requires assistance to ambulate ☐ Confusion, unable to go out of home alone
☐ Unable to safely leave home unassisted ☐ Severe SOB, SOB upon exertion
☐ Dependent upon adaptive device(s) ☐ Medical restrictions
☐ Other (specify) ________

SOC DATE 9 / 23 / 12
(If Initial Evaluation, complete Physical Therapy Care Plan)

PERTINENT BACKGROUND INFORMATION

OTHER DISCIPLINES PROVIDING CARE: ☐ SN ☐ OT ☐ ST ☐ MSW ☐ Aide

MEDICAL HISTORY

☐ Hypertension ☐ Cancer
☐ Cardiac ☐ Infection
☐ Diabetes ☐ Immunosuppressed
☐ Respiratory ☐ Open wound
☐ Osteoporosis ☐ Falls with injury
☐ Fractures ☐ Falls without injury
☐ Other (specify) ________

REASON FOR EVALUATION (Diagnosis/Problem)

Hx Ⓛ knee pain x 5 yrs; little relief c̄ PT

LIVING SITUATION

☒ Capable ☐ Able ☐ Willing caregiver available
☐ Limited caregiver support (ability/willingness)
☐ No caregiver available

HOME SAFETY BARRIERS:
☐ Clutter ☐ Throw rugs ☐ Bath bench/equipment ☐ Needs grab bar
☐ Needs railings ☐ Steps (number/condition) ________
☐ Other (specify) ________

PRIOR LEVEL OF FUNCTION

ADLs:
☒ Independent ☐ Needed assistance ☐ Unable
Equipment used: ________

IN-HOME MOBILITY (gait or wheelchair/scooter):
☒ Independent ☐ Needed assistance ☐ Unable
Equipment used: ________

COMMUNITY MOBILITY (gait or wheelchair/scooter):
☐ Independent ☐ Needed assistance ☐ Unable
Equipment used: ________

BEHAVIOR/MENTAL STATUS

☒ Alert ☐ Oriented ☐ Cooperative ☐ Confused ☐ Memory deficits
☐ Impaired judgement ☐ Other (specify) ________

PAIN

INTENSITY: 0 1 2 3 4 ⑤ 6 7 8 9 10
LOCATION: ________
AGGRAVATING FACTORS: ________
RELIEVING FACTORS: ________
BEST PAIN GETS: 2 WORST PAIN GETS: 8
ACCEPTABLE LEVEL OF PAIN: ________
CURRENT LEVEL OF PAIN: ________
IMPACT ON THERAPY POC? ☐ None ☐ (describe) ________

VITAL SIGNS/CURRENT STATUS

Blood Pressure: ________
Temperature: ________
Pulse: ________
Respirations: ________
O_2 saturation ____% (when ordered): ☐ at rest ☐ with activity
Skin: ________
Edema: ________
Vision: glasses
Sensation: ________
Communication: ________
Hearing: ________
Posture: ________
Endurance: ________

PATIENT NAME – Last, First, Middle Initial
Johnson, Thomas, J.

ID#

PHYSICAL THERAPY EVALUATION
☐ Continued on Reverse

Copyright © 2014, 2011, 2007 by Saunders, an imprint of Elsevier Inc. All rights reserved.

j. ______________________________

RELEASE OF MEDICAL INFORMATION

All information contained in the medical record is confidential, and the release of information is closely controlled. A properly completed and signed authorization form is required for the release of the following information.

PATIENT INFORMATION

Patient Name ______________________

Address ______________________ Social Security # ______________

City ____________ State ______ ZIP ________ Birth date ___/___/___

Phone (Home) ____________ Work ____________

RELEASE FROM:

Name ______________________

Address ______________________

City ____________ State ______ ZIP ______

RELEASE TO:

Name ______________________

Address ______________________

City ____________ State ______ ZIP ______

INFORMATION TO BE RELEASED:

1. GENERAL RELEASE:

___Entire Medical Record (excluding protected information)
___Hospital Records only (specify) ____________
___Lab Results only (specify) ____________
___X-ray Reports only (specify) ____________
___Other Records (specify) ____________

2. INFORMATION PROTECTED BY STATE/FEDERAL LAW:
If indicated below, I hereby authorize the disclosure and release of information regarding:

___Drug Abuse Diagnosis/Treatment
___Alcoholism Diagnosis/Treatment
___Mental Health Diagnosis/Treatment
___Sexually Transmitted Disease

PURPOSE/NEED FOR INFORMATION:

___Taking records to another doctor
___Moving
___Legal purposes
___Insurance purposes
___Worker's Compensation
___Other/Explain: ____________

METHOD OF RELEASE:

___US Mail
___Fax
___Telephone
___To Patient

PATIENT AUTHORIZATION TO RELEASE INFORMATION:

Authorization is valid for 60 days only from the date of my signature. I reserve the right to revoke this authorization at any time prior to 60 days (except for action that has already been taken) by notifying the medical office in writing.

I understand that my records are protected under HIPAA (Health Insurance Portability and Accountability Act) Standards for Privacy of Individually Identifiable Information (45 CFR Parts 160 and 164) unless otherwise permitted by federal law. Any information released or received shall not be further relayed to any other facility or person without my written authorization. I also understand that such information will not be given, sold, transferred, or in any way relayed to any other person or party not specified above without my further written authorization.

I hereby grant authorization to release the information listed above. I certify that this request has been made voluntarily and that the information given above is accurate to the best of my knowledge.

______________________ Signature of Patient/Legally Responsible Party ____________ Date

______________________ Witness Signature ____________ Date

OFFICE USE ONLY

Information indicated above released on ____________ Date

Explanation of information released: ______________________

____

Signature and credentials of individual releasing information: ______________________

Copyright © 2014, 2011, 2007 by Saunders, an imprint of Elsevier Inc. All rights reserved.

k. ______________________________

PATIENT INFORMATION **CONFIDENTIAL**

File no. 10140
Date 11-21-12

(PLEASE PRINT)

Name Carol (First) H (Middle) Jones (Last) Birth date 1-20-68 Home phone 740-555-1248

Address 743 Evergreen Terrace City Springfield State OH ZIP 12345

Check appropriate box: ☐ Minor ☐ Single ☒ Married ☐ Divorced ☐ Widowed ☐ Separated Gender: ☐ Male ☒ Female

Employer Rockford, Inc. Work phone 740-555-1234

Business address 1 Rockford Place City Shelbyville State OH ZIP 21346

Spouse or parent's name John Jones Employer Self-emp. Work phone 740-555-8654

If patient is a student, name of school/college N/A City ______ State ______

Whom may we thank for referring you? Henry Peterson, MD

Person to contact in case of emergency John Jones Phone 740-555-1248

RESPONSIBLE PARTY

Name of person responsible for this account Carol Jones Relationship to patient Self

Address 743 Evergreen Terrace City Springfield State OH ZIP 12345 Home phone 740-555-1248

Employer Rockford, Inc. Work phone 740-555-1234

Is this person currently a patient in our office? ☒ Yes ☐ No

INSURANCE INFORMATION

Name of insured Carol Jones Relationship to patient Self

Birth date 1-20-68 Social Security number 123-45-6789 Date employed 5-1-93

Name of employer Rockford, Inc. Work phone 740-555-1234

Address of employer 1 Rockford Place City Shelbyville State OH ZIP 21346

Insurance company Anthem BC/BS Group number 51045

Insurance company address 521 Anthem Drive City New Halberville State OH ZIP 21436

DO YOU HAVE ANY ADDITIONAL INSURANCE? ☐ YES ☒ NO **IF YES, COMPLETE THE FOLLOWING:**

Name of insured ______ Relationship to patient ______

Birth date ______ Social Security number ______ Date employed ______

Name of employer ______ Work phone ______

Address of employer ______ City ______ State ______ ZIP ______

Insurance company ______ Group number ______

Insurance company address ______ City ______ State ______ ZIP ______

X Carol Jones

SIGNATURE OF PATIENT OR PARENT IF MINOR

Copyright © 2014, 2011, 2007 by Saunders, an imprint of Elsevier Inc. All rights reserved.

1. ______________________________

DIAGNOSTIC IMAGING REPORT

Mt. Carmel Hospital,
Columbus, OH 43201

DATE REQUESTED	DATE TO BE DONE	TODAY'S DATE	DATE OF BIRTH
6/6/2012	6/10/2012	6/10/2012	8/19/1949
☐ WHEELCHAIR	☐ PORTABLE	☒ AMBULATORY	☐ CART

PATIENT: Vera Ruth

INSURANCE: Industrial

SEX	ROOM NO.	RESPONSIBLE PERSON OR EMPLOYER	RADIOLOGIST
F	OP	J.B. Warren, Inc.	Richard W. Adams, MD

CLINICAL INFORMATION AND PROVISIONAL DIAGNOSIS: Back injury

ATTENDING PHYSICIAN: Christopher Robb, MD

NURSE:

EXAMINATION REQUESTED (PINPOINT AREA OF CONCERN IF POSSIBLE): CT LUMBAR SPINE

TECHNIQUE:

CT of the lumbar spine without contrast was performed from L-3 through S-1.

FINDINGS:

The L3-4 level appears satisfactory without evidence of osseous proliferation or disc protrusion.

At the L4-5 level there is some increased density at the disc level, which may be more prominent on the left. This is partially obscured due to facet artifact crossing obliquely.

There does appear to be some retention of epidural fat plane. This, however, may represent left-sided disc bulge or protrusion with the appropriate corresponding clinical appearance. Osseous variation at this level is not identified.

At the L5-S1 level, significant variation is not apparent.

IMPRESSION:

Variation at the L4-5 level on the left, which may represent annular disc bulge or perhaps protrusion on the left. However, confirmation with myelography and/or Ampaque enhanced computed tomography of the lumbar spine should be suggested prior to any surgical intervention.

Richard W. Adams, MD

Richard W. Adams, MD

Copyright © 2014, 2011, 2007 by Saunders, an imprint of Elsevier Inc. All rights reserved.

m. ______________________________

COLLEGE HOSPITAL
4567 BROAD AVENUE
WOODLAND HILLS, MD 21532

PATHOLOGY REPORT

Date:	June 20, 2012	**Pathology No.:**	430211
Patient:	Molly Ramsdale	**Room No.:**	1308
Physician:	Harold B. Cooper, M.D.		
Specimen Submitted:	Tumor, right axilla		

FINDINGS

GROSS DESCRIPTION: Specimen A consists of an oval mass of yellow fibroadipose tissue measuring 4 x 3 x 2 cm. On cut section, there are some small, soft, pliable areas of gray apparent lymph node alternating with adipose tissue. A frozen section consultation at time of surgery was delivered as NO EVIDENCE OF MALIGNANCY on frozen section, to await permanent section for final diagnosis. Majority of the specimen will be submitted for microscopic examination.

Specimen B consists of an oval mass of yellow soft tissue measuring 2.5 x 2.5 x 1.5 cm. On cut section, there is a thin rim of pink to tan-brown lymphatic tissue and the mid portion appears to be adipose tissue. A pathological consultation at time of surgery was delivered as no suspicious areas noted and to await permanent sections for final diagnosis. The entire specimen will be submitted for microscopic examination.

MICROSCOPIC DESCRIPTION: Specimen A sections show fibroadipose tissue and nine fragments of lymph nodes. The lymph nodes show areas with prominent germinal centers and moderate sinus histiocytosis. There appears to be some increased vascularity and reactive endothelial cells seen. There is no evidence of malignancy.

Specimen B sections show adipose tissue and 5 lymph node fragments. These 5 portions of lymph nodes show reactive changes including sinus histiocytosis. There is no evidence of malignancy.

DIAGNOSIS: A & B: TUMOR, RIGHT AXILLA: SHOWING 14 LYMPH NODE FRAGMENTS WITH REACTIVE CHANGES AND NO EVIDENCE OF MALIGNANCY.

Stanley T. Nason, MD

Stanley T. Nason, MD

Copyright © 2014, 2011, 2007 by Saunders, an imprint of Elsevier Inc. All rights reserved.

n. ______________________________

PATIENT RECORD

Name: Morani, Betty
Number
Blood Type: A+
ALLERGIES/SENSITIVITY: Codeine, Sulfa

Prob. No.	Date	PROBLEM DESCRIPTION	Date Resolved	Index	Prob. No.	Date	PROBLEM DESCRIPTION	Date Resolved	Index
1	10/05	Hypertension - essential		✓					
2	10/05	Diabetes mellitus (mild)		✓					
3	1/08	L. Retinopathy	see below						
4	4/2012	Atherosclerosis with cerebral vascular insuffic.							
5	4/2012	Hearing loss							
6	1/2012	HBP Non-compliance	2/12						
3	1/2012	Bilat. Grade II Retinopathy							

Prob. No.	CONTINUING MEDICATIONS	Start	Stop	Prob. No.	CONTINUING MEDICATIONS	Start	Stop
1	Sinoserp 1 mg. b.i.d.	10/05	10/09				
2	Orinase 0.5 gm. daily	10/05	10/09				
1	Hydrodiuril 50 mg. A.M.	10/05					
2	1500 cal. diet low Na hi K	2/2012					

Periodic Health Examination	Dates	1/04	4/06	2/08	1/10							

Copyright © 2014, 2011, 2007 by Saunders, an imprint of Elsevier Inc. All rights reserved.

o. ______________________________

Home Health Agency — Visit Report

Date of Visit: 11/21/12 | Mileage Start: 7 | Finish: 9

Patient's Name: Clarence Castor

Financial: | Med. A: | Med. B: | GH: | VA: | Pvt: | Other: Hospice

BP: (L): 160/92 | (R): 160/92 | T: 97.7

P: (A): 78 | (R): 76 | Wt: 151 | R: 18

Area: | Diagnosis: Lung cancer

Pt. Instruction: Continue O_2 as needed

Procedures: | Age: 74

Comments/Observations: (Physical, mental, emotional, activity level, Environ., S/S, Treatments & Effects, Procedures, Med. Effects, Other)

Pt complaining of some difficulty breathing and swelling of his feet. Pt was given Proventil Atrovent neb tx and started on oxygen at 2 liters per nasal cannula. Tx was discussed with Dr. Shay.

Plan: monitor vitals every 2 hrs.

Supplies Used: O_2 @ 2 liters

Signature: D. Tilly, RN

Next Visit: 11/22/12	RN	PT	HHA	MSW	Other
	√				
Freq. of Visits: daily	√				

Travel Time: | Service Time:

Supervisory Visit:

LESSON 8

Filing Medical Records

Reading Assignment: Chapter 14—The Paper Medical Record
- Creating an Efficient Medical Records Management System
- Filing Procedures
- Filing Methods
- Organization of Files

Chapter 15—The Electronic Medical Record
- Technological Terms in Health Information
- Capabilities of EMR Systems

Patients: All

Learning Objectives:

- Alphabetize patient names for efficiency in filing medical records.
- List the necessary steps needed to prepare a paper medical record for filing.
- Describe the use of color coding to enhance paper medical record systems.
- Identify the filing systems used most frequently in the medical office for patient records.
- Discuss the differences between alphabetic and numeric filing systems.
- Determine which patients are established patients and which are new patients for preparing charts.
- Discuss the means for finding displaced paper medical records.
- Explain the most important function of primary features that EMR software may offer.

Overview:

Proper filing of medical records is essential in providing continuity of care for patients. You will determine if patients are new or established in preparation for filing and you will then alphabetize patients. You will be asked to differentiate between alphabetic and numeric filing systems and identify methods for locating misplaced medical information. One activity will involve answering questions about the different features with which typical EMR software comes.

Copyright © 2014, 2011, 2007 by Saunders, an imprint of Elsevier Inc. All rights reserved.

Exercise 1

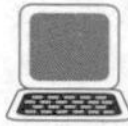

Online Activity—Preparing Patient Medical Records for Filing

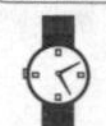

50 minutes

- Sign in to Mountain View Clinic.
- Select **Janet Jones** from the patient list.
- Click on **Reception**.
- Click on the **Computer**.
- Scroll down the appointment book to see both the morning and afternoon schedules.

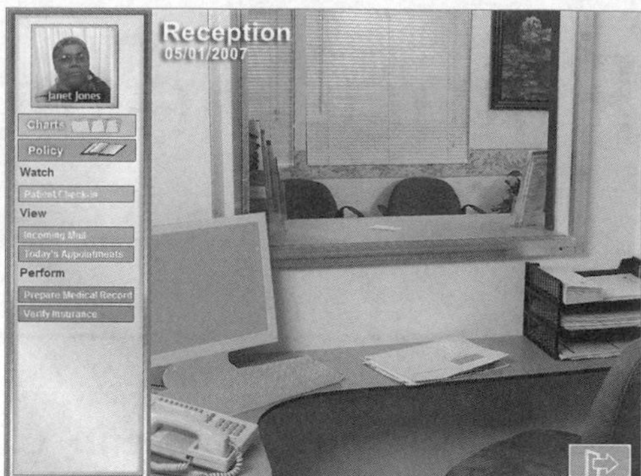

1. Look for each patient's name and note next to his or her name on the table above whether that patient is a new patient (NP) or an established patient (Est. Pt.) (*Note:* You will return to fill in the remaining columns of the table later in this exercise.)

Patient Name	New Patient (NP) or Established Patient (Est. Pt.)	First Date of Service mm/dd/yy	Last Date of Service mm/dd/yy
Janet Jones			
Wilson Metcalf			
Rhea Davison			
Shaunti Begay			
Jean Deere			
Renee Anderson			
Teresa Hernandez			
Louise Parlet			
Tristan Tsosie			
Jose Imero			
Jade Wong			
John R. Simmons			
Hu Huang			
Kevin McKinzie			
Jesus Santo			

Copyright © 2014, 2011, 2007 by Saunders, an imprint of Elsevier Inc. All rights reserved.

2. With the schedule of Today's Appointments still open, make a list below of the patients Dr. Hayler is to see in the morning. Place these patients in the correct order for their appointments and note whether the medical record can be pulled from the files of established patients or whether a new record should be prepared.

3. What medical records will need to be pulled from the files for Dr. Meyer's morning patients? Will any of these patients need to have a new record prepared? List these patients and their record needs below (in the order of their appointment times).

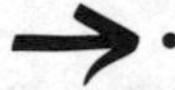

- Click **Finish** to return to the Reception area.
- Click on **Charts**.
- Click on the **Patient Medical Information** tab and select **1-Progress Notes**.
- Record the patient's first and last dates of service in columns 3 and 4 in the table in question 1. (*Important:* New patients will not have any forms in their chart. Use today's virtual date—5/1/07—as their first date of service; there will be no "last date of service" for new patients.)
- Click **Close Chart** to return to the Reception area.
- Click the exit arrow.
- Click **Return to Map** and select **Yes** at the pop-up menu to return to the office map.
- Repeat these instructions for each patient until you have completed the table in question 1.

Copyright © 2014, 2011, 2007 by Saunders, an imprint of Elsevier Inc. All rights reserved.

4. Using the table in question 1 as a reference, list the patients' names in alphabetic order in the left column below. In the right column indicate whether the medical records for each patient will be available in the file cabinet of established patients or whether the record will have to be organized and placed in the correct position as a new medical record.

Alphabetic List of Patients	New or Established Record?

5. As you pull the medical records for established patients, you will need to change the year on the medical records for these patients (unless the patient has already been seen in the current year). List the established patients below and indicate what year will need to be relabeled on their medical record (if this applies). Remember, today's virtual date is May 1, 2007.

Name of Established Patient	Year That Will Need to Be Relabeled

Copyright © 2014, 2011, 2007 by Saunders, an imprint of Elsevier Inc. All rights reserved.

6. At the end of the morning, the medical records need to be filed correctly to prevent loss and to ensure proper time management. Below, list in alphabetic order the names of patients who had morning appointments today and whose records will need to be refiled.

- Click the exit arrow.
- Click **Return to Map**, then click **Yes** at the pop-up menu to return to the office map or click Exit the Program.

Exercise 2

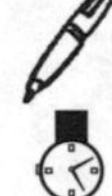

Writing Activity

25 minutes

Answer the following questions regarding paper medical records and capabilities of EMR systems.

1. Which of the following would *not* be used to help prevent misfiling of medical records?
   a. Colored letter tabs for use with names
   b. Colored tabs for the last year seen in the office
   c. Outguides
   d. Alphabetic tabs in the filing system

2. The two filing systems most often used in a medical office are

   ______________________ and ______________________ filing.

Copyright © 2014, 2011, 2007 by Saunders, an imprint of Elsevier Inc. All rights reserved.

3. Describe the differences in alphabetic and numeric filing systems.

4. Explain how color-coding enhances paper medical record systems?

5. List the five steps needed to prepare a paper medical record for filing.

   (1)

   (2)

   (3)

   (4)

   (5)

6. What steps can be followed for "finding" a misplaced paper medical record?

Copyright © 2014, 2011, 2007 by Saunders, an imprint of Elsevier Inc. All rights reserved.

7. Explain the primary function of the following features of EMR software systems.

   a. Specialty software

   b. Appointment scheduler

   c. Appointment reminder and confirmation

   d. Prescription writer

   e. Medical billing systems

Copyright © 2014, 2011, 2007 by Saunders, an imprint of Elsevier Inc. All rights reserved.

f. Charge capture

g. Eligibility verification

h. Referral management

i. Laboratory order integration

j. Patient portal

Copyright © 2014, 2011, 2007 by Saunders, an imprint of Elsevier Inc. All rights reserved.

LESSON 9

Insurance Forms and Verification

Reading Assignment: Chapter 7—Medicine and Law
- OSHA Record Keeping Regulations

Chapter 18—Basics of Diagnostic Coding
Chapter 19—Basics of Procedural Coding
Chapter 20—Basics of Health Insurance
Chapter 21—The Health Insurance Claim Form

Patients: Shaunti Begay, Louise Parlet, John R. Simmons, Janet Jones, Jose Imero

Learning Objectives:

- Apply managed care policies and procedures to office billing and coding.
- Use third party guidelines for preparing insurance claims and collecting copayments.
- Verify insurance information and initiate a referral for a patient.
- Determine which diagnosis should be coded, and which should not, from patient documentation in the chart.
- Proofread an insurance claim form and identify errors that will affect claims processing.

Overview:

In this lesson you will perform the necessary steps for preparing a clean claim for insurance purposes and collecting co-payments that are due to the practice. Completing these steps requires the correct use of managed care policies and procedures and the proper application of the office Policy Manual. A clean claim includes the appropriate diagnostic and procedural codes as well as the proper completion of the insurance claim form. You will proofread an insurance form and compare it with the information in the patient's chart and encounter form. You will indicate which boxes need corrections before the claim can be sent to the insurance company.

Copyright © 2014, 2011, 2007 by Saunders, an imprint of Elsevier Inc. All rights reserved.

Exercise 1

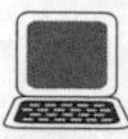

Online Activity—Verifying Insurance for a New Patient

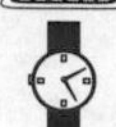

30 minutes

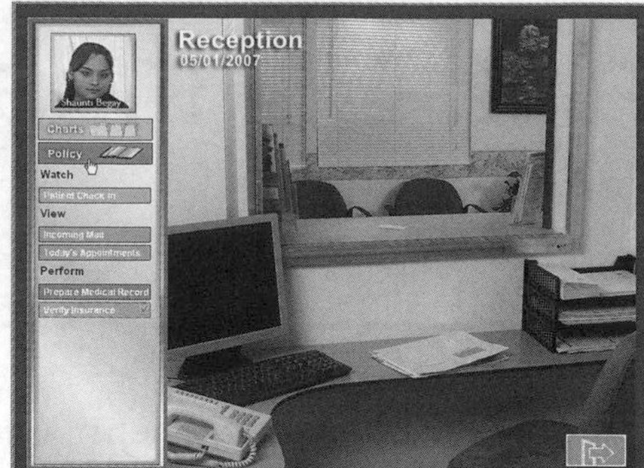

- Sign in to Mountain View Clinic.
- Select **Shaunti Begay** from the patient list.
- Click on **Reception**.
- Click on **Policy** to open the office Policy Manual.
- Type "payment" in the search bar and click on the magnifying glass.
- Read the section of the Policy Manual on the Telephone Policies, specifically concerning copays.
- Type "patient insurance policies" in the search bar and click on the magnifying glass.
- Read the section of the Policy Manual on the the policies that apply when patients have insurance coverage that is not accepted by the medical practice.

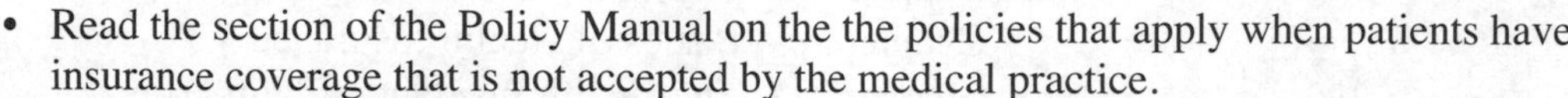

1. According to the Policy Manual, what information should be obtained from the patient when the appointment is made?

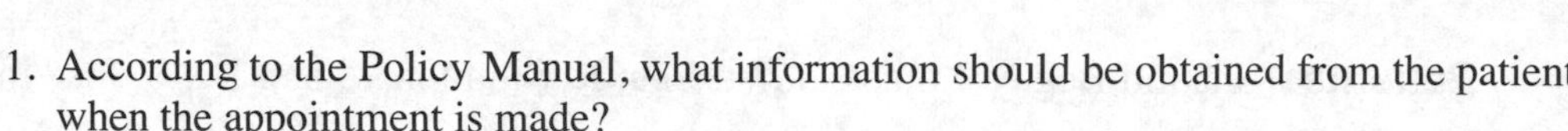

2. Why is it important for the medical assistant to verify whether the office is a preferred provider with the patient's insurance *at the time the appointment is made*?

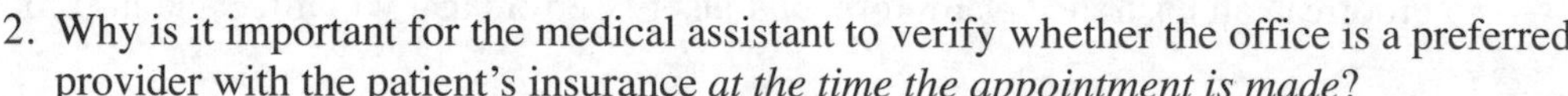

3. What does the Policy Manual state about collecting payments, copays, and percentages of charges for patient visits?

Copyright © 2014, 2011, 2007 by Saunders, an imprint of Elsevier Inc. All rights reserved.

- Click **Close Manual** to return to the Reception desk.
- Under the Watch heading, click on **Patient Check-In** and watch the video.
- Click the **X** on the video screen to close the video.
- Click on the **Insurance Card**.
- Identify the appropriate question to ask the patient regarding her insurance and click on **Ask**.
- Use the checkboxes to select which procedures are needed to verify the patient's insurance.
- Click **Finish** to return to the Reception area.

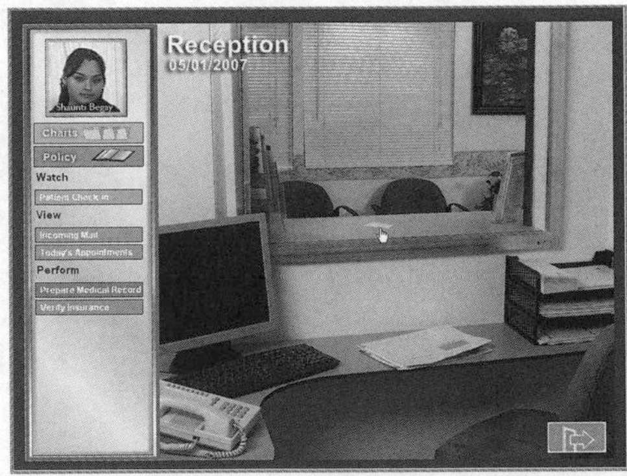

- Click on **Policy** to open the office Policy Manual.
- From the menu on the left side of the screen, click on the arrow next to **Coding/Billing Manual** to expand the menu.
- Click the arrow next to **Financial Policy** and select **Accepted Insurance Carriers** from the list to read that section of the Policy Manual.

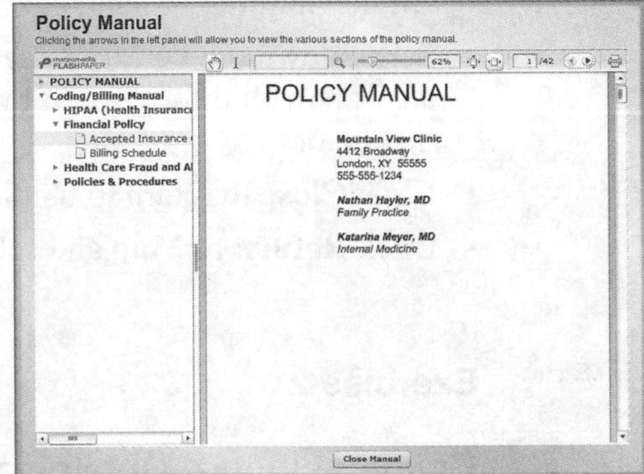

4. Was Kristin correct in stating that Mountain View Clinic was not a participating provider for Shaunti's insurance plan?

5. What did Shaunti's mother say about the information she gave the receptionist regarding their insurance coverage when she made the appointment?

Copyright © 2014, 2011, 2007 by Saunders, an imprint of Elsevier Inc. All rights reserved.

6. What steps should the medical assistant have taken to avoid the confusion that occurred when Shaunti checked in?

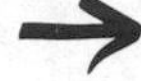

- Click **Close Manual** to return to the Reception area.
- Click the exit arrow.
- On the Summary Menu, click on **Look at Your Performance Summary**.
- Scroll down the Performance Summary to the Verify Insurance section and compare your answers with those chosen by the experts. The summary can be printed or saved for your instructor.
- Click **Close** to return to the Summary Menu.
- Click **Return to Map** and select **Yes** at the pop-up menu to return to the office map.

Exercise 2

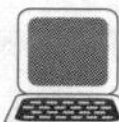

Online Activity—Obtaining a Referral for an Established Patient

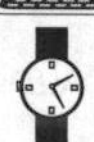

30 minutes

- Select **Louise Parlet** from the patient list.
- Click on **Check Out**.
- Under the Watch heading, click on **Patient Check-Out** and watch the video.

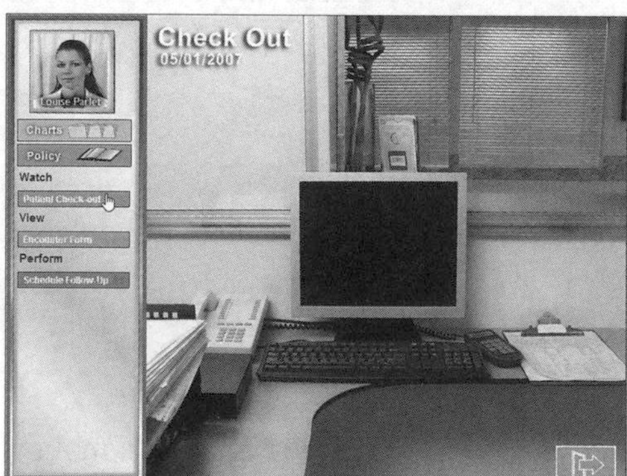

1. Why is it important that the medical assistant assist Ms. Parlet in obtaining approval from her insurance company for the referral to Dr. Lockett?

Copyright © 2014, 2011, 2007 by Saunders, an imprint of Elsevier Inc. All rights reserved.

2. After receiving the precertification verification number, how should the medical assistant handle the verification number?

- Click the **X** on the video screen to close the video.
- Click on **Charts**.
- Click on the **Patient Medical Information** tab and select **3-Progress Notes**.
- Read Dr. Hayler's notes regarding the examination.

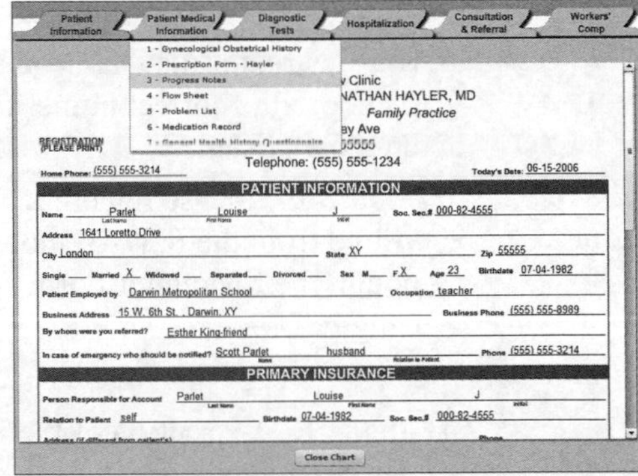

3. What instructions does Dr. Hayler give about the results of the lab work?

Critical Thinking Question

4. Do you think most insurance companies would reimburse a medical provider for a test if the test has already been completed at another facility?

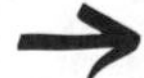

- Click **Close Chart** to return to the Check Out desk.
- Click the exit arrow.
- Click **Return to Map** and select **Yes** at the pop-up menu to return to the office map.

Copyright © 2014, 2011, 2007 by Saunders, an imprint of Elsevier Inc. All rights reserved.

Exercise 3

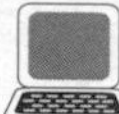

Online Activity—Choosing the Correct Diagnosis to Code for an Office Visit of a New Adult Patient

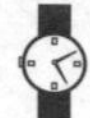

30 minutes

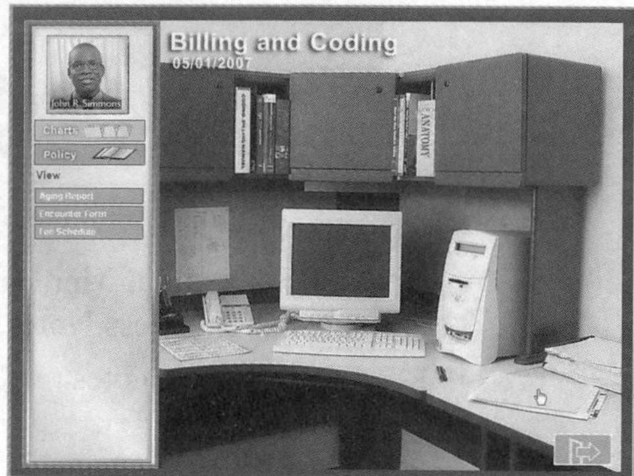

- Select **John R. Simmons** from the patient list.
- Click on **Billing and Coding**.
- Click on the **Encounter Form** clipboard.
- Your instructor may ask you to use the ICD-10 to choose the correct numeric codes for the diagnoses listed.
- ***Important:*** Please remember that your codes will be from the ICD-10, not ICD-9, even though the Encounter Form says the clinic is using ICD-9.

1. In the ICD-9 section of the Encounter Form, which diagnoses are checked off for Dr. Simmons' visit?

2. Which of these diagnoses should receive an ICD-9 code? If there are any diagnoses that should not be coded, explain why not.

3. When should the fecal occult Hemoccult test that the patient will collect at home be billed? Explain your answer.

Copyright © 2014, 2011, 2007 by Saunders, an imprint of Elsevier Inc. All rights reserved.

- Click **Finish** to return to the Billing and Coding area.
- Click on **Charts**.
- Click on the **Patient Information** and select **5-Insurance Cards**.

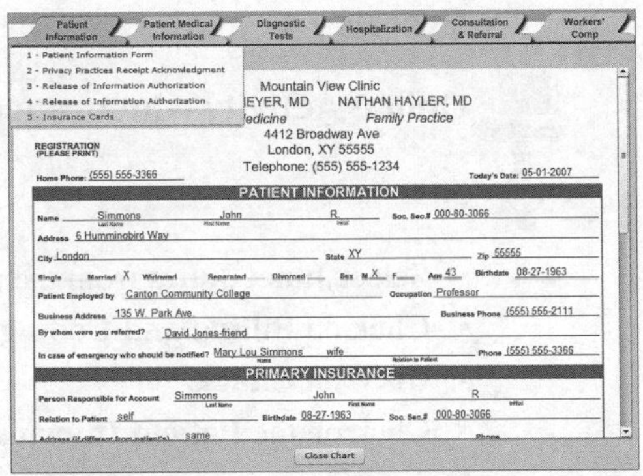

4. What is meant by PCP?

5. What is meant by POS?

6. Using the information on the insurance cards found in the medical record, what is the copay on the patient's insurance? What is the payment rate on the secondary insurance?

7. Look at the back of both of the insurance cards. What do you notice when comparing the cards?

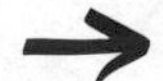

- Click **Close Chart** to return to the Billing and Coding area.
- Click the exit arrow.
- Click **Return to Map** and select **Yes** at the pop-up menu to return to the office map.

Copyright © 2014, 2011, 2007 by Saunders, an imprint of Elsevier Inc. All rights reserved.

Exercise 4

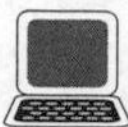

Online Activity—Insurance Versus Workers' Compensation Claims

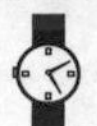

30 minutes

- Select **Janet Jones** from the patient list.
- Click on **Billing and Coding**.
- Click on **Charts**.
- Click on the **Patient Information** tab.

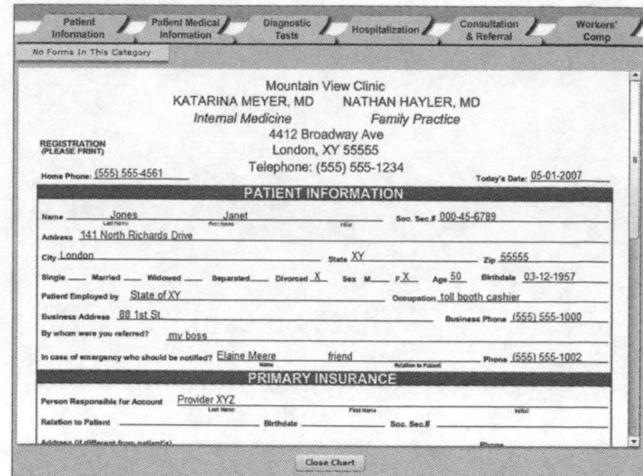

Patient Information | Patient Medical Information | Diagnostic Tests | Hospitalization | Consultation & Referral | Workers' Comp

No Forms In This Category

Mountain View Clinic
KATARINA MEYER, MD NATHAN HAYLER, MD
Internal Medicine *Family Practice*
4412 Broadway Ave
London, XY 55555
Telephone: (555) 555-1234

REGISTRATION (PLEASE PRINT)

Home Phone: (555) 555-4561 Today's Date: 05-01-2007

PATIENT INFORMATION

Name Jones Janet Soc. Sec.# 000-45-6789
Address 141 North Richards Drive
City London State XY Zip 55555
Single ___ Married ___ Widowed ___ Separated ___ Divorced X Sex M ___ F X Age 50 Birthdate 03-12-1957
Patient Employed by State of XY Occupation toll booth cashier
Business Address 88 1st St. Business Phone (555) 555-1000
By whom were you referred? my boss
In case of emergency who should be notified? Elaine Meere friend Phone (555) 555-1002

PRIMARY INSURANCE

Person Responsible for Account Provider XYZ
Relation to Patient ___ Birthdate ___ Soc. Sec.# ___
Address (if different from patient's) Phone

Close Chart

1. You will notice that in Ms. Jones' medical record, there is no information about private insurance coverage. Why is this important for this case?

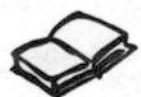

2. If a patient says that he or she is injured at the workplace, or have a work-related illness, what would the medical assistant need to do before escorting the patient to the examination room? Refer to the Workers' Compensation section in Chapter 20 and Chapter 7 of the textbook if you need help locating the answer.

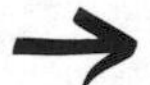

- Click on the **Workers' Comp** tab.

3. What information do you find under this tab in Ms. Jones' medical record?

Copyright © 2014, 2011, 2007 by Saunders, an imprint of Elsevier Inc. All rights reserved.

4. The top of the First Report of Injury states that this form is "approved as use for" two OSHA forms. What are the names of these forms?

5. If the workers' compensation carrier declares Ms. Jones' claim to be nonindustrial and refuses to pay it, is Mountain View Clinic required to write off the balance? *Use your critical thinking skills to answer this question.*

6. Can you give an example of an injury or a problem for which the insurance company might not pay if the patient had previous problems with the same or a similar diagnosis?

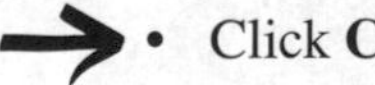

- Click **Close Chart** to return to the Billing and Coding area.
- Click the exit arrow.
- Click **Return to Map** and select **Yes** at the pop-up menu to return to the office map.

Copyright © 2014, 2011, 2007 by Saunders, an imprint of Elsevier Inc. All rights reserved.

Exercise 5

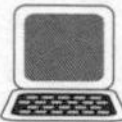

Other Activity—Proofreading and Critical Thinking Exercise

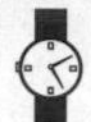

45 minutes

Jose Imero's insurance claim has been filled out by the medical assistant student. Your responsibility is to review the insurance form and make sure it is correct before billing the insurance company. There are several errors on the form. You will use the textbook, the Patient's Information Form, the Insurance Card, the Progress Notes, and the Encounter Form to ensure that everything on the form is correct. Review Chapter 21 in your textbook carefully before you begin this exercise, and use it as a tool as you review the insurance form.

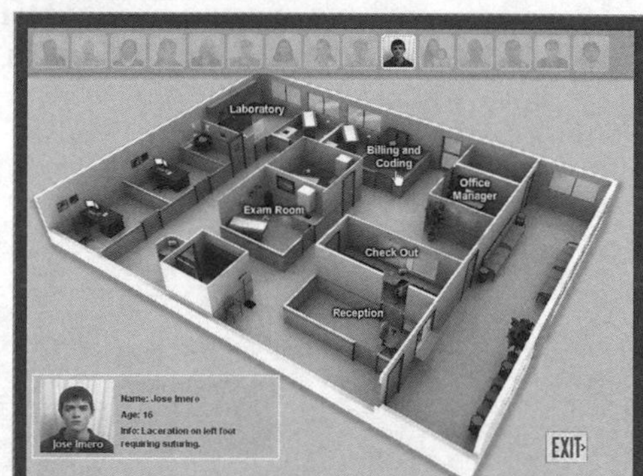

- Select **Jose Imero** from the patient list.
- Click on **Billing and Coding**.
- Click on **Charts**.
- Click on the **Patient Information** tab and select **1–Patient Information Form** to review the patient's demographic information.
- Click on the **Patient Information** tab and select **2–Insurance Cards** to verify that the insurance identification numbers are correct.
- When you get to Box 14 on the insurance claim form, click on the **Patient Medical Information** tab and select **1–Progress Notes**.
- Click **Close Chart** to return to the Billing and Coding area.
- When you get to Box 24 on the insurance claim form, click on the **Encounter Form** clipboard.
- Click **Finish** to return to the Billing and Coding area.
- Click on the **Fee Schedule** sheet to verify the insurance form has the correct amount for each service listed.
- Click **Finish** to return to the Billing and Coding area.

Important: The following instructions and notations will help as you go through the insurance form and make notations of errors.

It is indicated on Jose Imero's registration form that he is a student. For this exercise, consider his status as full-time student.

- Boxes 24 i and j should be left blank.
- For Box 25, you can locate the federal tax ID number on the Encounter Form at the top right-hand side.
- For Box 31, the office will file the claim the same date as the service was provided.
- For Box 33, the NPI number is 1234567899.

Copyright © 2014, 2011, 2007 by Saunders, an imprint of Elsevier Inc. All rights reserved.

1500

HEALTH INSURANCE CLAIM FORM

APPROVED BY NATIONAL UNIFORM CLAIM COMMITTEE 08/05

PICA | PICA

CARRIER

1. MEDICARE (Medicare #) / MEDICAID (Medicaid #) / TRICARE CHAMPUS (Sponsor's SSN) / CHAMPVA (Member ID#) / GROUP HEALTH PLAN (SSN or ID) [X] / FECA BLK LUNG (SSN) / OTHER (ID)

1a. INSURED'S I.D. NUMBER (For Program in Item 1): YAM 150221114

2. PATIENT'S NAME (Last Name, First Name, Middle Initial): Imero, Jose

3. PATIENT'S BIRTH DATE (MM DD YY): 03 15 91 — SEX: M [X] F [ ]

4. INSURED'S NAME (Last Name, First Name, Middle Initial): IMERO ANTONIO

5. PATIENT'S ADDRESS (No., Street): 253 Lindhurst Way — CITY: London — STATE: XY — ZIP CODE: 55555 — TELEPHONE (Include Area Code): (555) 555-5455

6. PATIENT RELATIONSHIP TO INSURED: Self [ ] Spouse [ ] Child [X] Other [ ]

7. INSURED'S ADDRESS (No., Street): 4628 Mission Way — CITY: Trumball — STATE: YZ — ZIP CODE: 99999 — TELEPHONE (Include Area Code): (555) 555-7878

8. PATIENT STATUS: Single [ ] Married [ ] Other [ ] — Employed [ ] Full-Time Student [X] Part-Time Student [ ]

9. OTHER INSURED'S NAME (Last Name, First Name, Middle Initial)

a. OTHER INSURED'S POLICY OR GROUP NUMBER

b. OTHER INSURED'S DATE OF BIRTH (MM DD YY) — SEX: M [ ] F [ ]

c. EMPLOYER'S NAME OR SCHOOL NAME

d. INSURANCE PLAN NAME OR PROGRAM NAME

10. IS PATIENT'S CONDITION RELATED TO:

a. EMPLOYMENT? (Current or Previous): YES [ ] NO [X]

b. AUTO ACCIDENT?: YES [ ] NO [X] — PLACE (State)

c. OTHER ACCIDENT?: YES [X] NO [ ]

10d. RESERVED FOR LOCAL USE

11. INSURED'S POLICY GROUP OR FECA NUMBER: 1822

a. INSURED'S DATE OF BIRTH (MM DD YY): 12 12 74 — SEX: M [X] F [ ]

b. EMPLOYER'S NAME OR SCHOOL NAME: Sunshine Foods

c. INSURANCE PLAN NAME OR PROGRAM NAME: Blue Cross/Blue Shield

d. IS THERE ANOTHER HEALTH BENEFIT PLAN?: YES [ ] NO [X] *If yes*, return to and complete item 9 a-d.

READ BACK OF FORM BEFORE COMPLETING & SIGNING THIS FORM.

12. PATIENT'S OR AUTHORIZED PERSON'S SIGNATURE I authorize the release of any medical or other information necessary to process this claim. I also request payment of government benefits either to myself or to the party who accepts assignment below.

SIGNED Signature on File DATE

13. INSURED'S OR AUTHORIZED PERSON'S SIGNATURE I authorize payment of medical benefits to the undersigned physician or supplier for services described below.

SIGNED Signature on File

PATIENT AND INSURED INFORMATION

14. DATE OF CURRENT (MM DD YY): 05 01 07 — ILLNESS (First symptom) OR INJURY (Accident) OR PREGNANCY(LMP)

15. IF PATIENT HAS HAD SAME OR SIMILAR ILLNESS, GIVE FIRST DATE MM DD YY

16. DATES PATIENT UNABLE TO WORK IN CURRENT OCCUPATION FROM MM DD YY TO MM DD YY

17. NAME OF REFERRING PROVIDER OR OTHER SOURCE — 17a. — 17b. NPI

18. HOSPITALIZATION DATES RELATED TO CURRENT SERVICES FROM MM DD YY TO MM DD YY

19. RESERVED FOR LOCAL USE

20. OUTSIDE LAB?: YES [ ] NO [X] — $ CHARGES

21. DIAGNOSIS OR NATURE OF ILLNESS OR INJURY (Relate Items 1, 2, 3 or 4 to Item 24E by Line)

1. Open Wound L foot 8 cm w/ complications
2.
3.
4.

22. MEDICAID RESUBMISSION CODE — ORIGINAL REF. NO.

23. PRIOR AUTHORIZATION NUMBER

	24. A. DATE(S) OF SERVICE From MM	DD	YY	To MM	DD	YY	B. PLACE OF SERVICE	C. EMG	D. PROCEDURES, SERVICES, OR SUPPLIES (Explain Unusual Circumstances) CPT/HCPCS	MODIFIER	E. DIAGNOSIS POINTER	F. $ CHARGES	G. DAYS OR UNITS	H. EPSDT Family Plan	I. ID. QUAL.	J. RENDERING PROVIDER ID. #
1	05	05	07	05	01	07	11		Est. visit, Level II		laceration	45 00	1	N	NPI	
2									Tetanus		laceration	15 00	1	N	NPI	
3									Immun. Single		laceration	25 00	1	N	NPI	
4									Surgical Tray		laceration	15 00	1	N	NPI	
5									Wound Repair		laceration	175 00	1	N	NPI	
6															NPI	

25. FEDERAL TAX I.D. NUMBER: 123456789 — SSN [ ] EIN [ ]

26. PATIENT'S ACCOUNT NO.

27. ACCEPT ASSIGNMENT? (For govt. claims, see back): YES [X] NO [ ]

28. TOTAL CHARGE: $ 275 00

29. AMOUNT PAID: $ 25 00

30. BALANCE DUE: $ 250 00

31. SIGNATURE OF PHYSICIAN OR SUPPLIER INCLUDING DEGREES OR CREDENTIALS (I certify that the statements on the reverse apply to this bill and are made a part thereof.)

SOF

SIGNED — DATE 05012007

32. SERVICE FACILITY LOCATION INFORMATION

44 BROADWAY
LONDON, XY, 55555

a. NPI b.

33. BILLING PROVIDER INFO & PH # ( )

NATHAN HAYLER MD
4412 BROADWAY
LONDON, XY, 55555

a. 1234567899 b.

PHYSICIAN OR SUPPLIER INFORMATION

NUCC Instruction Manual available at: www.nucc.org

APPROVED OMB-0938-0999 FORM CMS-1500 (08/05)

Copyright © 2014, 2011, 2007 by Saunders, an imprint of Elsevier Inc. All rights reserved.

1. Below, list any errors you found as you reviewed Jose Imero's insurance claim form.

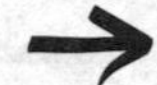

- Click the exit arrow.
- Click **Return to Map**, then click **Yes** at the pop-up menu to return to the office map or click Exit the Program.

Copyright © 2014, 2011, 2007 by Saunders, an imprint of Elsevier Inc. All rights reserved.

LESSON 10

Bookkeeping

Reading Assignment: Chapter 22—Professional Fees, Billing, and Collection
- How Fees Are Determined
- Bookkeeping Computations Used on Patient Accounts
- Comparison of Manual and Computerized Bookkeeping Systems
- Special Bookkeeping Entries
- Payment Options
- Collection Techniques
- Using Outside Collection Assistance

Chapter 23—Banking Services and Procedures
Chapter 24—Financial and Practice Management
- What Is Accounting?

Patients: All

Learning Objectives:

- Post daily entries on the day sheet and prepare bank deposits at the end of the day.
- Process credit balances, NSF checks, and checks from collection agencies.
- Process credit balances and complete necessary steps to process a refund, including preparation of a check.
- Reconcile a bank statement.
- Maintain a petty cash fund.
- Discuss the maintenance of records for accounting and banking purposes.
- Discuss the importance of managing accounts payable promptly.

Overview:

In this lesson the basic bookkeeping procedures will be accomplished. All patients will be added to the day sheet, along with the payments and the NSF check received in today's mail. A deposit record will be prepared. The steps for reconciliation of the bank statement and maintenance of records for accounting purposes will also be covered.

Copyright © 2014, 2011, 2007 by Saunders, an imprint of Elsevier Inc. All rights reserved.

Exercise 1

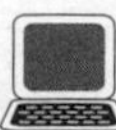

Online Activity—Posting Charges to Ledger Cards

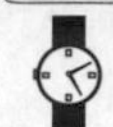

30 minutes

- Sign in to Mountain View Clinic.
- Select **Jade Wong** from the patient list.
- Click on **Billing and Coding**.
- Click on the **Encounter Form** clipboard and **Fee Schedule** sheet as needed to complete the following questions.

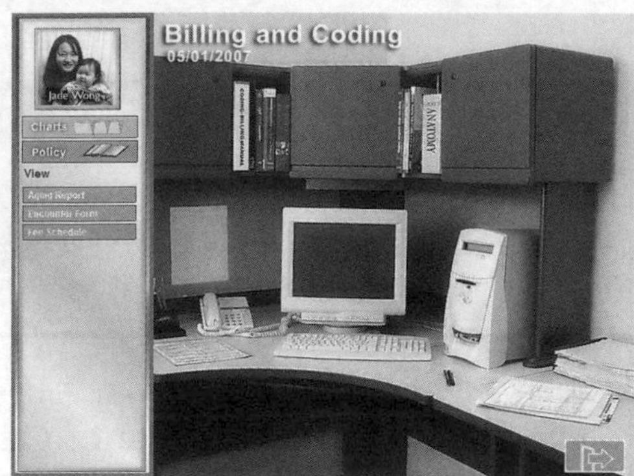

Copyright © 2014, 2011, 2007 by Saunders, an imprint of Elsevier Inc. All rights reserved.

1. a. Using the Encounter Form for Jade Wong, begin completing the blank ledger card below.
   b. In the column marked Professional Service, list each individual service provided, but do not enter any fee or balance information.
   c. After the last service has been entered, be sure to record that the co-pay was collected and enter the amount in the Payment column.
   d. Fill in the fees charged for the listed services and calculate the balances.

Important: The balance should be corrected line by line as each service or payment is added or subtracted.

Mountain View Clinic

Patient Ledger

Patient Name:

Insurance Type:

Date	Professional Service	Fee ($)	Payment ($)	Adj. ($)	Prev. Bal. ($)	New Balance ($)
	Totals:					

2. After filling in the services, fees, and payments for Jade's current visit, should the ledger card be totaled as indicated at the bottom of the card? Refer to the textbook, if needed, and explain your answer.

Copyright © 2014, 2011, 2007 by Saunders, an imprint of Elsevier Inc. All rights reserved.

3. How did the medical assistant know what Jade's copay was?

- Click **Finish** to return to the Billing and Coding area.
- Click the exit arrow.
- Click **Return to Map** and select **Yes** at the pop-up menu to return to the office map.

Exercise 2

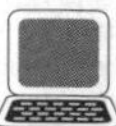

Online Activity—Posting Entries to a Day Sheet

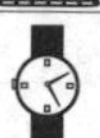

60 minutes

1. In this activity you will post charges and payments for the patients who were seen in the office today, using the day sheet on the next page. Note that the distribution column indicates which physician, Dr. Hayler or Dr. Meyer, provided care to the patient. The amount of money the patient paid should be written in one of those columns in addition to the payment column.

   a. In the Patient Name column on the blank day sheet below, list the patients in the following order: Jade Wong, Louise Parlet, Hu Huang, Rhea Davison, Jesus Santo, Jean Deere, Tristan Tsosie, Wilson Metcalf, Renee Anderson, Jose Imero, Shaunti Begay, Janet Jones, Kevin McKinzie, John R. Simmons, and Teresa Hernandez.

   b. Select **Jade Wong** from the patient list. Then click on **Check Out** on the office map. Once in the Check Out area, click on the **Encounter Form** clipboard.

   c. Using one line per patient, complete each column on the day sheet using the Total Charges, Previous Balance, and Amount Received information listed on the Encounter Form. Refer back to the ledger card in Exercise 1 to confirm your totals. (Note: Unlike the ledger card, the Professional Service column on the day sheet is a summary description of the visit.)

   d. For the purposes of this exercise, also make a note next to each patient's name to indicate whether the patient paid by cash, check, or credit card. If payment was made by check, include the check number.

   e. Click **Finish** to close the Encounter Form. Click the exit arrow, then click **Return to Map** and select **Yes** at the pop-up menu to return to the office map and select the next patient.

   Repeat the above steps by selecting each patient and opening his or her Encounter Form at Check Out.

   f. When you finish recording the information for the last patient on the list, remain at the office map to continue with the next question.

Copyright © 2014, 2011, 2007 by Saunders, an imprint of Elsevier Inc. All rights reserved.

Mountain View Clinic
Daysheet

Date	Professional Service	Fee	Payment	Adjustment	New Balance	Old Balance	Patient's Name	Distribution	
								Dr. Hayler	Dr. Meyer
	TOTALS						TOTALS		

Copyright © 2014, 2011, 2007 by Saunders, an imprint of Elsevier Inc. All rights reserved.

- Click on **Reception**.
- Click on the **Stackable Trays**.
- Click the numbers or arrows at the top of the page to examine and read each piece of mail.

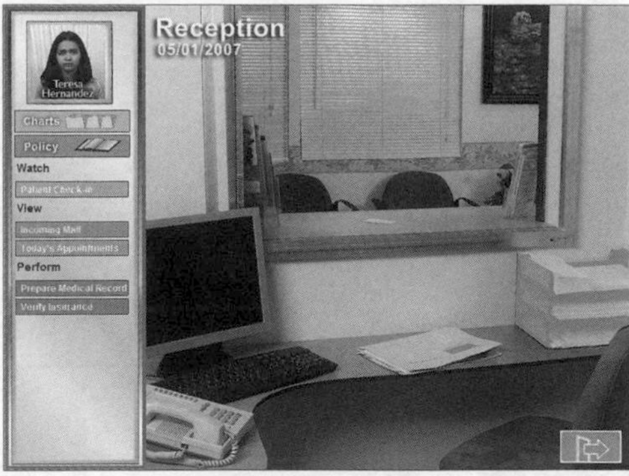

2. a. On the blank day sheet on the next page, record any payments received by the clinic and any charges paid by the clinic in the appropriate columns.

   b. Be sure to include a description of the payment/charge and the patient's name.

   c. For the purposes of this exercise, make a note of the bank and check number next to the name of any patient who paid by check.

   d. To complete the remaining columns, click **Finish** to return to the Reception area.

   e. Click the exit arrow, then click **Return to Map** and select **Yes** at the pop-up menu to return to the office map

   f. Click on **Office Manager** and then on the **Day Sheet** document to find any previous balance information. Recalculate the balance and record in the New Balance column.

   g. Mark Bonsel's previous account balance was zero ("0") before you received the NSF check. The NSF check shows that it was paid on April 7, 2007, but it does not indicate what it was for, other than a balance. Assume it was for a Level II New Patient Visit, which would be $65.00 on the date of April 7, 2007.

   h. *Note:* A copy of Sarah Anita's EOB from Blue Cross/Blue Shield was received in the mail. The insurance payment and adjustment were already posted on the day sheet and her ledger in the office manager's section of the Office. The copy of the EOB in the mail will not need posting again.

   i. Recalculate the balance and record it in the New Balance column.

Copyright © 2014, 2011, 2007 by Saunders, an imprint of Elsevier Inc. All rights reserved.

Mountain View Clinic
Daysheet

Date	Professional Service	Fee	Payment	Adjustment	New Balance	Old Balance	Patient's Name	Distribution	
								Dr. Hayler	Dr. Meyer
	TOTALS						TOTALS		

Copyright © 2014, 2011, 2007 by Saunders, an imprint of Elsevier Inc. All rights reserved.

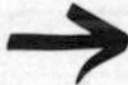

- Click **Finish** to return to the manager's office.
- Remain in the Office Manager area to continue to Exercise 4.

Exercise 3

Writing Activity—Preparing a Bank Deposit

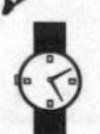

15 minutes

Using the information recorded in the completed day sheets in Exercise 2, you will now prepare a bank deposit (both front and back) for the accounts receivable for the day. Be sure the total on the deposit slip balances with the total of receivables on the day sheet.

1. Below, complete the front side of the deposit slip.

DEPOSIT SLIP

Clarion National Bank
90 Grape Vine Road
London, XY 55555-0001

Mountain View Clinic
4412 Broadway
London, XY 55555

Date: ______________________

____
SIGN HERE IN TELLER'S PRESENCE FOR CASH RECEIVED

CASH			TOTAL
	Currency	$_____	
	Coin	$_____	$_____
	Total Cash		$_____
CHECKS	See other side for detail		$_____
- CASH REC'D			$_____
NET DEPOSIT			$_____

Copyright © 2014, 2011, 2007 by Saunders, an imprint of Elsevier Inc. All rights reserved.

2. Below, complete the back portion of the bank deposit slip. (*Note:* The bank number cannot be obtained from the day sheet. For the purposes of this exercise, use the check number as a substitute.)

BANK DEPOSIT DETAIL

PAYMENTS						
BANK NUMBER	BY CHECK OR PMO		BY COIN OR CURRENCY		CREDIT CARD	
TOTALS						

CURRENCY		
COIN		
CHECKS		
CREDIT CARDS		
TOTAL RECEIPTS		
LESS CREDIT CARD $		
TOTAL DEPOSIT		

DEPOSIT DATE ____________________

Copyright © 2014, 2011, 2007 by Saunders, an imprint of Elsevier Inc. All rights reserved.

Exercise 4

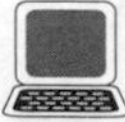

Online Activity—Processing Credit Balances

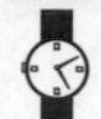

20 minutes

- Click on **Day Sheet** document.

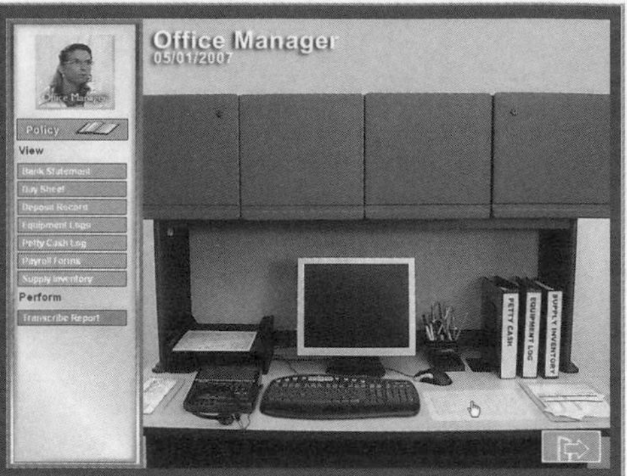

1. Two patients listed on the day sheet have overpaid, which resulted in a credit balance denoted by a parenthesis around the amount that was overpaid. Betsy Dunworthy overpaid by $20.00 and her refund was already processed. What is the name of the other patient who should receive a refund, and how much money should he receive?

2. Using the blank check below, process the outstanding refund for payment.

173975

DATE:	
TO:	
FOR:	
ACCOUNT NO.	
AMOUNT PAID	$

MOUNTAIN VIEW CLINIC
4412 Broadway
London, XY 55555

173975

94-72/1224

Date: ______________________

Pay to the order of: ______________________

______________________ Dollars $

Clarion National Bank
Member FDIC
90 Grape Vine Road
London, XY 55555-0001

____
Authorized Signature

⑈005503⑈ 446782011⑈ 678800470

- Click **Finish** to return to the manager's office.

Copyright © 2014, 2011, 2007 by Saunders, an imprint of Elsevier Inc. All rights reserved.

Exercise 5

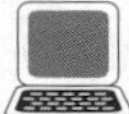

Online Activity—Maintaining Petty Cash Fund

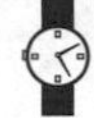

30 minutes

- Click on the **Petty Cash Binder**.

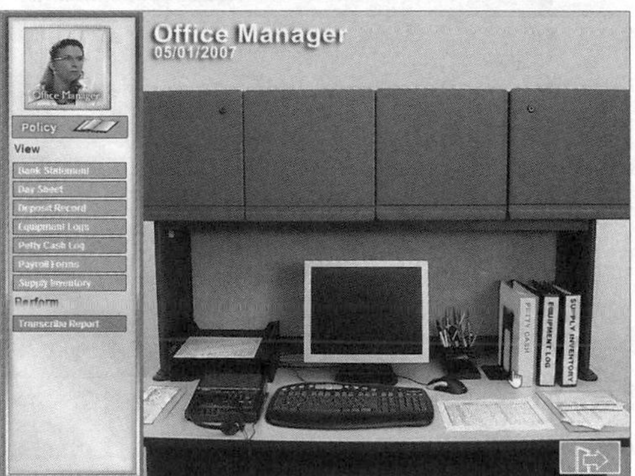

1. Petty cash was used to pay for the mailing of a certified letter. What is the receipt number and date from this transaction?

2. On 5/1/07, the administrative medical assistant was asked to obtain soft drinks for an office celebration to be held that afternoon. These were bought at Sav-A-Grocery for the amount of $24.56. She also mailed a large package at the post office. The cost for mailing the package was $15.08. Using the form below, fill out the first petty cash voucher.

Date: ______________________ No.: _____

PETTY CASH VOUCHER

For: ____

Charge to: ____

____

Approved by: Received by:

______________________ ______________________

Authorized Signature

Copyright © 2014, 2011, 2007 by Saunders, an imprint of Elsevier Inc. All rights reserved.

3. Now fill out the second petty cash voucher.

Date: ______________________ No.: ______

PETTY CASH VOUCHER

For: ____

Charge to: ______________________________________

____

Approved by: Received by:

______________________ ______________________

Authorized Signature

4. Using the completed petty cash vouchers from questions 2 and 3, update the petty cash log below accordingly. Be sure to distribute the expenses to the proper expense column.

NO.	DATE	DESCRIPTION	AMOUNT	OFFICE EXP.	AUTO.	MISC.	BALANCE
	2/16/2007	Fund Established (check #217)					200.00
101	2/24/2007	Certified Letter	3.74	3.74			196.26
102	3/1/2007	Staff Meeting/Lunch	24.60			24.60	171.66
103	3/6/2007	Coffee	4.32			4.32	167.34
104	3/8/2007	Tympanic Thermometer	38.00	38.00			129.34
105	3/8/2007	Parking Fee	6.00		6.00		123.34
106	4/1/2007	Staff Meeting/Lunch	27.43			27.43	95.91
107	4/13/2007	Miscellaneous Supplies	9.01	9.01			86.90
108	4/21/2007	Patient Birthday Cards	12.17	12.17			74.73

Copyright © 2014, 2011, 2007 by Saunders, an imprint of Elsevier Inc. All rights reserved.

5. Office policy states that petty cash should be replenished when the amount falls below $50. Use the blank check below to replenish the petty cash fund to the full $200 balance as required by the office policy. Then, using the updated petty cash log in question 4, verify the petty cash fund balances by totaling all the columns, and add this transaction to the log.

173976

DATE: ______________
TO: ______________
FOR: ______________
ACCOUNT NO. ______________
AMOUNT PAID $

MOUNTAIN VIEW CLINIC
4412 Broadway
London, XY 55555

173976
94-72/1224

Date: ______________

Pay to the order of: ______________

______________ Dollars $

Clarion National Bank
Member FDIC
90 Grape Vine Road
London, XY 55555-0001

____
Authorized Signature

||■ 005503 ||■ 446782011 ||■ 678800470

- Click **Finish** to return to the manager's office.
- Click the exit arrow.
- Click **Return to Map** and select **Yes** at the pop-up menu to return to the office map.
- Select **Jose Imero** from the patient list.
- Click on **Check Out**.
- Under the Watch heading, click on Patient Check-Out and watch the video.

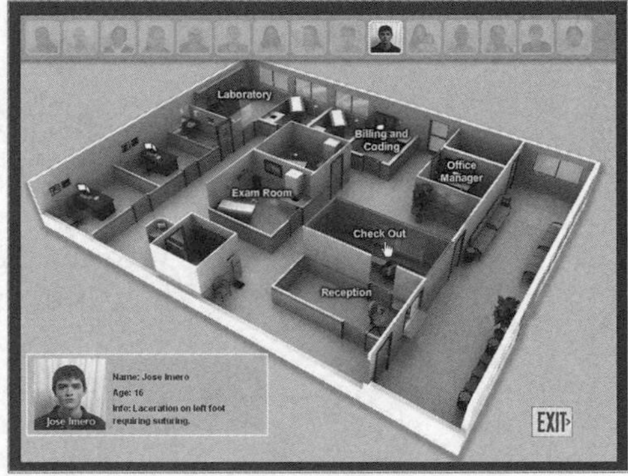

6. What are the ethical implications of Kristin asking another medical assistant for money from petty cash?

- Click the **X** on the video screen to close the video.
- Click the exit arrow.
- Click **Return to Map** and select **Yes** at the pop-up menu to return to the office map.

Copyright © 2014, 2011, 2007 by Saunders, an imprint of Elsevier Inc. All rights reserved.

Exercise 6

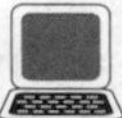

Online Activity—Managing Accounts Payable

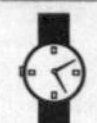

30 minutes

- Click on **Reception**.
- Click on the **Stackable Trays**.
- Click the numbers or arrows at the top of the page to examine and read pieces 8 and 9.

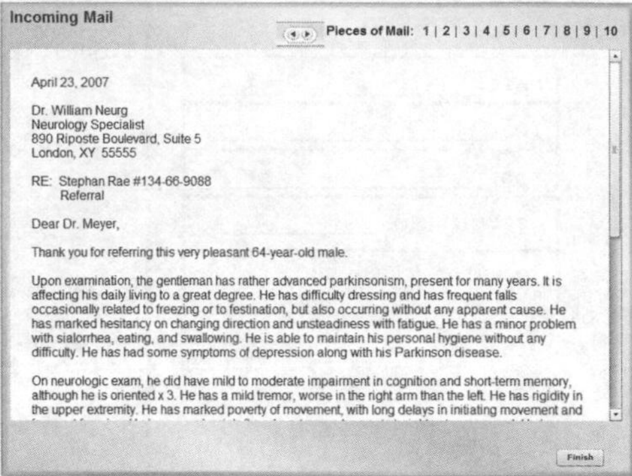

April 23, 2007

Dr. William Neurg
Neurology Specialist
890 Riposte Boulevard, Suite 5
London, XY 55555

RE: Stephan Rae #134-66-9088
Referral

Dear Dr. Meyer,

Thank you for referring this very pleasant 64-year-old male.

Upon examination, the gentleman has rather advanced parkinsonism, present for many years. It is affecting his daily living to a great degree. He has difficulty dressing and has frequent falls occasionally related to freezing or to festination, but also occurring without any apparent cause. He has marked hesitancy on changing direction and unsteadiness with fatigue. He has a minor problem with sialorrhea, eating, and swallowing. He is able to maintain his personal hygiene without any difficulty. He has had some symptoms of depression along with his Parkinson disease.

On neurologic exam, he did have mild to moderate impairment in cognition and short-term memory, although he is oriented x 3. He has a mild tremor, worse in the right arm than the left. He has rigidity in the upper extremity. He has marked poverty of movement, with long delays in initiating movement and

1. Indicate whether each of the following statements is true or false.

   a. ________ When accounts payable arrive, the date for payment with discounts should be noted.

   b. ________ It really does not matter what day of the month an accounts payable payment is made, as long as it is paid before the next billing cycle.

   c. ________ Invoices should be marked with the date and check number, as well as the initials of the person preparing the check.

   d. ________ All accounts payables should be checked against invoices and packing slips before payment is made.

   e. ________ All vendors will present invoices before payment is due.

Copyright © 2014, 2011, 2007 by Saunders, an imprint of Elsevier Inc. All rights reserved.

2. What information does the accounts payable person need to correctly process and post the payment of the invoices (pieces 8 and 9 of the incoming mail)? Select all that apply.

_____ Invoice number

_____ Company name

_____ Name of the customer service representative

_____ Date of check

_____ Account number

_____ Company address

_____ Company phone number

_____ Name of the company's bank

_____ Company's bank account number

_____ Type of expense

_____ Amount of the check

_____ Invoice date

_____ Check number

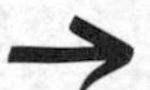

- Click **Finish** to return to the Reception area.
- Click the exit arrow.
- Click **Return to Map** and select **Yes** at the pop-up menu to return to the office map.

Exercise 7

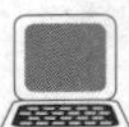

Online Activity—Reconciling a Bank Statement

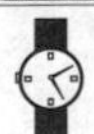

30 minutes

The clinic's bank statement arrives in today's mail. This is found in the manager's office. She is extremely busy and asks that you take the time to reconcile the statement for her.

- Click on **Office Manager**.
- Click on the **Bank Statement** file folder.

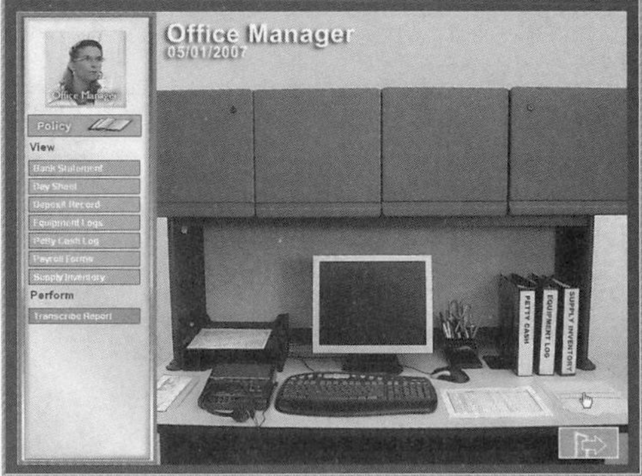

Copyright © 2014, 2011, 2007 by Saunders, an imprint of Elsevier Inc. All rights reserved.

1. a. Using the check ledger below, review the bank statement and check off each deposit, check, withdrawal, ATM transaction, or credit listed on the statement.

   b. If the statement shows any interest paid to the account, any service charges, bank fees, automatic payments, or ATM transactions withdrawn from the account that are not listed on the check ledger, make an entry for those items now and recalculate the account balance in the ledger.

No.	Date	Description	Payment/ Debit	Ref	Deposit/ Credit	Balance
1216	3/5/2007	Rocke Medical	$625.00			$9,264.35
1217	3/5/2007	Wal Store	$38.46			$9,225.89
1218	3/6/2007	Lorenz Equipment	$1,006.00			$8,219.89
1219	3/8/2007	Office Station	$199.43			$8,020.46
	3/10/2007	Dep. Daily Trans			$1,050.00	$10,833.46
1220	3/10/2007	West Electric	$93.99			$7,926.47
	3/12/2007	Dep. Daily Trans			$2,008.00	$9,934.47
1221	3/12/2007	Office Depot	$102.01			$9,832.46
1222	3/12/2007	Video Inc.	$49.00			$9,783.46
	3/15/2007	Dep. Daily Trans			$1,002.00	$11,835.46
1223	3/17/2007	Bonus	$200.00			$12,560.46
1224	3/17/2007	Bonus	$200.00			$12,360.46
1225	3/17/2007	Bonus	$200.00			$12,160.46
	3/20/2007	Dep. Daily Trans			$925.00	$12,760.46
1226	3/21/2007	Jamison Medical	$2,024.20			$10,136.26
1227	3/22/2007	Healthy Living Magazine	$32.95			$10,103.31
1228	3/22/2007	Greater London Electric	$422.00			$9,681.31
1229	3/24/2007	Office Station	$344.70			$9,336.61
1230	3/25/2007	Summer Oxygen	$230.99			$9,105.62
	3/27/2007	Dep. Daily Trans			$1,550.00	$10,655.62

Copyright © 2014, 2011, 2007 by Saunders, an imprint of Elsevier Inc. All rights reserved.

2. Now complete the bank reconciliation worksheet below.

THIS WORKSHEET IS PROVIDED TO HELP YOU BALANCE YOUR ACCOUNT

1. Go through your register and mark each check, withdrawal, Express ATM transaction, payment, deposit or other credit listed on your statement. Be sure that your register shows any interest paid into your account, and any service charges, bank fees, automatic payments, or Express Transfers withdrawn from your account during this statement period.

2. Using the chart below, list any outstanding checks, Express ATM withdrawals, payments or any other withdrawals (including any from previous months) that are listed in your register but are not shown on this statement.

3. Balance your account by filling in the spaces below.

ITEMS OUTSTANDING		
NUMBER	AMOUNT	
TOTAL		

ENTER

The ENDING BALANCE shown on this statement ---------------------------------- $ ______ __

ADD

Any deposits listed in your register or transfers into your account which are not shown on this statement
$ ________ __
$ ________ __
$ ________ __
+$ ________ __

TOTAL-- + $ ______ __

CALCULATE THE SUBTOTAL -- $ ______ __

SUBTRACT

The total outstanding checks and Withdrawals from the chart at the left --- $ ______ __

CALCULATE THE ENDING BALANCE

This amount should be the same as The current balance shown in your Check register -- $ ______ __

- Click **Finish** to return to the manager's office.
- Click the exit arrow.
- Click **Return to Map** and select **Yes** at the pop-up menu to return to the office map or click **Exit the Program**.

Copyright © 2014, 2011, 2007 by Saunders, an imprint of Elsevier Inc. All rights reserved.

LESSON 11

Payroll Procedures

Reading Assignment: Chapter 24—Management of Practice Finances
- Payroll Records

Patients: None

Learning Objectives:

- Process the employee payroll.
- Locate federal tax withholding resources by using the Internet

Overview:

For administrative medical assistants, the task of preparing an employee payroll may be a routine function. This lesson will give you practice in preparing payroll for employees.

Copyright © 2014, 2011, 2007 by Saunders, an imprint of Elsevier Inc. All rights reserved.

Exercise 1

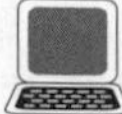

Online Activity—Processing Payroll

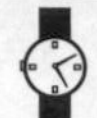

20 minutes

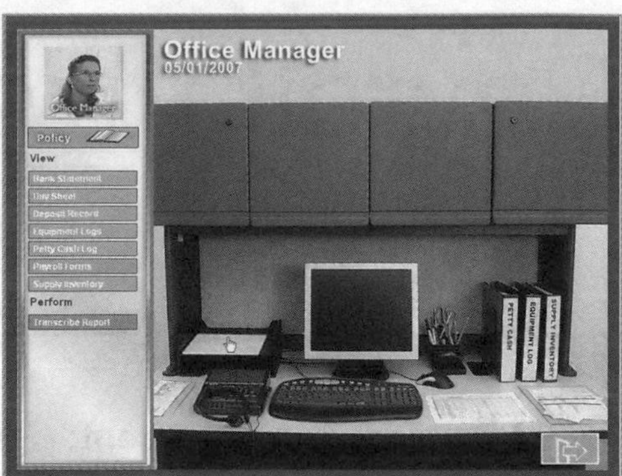

- Sign in to Mountain View Clinic.
- Click on **Office Manager**.
- Click on the **Stackable Trays**.
- The time sheet for employee Cathy Wright will appear first. Review and confirm that the number of hours have been calculated correctly.
- Next, click on the down arrow next to Person and select **Susan Bronski**.
- Review Susan Bronski's and confirm that the number of hours have been calculated correctly.

1. Cathy Wright's total number of hours worked: __________

   Susan Bronski's total number of hours worked: __________

2. Cathy Wright has been employed by the clinic for 10 years. Her salary is $18.00 per hour for the first 80 hours and $27.00 per hour for any hours over 80 during the 2-week pay period. Compute the gross pay for Cathy for the 2-week period.

3. Susan Bronski is a relatively new employee who is making $15.00 per hour for the first 80 hours and $20 per hour for hours over 80. Complete the gross pay for Susan for the 2-week period.

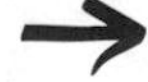

- Now review the W-4 form filled out by each employee.
- To view Cathy Wright's W-4 form, first make sure her name is selected from the drop-down menu next to Person. Next, click on the down arrow next to Form and select W-4. Review her form.
- To view Susan Bronski's W-4 form, select her name from the drop-down menu next to Person.

Copyright © 2014, 2011, 2007 by Saunders, an imprint of Elsevier Inc. All rights reserved.

4. Cathy Wright elected to have her federal taxes withheld under which designation?

_____ Single

_____ Married

_____ Married, but withhold at the higher single rate

5. The number of allowances claimed by Cathy Wright is __________.

6. Did Cathy Wright elect to have any additional money withheld from her paycheck for federal taxes? If yes, how much?

7. Susan Bronski will have her federal taxes withheld under which designation?

_____ Single

_____ Married

_____ Married, but withhold at the higher single rate

8. The number of allowances claimed by Susan Bronski is __________.

9. Did Susan Bronski elect to have any additional money withheld from her paycheck for federal taxes? If yes, how much?

Exercise 2

Writing Activity—Calculating Net Pay

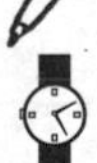

30 minutes

The IRS updates the federal tax tables each year. The tables we are using for this activity are 2010 tables for Single and Married Persons BiWeekly Payroll (you will choose which table to use based on the employee's filing status). Go to the Evolve course website. Click on Course Documents to view the 2010 tax tables. If you are instructed by your teacher to obtain the most recent copy of the schedules, go to the IRS website at www.irs.gov. Each state may have its own amount for the state withholding, but for this exercise we will use 1%.

Copyright © 2014, 2011, 2007 by Saunders, an imprint of Elsevier Inc. All rights reserved.

1. Calculate the total withholding allowance for Cathy Wright and Susan Bronski.

   Total withholding allowance for Cathy Wright: _______________

   Total withholding allowance for Susan Bronski: _______________

2. Now subtract the total withholding allowance from each employee's gross pay to calculate the adjusted gross pay.

   Cathy Wright's adjusted gross pay: _______________

   Susan Bronski's adjusted gross pay: _______________

3. Account for the following additional deductions for Cathy Wright: Medicare = 1.45%, Social Security = 6.2%, Health Insurance = $125 per pay period, State Income Tax = 1%, Retirement Plan = $150 per pay period.

Federal Income Tax	
Medicare	
Social Security	
Health Insurance	
State Income Tax	
Retirement Plan	

4. What is the net pay for Cathy Wright?

5. a. Using the correct tax table, calculate the correct deductions for Susan Bronski, who will file as head of household.
   b. Account for the following additional deductions for Susan Bronski: Medicare = 1.45%, Social Security = 6.2%, Health Insurance = $175 per pay period, State Income Tax = 1%, Savings Plan = $50 per pay period, Additional Tax Withholding from W-4 = $190.00.

Federal Income Tax	
Medicare	
Social Security	
Health Insurance	
State Income Tax	
Savings Deduction	
Additional Tax Withholding	

Copyright © 2014, 2011, 2007 by Saunders, an imprint of Elsevier Inc. All rights reserved.

6. What is the net pay for Susan Bronski?

Exercise 3

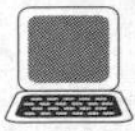

Online Activity—Writing the Check for Payroll

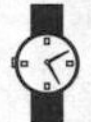

15 minutes

You are now ready to prepare and issue the payroll checks for Cathy Wright and Susan Bronski. To obtain the correct ending date for the pay period, return to the employees' time sheets by clicking on Payroll Forms in the manager's office. Date the checks for the Monday following the end of the pay period.

1. Prepare Cathy Wright's payroll check below.

PERIOD ENDING	EARNINGS			DEDUCTIONS										NET PAY
HOURS WORKED REG. OT	REGULAR	OVERTIME	TOTAL	FEDERAL INCOME TAX	FICA TAX	STATE INCOME TAX	SDI TAX	HEALTH INS.	SAVINGS	MEDICARE	MISC DED.	TOTAL DED.	AMOUNT

CHECK # 173977 Employee:

MOUNTAIN VIEW CLINIC
4412 Broadway
London, XY 55555

173977

94-72/1224

Date: ____________

Pay to the order of: ____________

____________ Dollars $

Clarion National Bank
Member FDIC
90 Grape Vine Road
London, XY 55555-0001

Authorized Signature

⑈005503⑈ 446782011⑈ 678800470

Copyright © 2014, 2011, 2007 by Saunders, an imprint of Elsevier Inc. All rights reserved.

2. Prepare Susan Bronski's payroll check below.

PERIOD ENDING	EARNINGS			DEDUCTIONS									NET PAY
HOURS WORKED REG. OT	REGULAR	OVERTIME	TOTAL	FEDERAL INCOME TAX	FICA TAX	STATE INCOME TAX	SDI TAX	HEALTH INS.	SAVINGS	MEDICARE	MISC DED.	TOTAL DED.	AMOUNT

CHECK # 173978 **Employee:**

MOUNTAIN VIEW CLINIC
4412 Broadway
London, XY 55555

173978

94-72/1224

Date: ____________________

Pay to the order of: ____________________

____________________ *Dollars* $

Clarion National Bank
Member FDIC
90 Grape Vine Road
London, XY 55555-0001

____
Authorized Signature

⑈005503⑈ 446782011⑈ 678800470

Copyright © 2014, 2011, 2007 by Saunders, an imprint of Elsevier Inc. All rights reserved.

LESSON 12

Standard Precautions and Biohazardous Materials

Reading Assignment: Chapter 27—Infection Control
- OSHA Standards for the Healthcare Setting

Patients: Shaunti Begay, Hu Huang, Tristan Tsosie

Learning Objectives:

- Recognize what materials are biohazardous.
- Indicate the proper disposal of used medical equipment and supplies.
- Identify the proper practice of standard precautions.
- Understand how to apply OSHA standards.
- Apply critical thinking skills to answer questions regarding biohazardous waste.
- Understand the importance of an infection control plan and its impact on preventing the spread of disease in the medical facility.

Overview:

In this lesson standard precautions (as dictated by OSHA regulations) will be discussed. You will learn to distinguish acceptable practices from those practices that could cause injury to patients and staff. Included in the practice of standard precautions is the disposal of biohazardous waste. (*Note:* Although medical asepsis, including handwashing, is an important factor in infection control, this topic is covered in another lesson and will not be addressed here.)

Copyright © 2014, 2011, 2007 by Saunders, an imprint of Elsevier Inc. All rights reserved.

Exercise 1

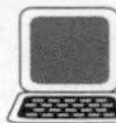

Online Activity—Infection Control in the Medical Office Using OSHA Standards

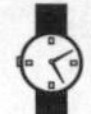

20 minutes

- Sign in to Mountain View Clinic.
- Select **Shaunti Begay** from the patient list.
- Click on **Exam Room**.
- Click on **Policy** to open the office Policy Manual.
- Type "OSHA" and click on the magnifying glass.
- Read the section of the Policy Manual on OSHA Bloodborne Pathogens.

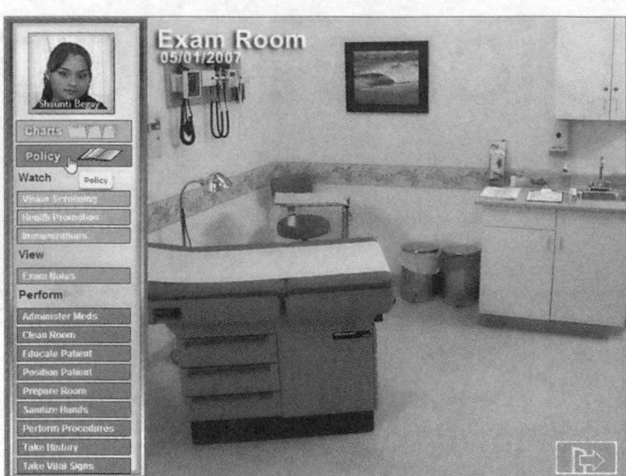

1. Name four body fluids that would be considered biohazardous waste in this medical office.

Critical Thinking Question

2. What additional body secretion is not included in the list of biohazardous waste?

3. According to the Policy Manual, what are universal precautions?

4. What are work practice controls?

Copyright © 2014, 2011, 2007 by Saunders, an imprint of Elsevier Inc. All rights reserved.

5. What are engineering controls?

6. What does PPE stand for?

7. OSHA requires that specific housekeeping procedures be followed to ensure the work site is maintained and in a clean and sanitary condition. Using your textbook, list some specific examples of these procedures in regard to the Bloodborne Pathogens Standard.

→ • Click **Close Manual** to return to the Exam Room.

• Remain in the Exam area with Shaunti Begay as your patient to continue to the next exercise.

Copyright © 2014, 2011, 2007 by Saunders, an imprint of Elsevier Inc. All rights reserved.

Exercise 2

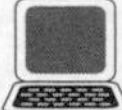

Online Activity—Application of OSHA Standards

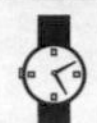

30 minutes

- Under the Watch heading, click on **Immunization** and watch the video.
- Pause the video at the first fade-out by clicking the pause button.

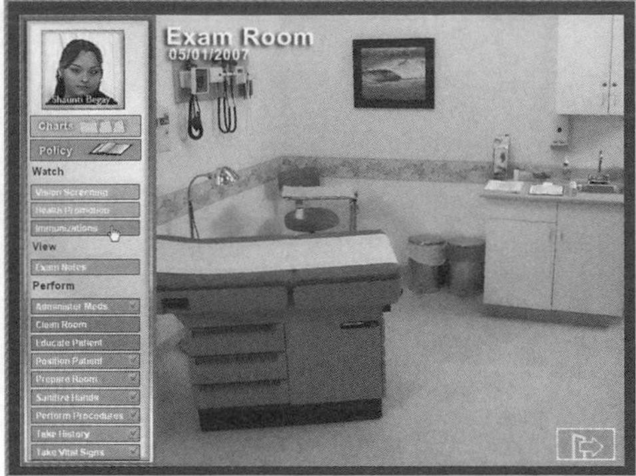

1. Did the medical assistant wear the proper PPE for giving an injection? Explain your answer.

2. Assume the gloves used by the medical assistant became contaminated with blood and are visibly soiled. In this case, which trash receptacle should the medical assistant use for disposal of gloves?

3. Where did the medical assistant dispose of the used needle and syringe?

4. What engineering controls did you see in the video?

Copyright © 2014, 2011, 2007 by Saunders, an imprint of Elsevier Inc. All rights reserved.

- Click the **X** on the video screen to close the video.
- Click the exit arrow.
- Click **Return to Map** and select **Yes** at the pop-up menu to return to the office map.
- Select **Hu Huang** from the patient list.
- Click on **Reception**.
- Under the Watch heading, click on **Patient Check-In** and watch the video.

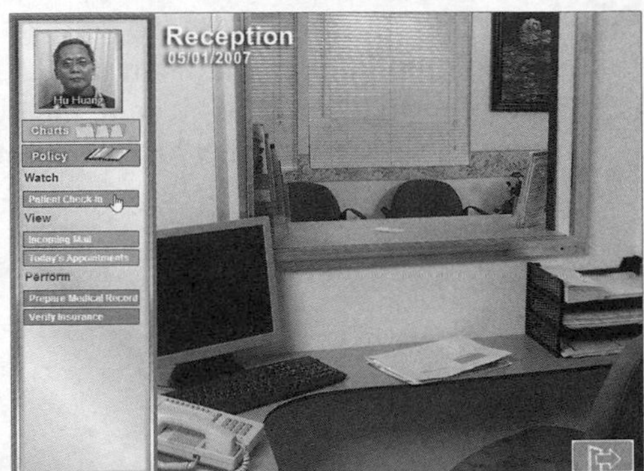

5. Mr. Huang has a productive cough when he approaches the Reception area. He lays a contaminated tissue on the counter just before Kristin takes him to a room. Should she have left the area without disinfecting the counter? Explain your answer.

6. Explain the proper disposal of contaminated tissues.

7. Which of the following are proper steps in infection control that should be observed during the check-in of Mr. Huang? Select all that apply.

_____ Provide tissues as shown in the video.

_____ Allow Mr. Huang to stay in the waiting room.

_____ Throw the tissue in the trash at the desk so that the contamination cannot spread.

_____ Apply gloves before handling the used tissues.

_____ Provide Mr. Huang with a means of disposing of the used tissues in biohazard waste.

_____ Wash hands after disinfecting the counter.

_____ Don a gown and mask when caring for Mr. Huang.

Copyright © 2014, 2011, 2007 by Saunders, an imprint of Elsevier Inc. All rights reserved.

8. Based on the video you watched, how do you think the patients in the waiting room probably felt when the medical assistant stated that Hu Huang might have an infectious disease that could be given to the other patients. Do you think Kristin handled the check-in in an ethical manner? Explain your answer.

9. If Kristin had not placed the patient in the examination room, would you expect patients to complain verbally about Mr. Huang's persistent cough? Would there be times you could not move a patient into a separate room?

10. Indicate whether each of the following statements is true or false.

    a. _________ Because Mr. Huang laid his contaminated tissue on the counter, OSHA standards would require that Kristin disinfect the counter before allowing another patient to register.

    b. _________ Ideally, after Mr. Huang laid his tissue on the counter, Kristin should have donned gloves and removed the tissue before moving the patient to a room.

    c. _________ Ideally, in offices where patients may have infectious diseases, a biohazard waste bag should be placed at the check-in window for situations similar to what you saw in the video.

    d. _________ Ideally, the check-in desk should have unsterile gloves available for removing biohazardous waste.

    e. _________ Because Kristin did not touch the contaminated tissues, she does not need to sanitize her hands.

    f. _________ The better method of sanitization of Kristin's hands would be washing.

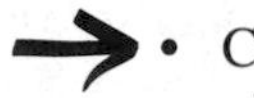

- Click the **X** on the video screen to close the video.
- Click the exit arrow.
- Click **Return to Map** and select **Yes** at the pop-up menu to return to the office map.
- Click on **Exam Room**.
- Click on the **Exam Notes** file folder and read the documentation for Hu Huang's visit.

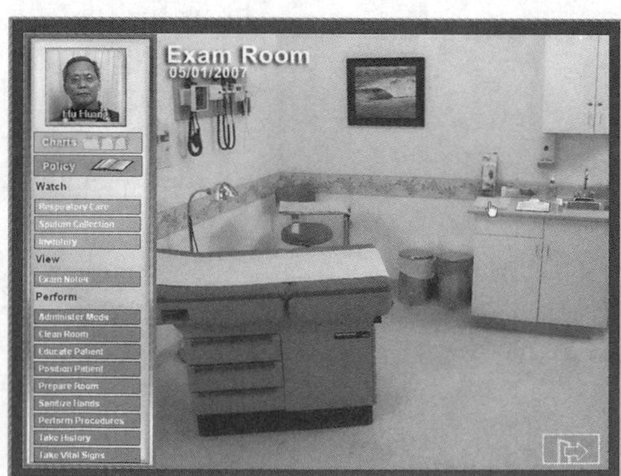

Copyright © 2014, 2011, 2007 by Saunders, an imprint of Elsevier Inc. All rights reserved.

- Click **Finish** to return to the Exam Room.
- Click on the **Waste Receptacles**.
- Use the checkboxes to select the appropriate steps necessary to clean the Exam Room after the patient's exam.
- Click **Finish** to return to the Exam Room.
- Click on the exit arrow.
- On the Summary Menu, click on **Look at Your Performance Summary**.
- Scroll down the Performance Summary to the Clean Room section and compare your answers with those chosen by the experts. The summary can be saved or printed for your instructor.
- Click **Close** to return to the Summary Menu.
- Click **Return to Map** and select **Yes** at the pop-up menu to return to the office map.

Exercise 3

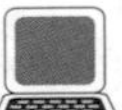

Online Activity—Applying Knowledge of Federal Regulations (OSHA)

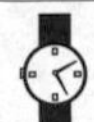

15 minutes

- Select **Tristan Tsosie** from the patient list.
- Click on **Exam Room**.
- Under the Watch heading, click on **Throat Specimen** and watch the video.

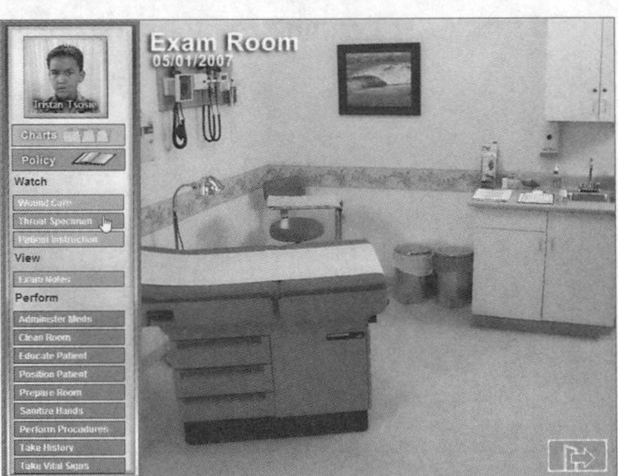

1. Which of the following PPE were used by Cathy when she obtained a throat culture? Select all that apply.

_____ Sterile gloves

_____ Unsterile gloves

_____ Face shield

_____ Sterile gown

_____ Disposable gown

_____ Goggles

Copyright © 2014, 2011, 2007 by Saunders, an imprint of Elsevier Inc. All rights reserved.

2. Indicate whether each of the following statements is true or false.

   a. ________ Cathy followed OSHA policy regarding the PPE needed for obtaining a throat culture.

   b. ________ The supplies used to collect the throat specimen should be disposed of in the biohazard waste container.

   c. ________ The gown and mask may be used again with another patient since Tristan did not cough.

   d. ________ The personal protective equipment (PPE) used by Cathy must be provided by her employer.

   e. ________ It is acceptable to push trash down in a biohazard bag, to make more room for more trash.

   f. ________ Each medical office must have its own infection control system.

   g. ________ Compliance with OSHA standards is required by law.

3. Do you feel that Cathy handled the use of PPE in an acceptable manner when talking with Tristan? Explain your reasoning.

→ • Click the **X** on the video screen to close the video.
- Click the exit arrow.
- Click **Return to Map** and select **Yes** at the pop-up menu to return to the office map or click **Exit the Program**.

Copyright © 2014, 2011, 2007 by Saunders, an imprint of Elsevier Inc. All rights reserved.

LESSON 13

Handwashing

Reading Assignment: Chapter 27—Infection Control
- Aseptic Techniques: Prevention of Disease Transmission
- Hand Washing
- Role of Medical Assistant in Asepsis

Patients: Jean Deere, Louise Parlet, Kevin McKinzie

Learning Objectives:

- Discuss the rationale for handwashing versus hand sanitization.
- Identify the specific circumstances in which handwashing is appropriate.
- Identify the specific circumstances in which hand sanitization is appropriate.
- Examine the policy manual regarding policies of infection control for this office.
- Use the Internet to research titles specific to medical assisting practice.

Overview:

Handwashing has been a foundation of infection control for over a century. This practice is still essential today. Handwashing not only protects the patient from cross contamination but also protects the healthcare worker. The Centers for Disease Control and Prevention (CDC) has designated when an alcohol-based hand rub may be used for hand sanitization.

In this lesson, we review the circumstances in which each of these means of hand hygiene are appropriate. After looking at the CD scenarios, you will continue to look at each patient in the VMO and use critical thinking skills to decide whether the medical assistant should wash his or her hands or use an alcohol-based hand rub.

Copyright © 2014, 2011, 2007 by Saunders, an imprint of Elsevier Inc. All rights reserved.

Exercise 1

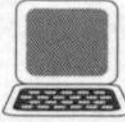

Online Activity—Handwashing/Hand Sanitization

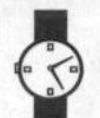

40 minutes

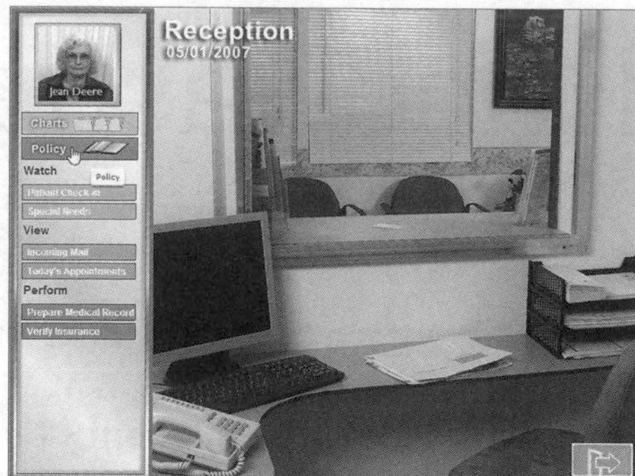

- Sign in to Mountain View Clinic.
- Select **Jean Deere** from the patient list.
- Click on **Reception**.
- Click on **Policy** to open the office Policy Manual.
- Type "handwashing" in the search bar and click once on the magnifying glass.
- Read the section of the Policy Manual on hand-washing.
- Since the office follows the CDC guidelines, go to http://www.cdc.gov and search for "hand hygiene in healthcare settings." The CDC currently has guidelines in PDF format. View these to see current recommendations. If you need assistance, your instructor can help you narrow down the search based on current information to the links.

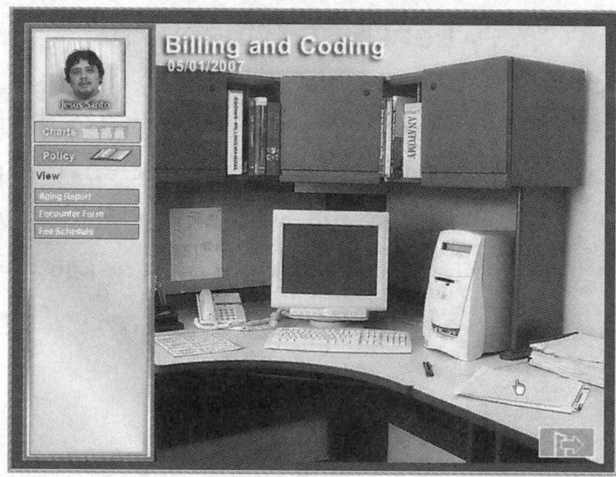

- Click on **Close Manual** to return to Reception area.
- Click the exit arrow.
- Click **Return to Map** and select **Yes** at the pop-up menu to return to the office map.
- Select **Jesus Santo** from the patient list.
- Click on **Billing and Coding**.
- Click on the **Encounter Form** clipboard and read the documentation for this visit.

1. Mr. Santo was in the examination room just before Jean Deere. Based on the diagnosis listed on the Encounter Form for Mr. Santo and your review of the CDC guidelines for hand hygiene, what would be the correct method of hand hygiene to use between patients?

Copyright © 2014, 2011, 2007 by Saunders, an imprint of Elsevier Inc. All rights reserved.

- Click **Finish** to return to the Billing and Coding area.
- Click the exit arrow.
- Click **Return to Map** and select **Yes** at the pop-up menu to return to the office map.
- Select **Jean Deere** from the patient list.
- Click on **Exam Room**.
- Under the Watch heading, click on **Room Preparation** and watch the video.

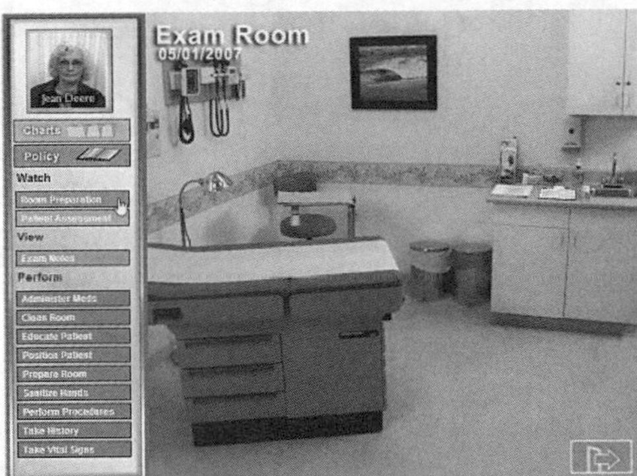

2. Why did the medical assisting extern need to wash her hands before preparing the room for a patient?

3. According to CDC policy, if the patient seen before Jean Deere did not have a diagnosis with the possibility of disease transmission, what would have been the appropriate form of hand sanitization?

4. If a medical assistant wears gloves, is it necessary to perform hand hygiene when the gloves are removed, before working with the next patient?

Thought Question

5. What potential risk do artificial fingernails or natural nails longer than ¼ inch present in the healthcare setting? To assist in your answer, you may go to the CDC website link at http://www.cdc.gov/mmwr/preview/mmwrhtml/rr5116a1.htm to view the CDC's recommendations. Scroll down the page to find Recommendations; then go to number 6.

Copyright © 2014, 2011, 2007 by Saunders, an imprint of Elsevier Inc. All rights reserved.

Critical Thinking Question

6. Laney will be starting her medical assisting externship in a few days. She has been advised that she will need to remove her artificial nails before she can begin working as an extern. Laney is upset about this requirement as the nails were expensive. She mentions that she doesn't understand why she needs to remove the nails when she'll be working with gloves on. What would you say to Laney to convince her of the importance of having the artificial nails removed?

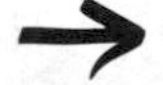

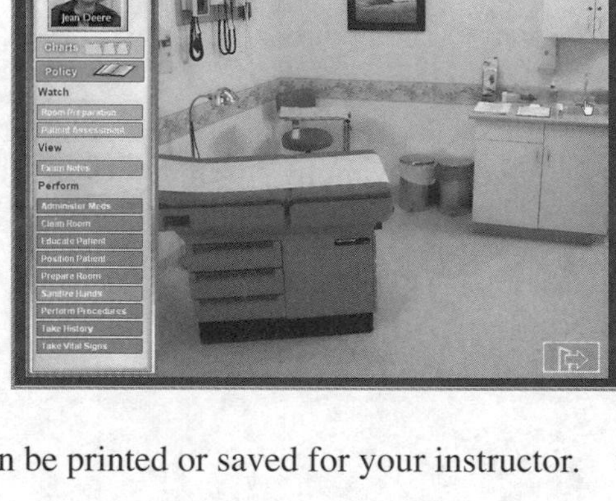

- Click the **X** on the video screen to close the video.
- Click on the **Sink**.
- Select the correct method of hand sanitization following Jean Deere's examination.
- Click **Finish** to return to the Exam Room.
- Click the exit arrow.
- On the Summary Menu, click on **Look at Your Performance Summary**.
- Scroll down the Performance Summary to the Sanitize Hands section and compare your answers with those chosen by the experts. The summary can be printed or saved for your instructor.
- Click **Close** to return to the Summary Menu.
- On the Summary Menu, click **Return to Map** and select **Yes** at the pop-up menu to return to the office Map.

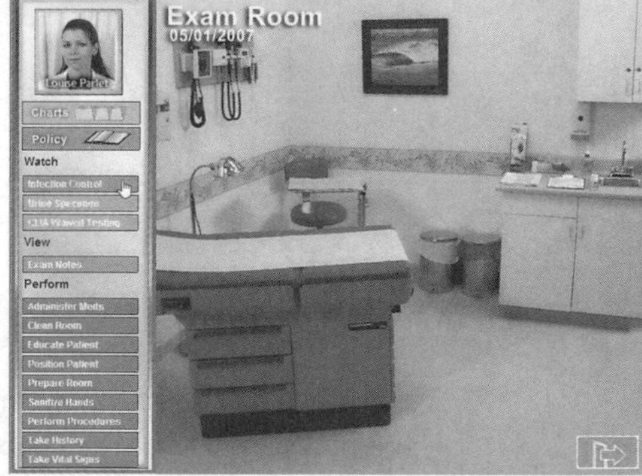

- Select **Louise Parlet** from the patient list.
- Click on **Exam Room**.
- Under the Watch heading, click on **Infection Control** and watch the video.

Copyright © 2014, 2011, 2007 by Saunders, an imprint of Elsevier Inc. All rights reserved.

7. Would it have been acceptable for the medical assisting extern to clean the table without gloves if she had sanitized her hands before and immediately after disposing of the table paper and gown? Why or why not?

8. After the extern has cleaned the examination table and removed gloves, what is the appropriate means of hand hygiene?

Exercise 2

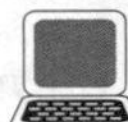

Online Activity—Hand Sanitization with Possible Infectious Disease

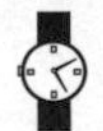

20 minutes

- Select **Kevin McKinzie** from the patient list.
- Click on **Check Out**.
- Click on **Charts**
- Click on the **Patient Medical Information** tab and select **1-Progress Notes**.

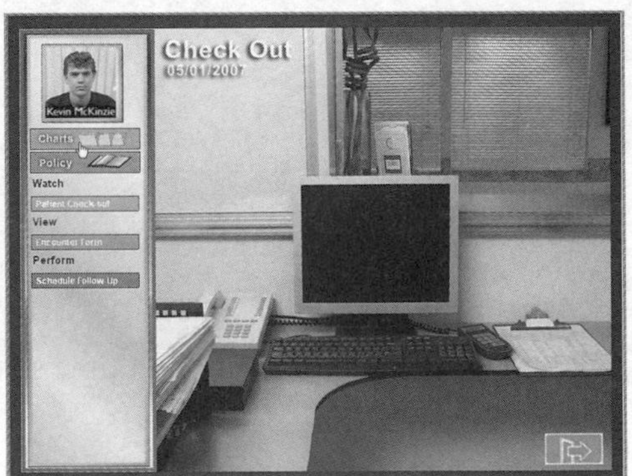

1. What is the possible diagnosis for this patient?

Copyright © 2014, 2011, 2007 by Saunders, an imprint of Elsevier Inc. All rights reserved.

2. With this diagnosis, what would be the safest means of hand hygiene following patient care?

3. _________ According to the CDC, the use of gloves is not necessary when good hand hygiene is used. (True or False)

4. According to the CDC guidelines, when is handwashing always necessary in the medical office? (*Hint:* Refer to the textbook if you need help.)

5. According to the CDC guidelines, when may an alcohol-based handwash be used for hand sanitization?

6. For what length of time should a handwash be performed at the beginning of the day?

7. The CDC has recommended the use of alcohol-based hand rubs instead of handwashing in some instances. What are the advantages of alcohol-based hand rubs? (*Hint:* Refer to the textbook if you need assistance.)

Copyright © 2014, 2011, 2007 by Saunders, an imprint of Elsevier Inc. All rights reserved.

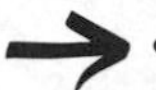

- Click **Close Chart** to return to the Check Out area.
- Click the exit arrow.
- On the Summary Menu, click **Return to Map** and select **Yes** at the pop-up menu to return to the office map.

Exercise 3

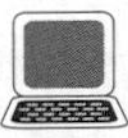

Online Activity—Handwashing and Hand Sanitization

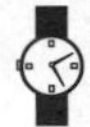

45 minutes

For additional practice, you will review the progress notes of all the patients in the VMO and decide whether hand sanitization with traditional handwashing would be best or if an alcohol-based hand rub would be appropriate. Your instructor may assign all of the patients or just a few.

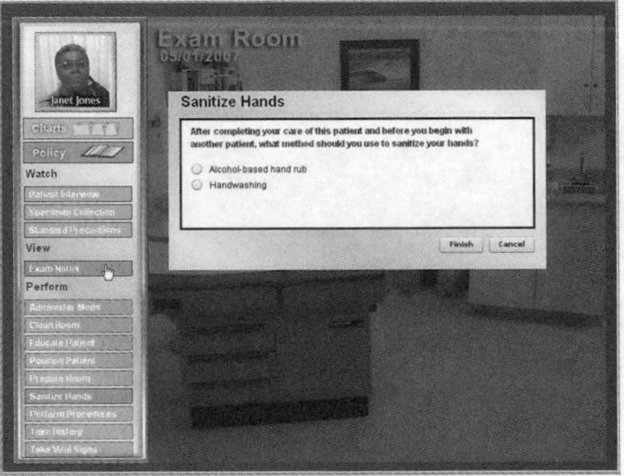

- Select **Janet Jones** from the patient list..
- Click on **Exam Room**.
- Click on the **Sink**.
- Click on the **Exam Notes** file folder and read the documentation for Janet Jones' visit.
- Click **Finish** to close the Exam Notes and return to the Sanitize Hands window.
- Select the correct method of hand sanitization following the patient's exam.
- Click **Finish** to return to the Exam Room.
- Click the exit arrow.
- On the Summary Menu, click on **Look at Your Performance Summary**.
- Scroll down the Performance Summary to the Sanitize Hands section and compare your answers with those chosen by the experts. The summary can be printed or saved for your instructor.
- Click **Close** to return to the Summary Menu.
- On the Summary Menu, click **Return to Map** and select **Yes** at the pop-up menu to return to the office map.
- Repeat these steps for all the patients in the VMO and compare your answers with the experts.

Copyright © 2014, 2011, 2007 by Saunders, an imprint of Elsevier Inc. All rights reserved.

LESSON 14

Obtaining and Documenting a Health History

Reading Assignment: Chapter 28—Patient Assessment

Patients: Kevin McKinzie, Hu Huang, Tristan Tsosie, Wilson Metcalf

Learning Objectives:

- List the components of the health history and understand the importance of each.
- Identify the questions that should be included during a health history.
- Indicate the accurate method of documenting a health history in a medical record.
- Demonstrate accurate written communication skills.
- Explain the difference between signs and symptoms.
- Differentiate between objective and subjective symptoms.
- Explain the need for confidentiality when obtaining a health history.

Overview:

In this lesson you will learn the proper questions to ask to obtain an accurate health history and the proper method of documenting the information you obtain. Kevin McKinzie is a new patient, whereas Hu Huang is an established patient who has just returned from a visit to China. Both of these patients have specific indications for obtaining an accurate medical history. In both cases, it is especially important for the medical assistant to recognize and respond to verbal and nonverbal communication appropriately.

Copyright © 2014, 2011, 2007 by Saunders, an imprint of Elsevier Inc. All rights reserved.

Exercise 1

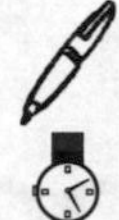

Writing Activity—Background for Obtaining a Health History

30 minutes

1. What components should be included when you obtain a health history?

2. When obtaining a patient's past medical history, why is it important that the medical assistant review this information with the patient rather than just rely on what the patient writes on the form?

3. Why would the physician need to know any previous surgical procedures a patient has undergone and where these procedures were done?

4. What is included in a social history?

5. Why is it important to include educational background in a medical history?

Copyright © 2014, 2011, 2007 by Saunders, an imprint of Elsevier Inc. All rights reserved.

6. Why are environmental factors important to include in a medical history?

7. Define *chief complaint* or *present illness*.

8. While listening to the chief complaint, what should the medical assistant remember to do during the documentation?

9. Subjective findings are called ____________________, whereas objective findings are called ____________________. Symptoms of the greatest significance in identifying a disease are called ____________________ symptoms.

10. How are subjective symptoms obtained?

11. How are objective symptoms obtained?

Copyright © 2014, 2011, 2007 by Saunders, an imprint of Elsevier Inc. All rights reserved.

12. Why is it important that the medical assistant ask questions of the patient in a private area rather than in the reception area?

Exercise 2

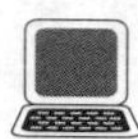

Online Activity—Obtaining a Medical History from a New Patient

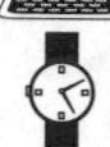

30 minutes

- Sign in to Mountain View Clinic.
- Select **Kevin McKinzie** from the patient list.
- Click on **Reception**.
- Under the Watch heading, select **Patient Check-In** and watch the video.

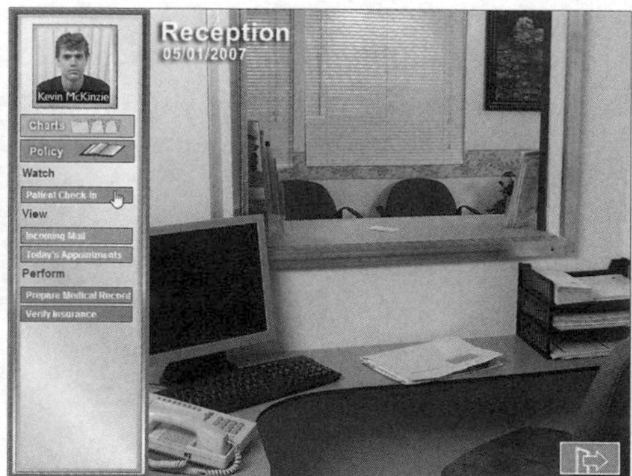

1. Kevin McKinzie brings a history form to the medical office with him. What are the disadvantages of having the patient complete the medical history at home?

2. The administrative medical assistant takes the medical history and places it in a chart without reviewing it for completeness. Is this good practice? Explain your answer.

Copyright © 2014, 2011, 2007 by Saunders, an imprint of Elsevier Inc. All rights reserved.

3. If the history was not complete, would it be appropriate for the medical assistant to gather additional information at the window?

4. Would you have handled the check-in of Mr. McKinzie differently? If yes, explain how. Did the medical assistant respond adequately to the patient's verbal and nonverbal communication?

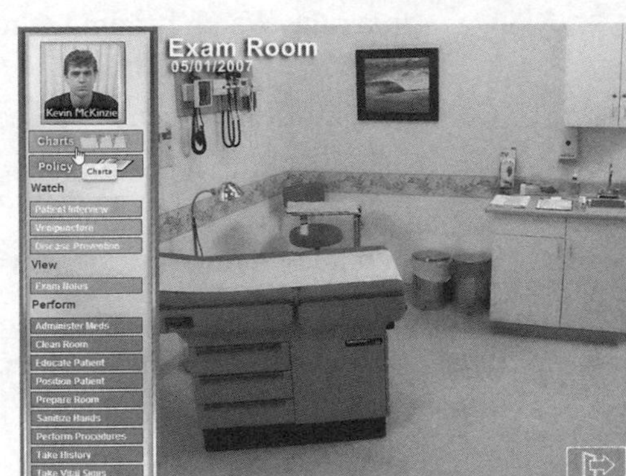

- Click the **X** on the video screen to close the video.
- Click the exit arrow.
- Click **Return to Map** and select **Yes** at the pop-up menu to return to the office map.
- Click on **Exam Room**.
- Click on **Charts**.
- Click on the **Patient Medical Information** tab and select **1-General Health History Questionnaire**.
- Using the arrow at the top right of the questionnaire, turn to page 2 and review the information.

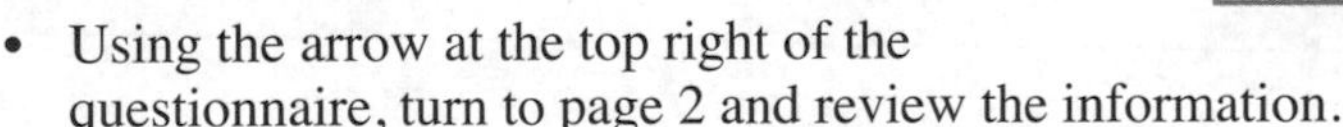

5. What is the patient's chief complaint as documented under Current Medical History?

6. What are two areas of Mr. McKinzie's social history that could have a bearing on this illness?

- Again using the arrow at the top of the screen, turn to page 3 of the questionnaire and review the information.

Copyright © 2014, 2011, 2007 by Saunders, an imprint of Elsevier Inc. All rights reserved.

Critical Thinking Question

7. What, if any, familial history is relevant to his chief complaint?

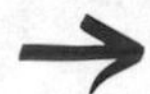

- Click on the **Patient Information** tab and select **1-Patient Information Form**.
- Read the Patient Information Form to find Mr. McKinzie's type of employment.
- Click **Close Chart** to return to the Exam Room.
- Click on the **Exam Notes** folder and read the clinical diagnoses as documented by Dr. Hayler.
- Click **Finish** to return to the Exam Room.
- Under the Watch heading, click on **Patient Interview** and watch the video.
- Click the **X** on the video screen to close the video.
- Under the Watch heading, click on **Disease Prevention** and watch the video.

8. What are the indications for patient education and infection control for these clinical diagnoses?

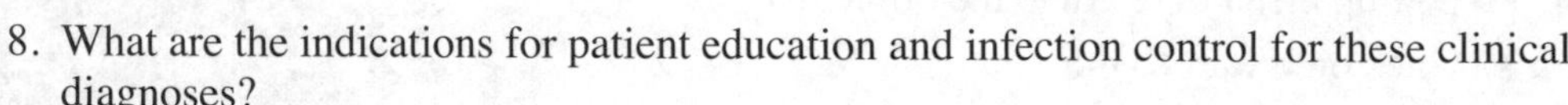

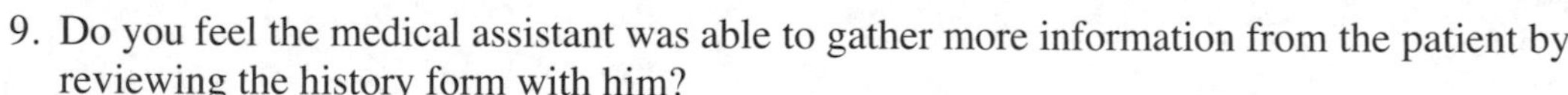

9. Do you feel the medical assistant was able to gather more information from the patient by reviewing the history form with him?

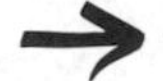

- Click the **X** on the video screen to close the video.
- Click the exit arrow.
- Click **Return to Map** and select **Yes** at the pop-up menu to return to the office map.

Copyright © 2014, 2011, 2007 by Saunders, an imprint of Elsevier Inc. All rights reserved.

Exercise 3

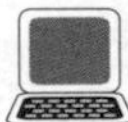

Online Activity—Documentation of the Chief Complaint for an Established Patient

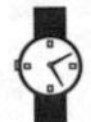

30 minutes

- Select **Hu Huang** from the patient list.
- Click on **Exam Room**.
- Under the Watch heading, select **Respiratory Care** to view and watch the video.
- Click the **X** on the video screen to close the video.
- Click on the **Exam Notes** folder.

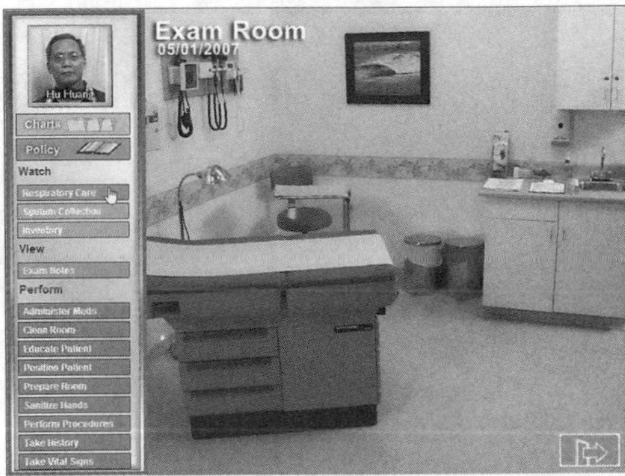

1. What is your assessment of the verbal and nonverbal communication that Charlie conducted with Mr. Huang in the video?

2. Why do you think Charlie seemed a little "stiff" with his body language?

3. What is the chief complaint for Mr. Huang?

4. Which of the symptoms listed are subjective symptoms?

Copyright © 2014, 2011, 2007 by Saunders, an imprint of Elsevier Inc. All rights reserved.

5. What are the objective symptoms?

6. What other information could be placed in the History section of the Progress Notes?

7. Why was it important to obtain the information that Mr. Huang had been in China for several months?

- Click **Finish** to return to the Exam Room.
- Click on **Chart**.
- Click on the **Patient Medical Information** tab and select **1-Progress Notes**.
- Read the documentation from all of Mr. Huang's previous visits.

8. After reading the Progress Notes for all his visits, what questions would have been appropriate for the medical assistant to ask Mr. Huang regarding medication compliance?

9. Indicate whether each of the following statements is true or false regarding documentation of patient history in Progress Notes on established patients.

   a. ________ The chief complaint for an established patient should be documented in Progress Notes unless a new history/physical exam form is being completed.

   b. ________ When documenting the chief complaint in the medical record of an established patient, the same questions of when, where, how, and how long should be asked.

Copyright © 2014, 2011, 2007 by Saunders, an imprint of Elsevier Inc. All rights reserved.

c. __________ After the physician identifies a diagnosis, it is permissible for the medical assistant to use that diagnosis in documentation of the chief complaint.

d. __________ Proper spelling is not as important when documenting the care of an established patient since the physician has already spelled the medical terminology correctly in earlier Progress Notes.

e. __________ Only clinical medical assistants document in medical records.

f. __________ If the medical office has specific guidelines concerning documentation, these are not as important as those taught in class and should not be followed.

g. __________ When documenting in any medical record, the extern or medical assisting student should sign the medical record with the indication of student medical assistant (SMA).

h. __________ The medical assistant should document both objective and subjective symptoms in the medical record.

i. __________ If the physician has used a local abbreviation in the medical record, it is acceptable for the medical assistant to also use this abbreviation.

- Click **Close Chart** to return to the Exam Room.
- Click the exit arrow.
- Click **Return to Map** and select **Yes** at the pop-up menu to return to the office map.

Exercise 4

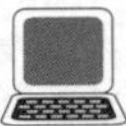

Online Activity—Documentation by Administrative Medical Assistants

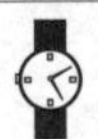

15 minutes

- Select **Tristan Tsosie** from the patient list.
- Click on **Reception**.
- Under the Watch heading, click on **Patient Check-In** and watch the video.

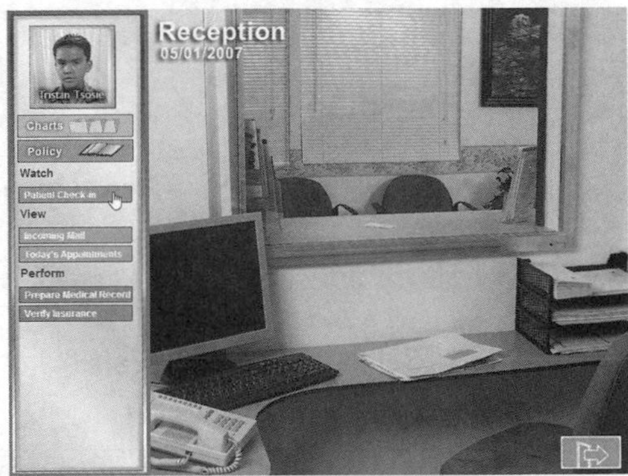

1. What important subjective symptoms does Tristan's sister report to the administrative medical assistant?

Copyright © 2014, 2011, 2007 by Saunders, an imprint of Elsevier Inc. All rights reserved.

- Click the **X** on the video screen to close the video.
- Click the exit arrow.
- Click **Return to Map** and select **Yes** at the pop-up menu to return to the office map.
- Click on **Check Out**.
- Click on **Charts**.
- Click on the **Patient Medical Information** tab and select **1-Progress Notes**.
- Read the initial documentation written by Dana Brick, CMA.

2. Dana is a clinical medical assistant, and Kristin is an administrative medical assistant. Did the correct medical assistant document the information from the sister in the medical record?

3. How did you feel about the verbal and nonverbal communication between Kristin and Tristan and his sister during check-in? If you think there was a problem, how could it have been better handled?

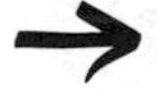

- Click **Close Chart** to return to the Check Out area.
- Click the exit arrow.
- Click **Return to Map** and select **Yes** at the pop-up menu to return to the office map.

Exercise 5

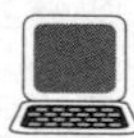

Online Activity—Practicing Documentation of History and Chief Complaint

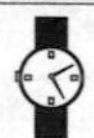

50 minutes

- Select **Wilson Metcalf** from the patient list.
- Click on **Check Out**.
- Click on **Charts**.
- Click on the **Patient Medical Information** tab and select **1-Progress Notes**.
- Read the Progress Notes for Wilson Metcalf beginning with his initial visit to the office on 1/4/2007.

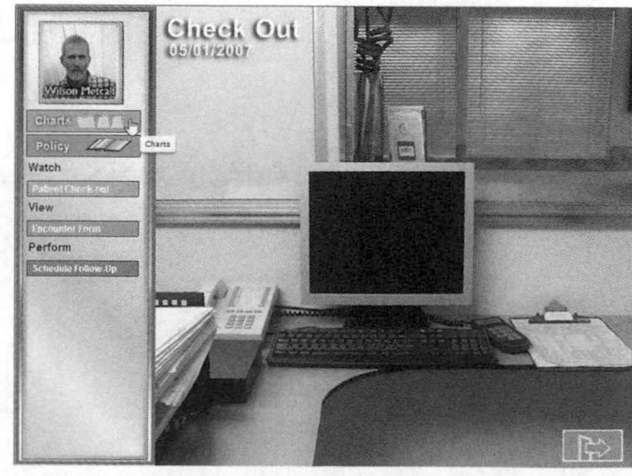

Copyright © 2014, 2011, 2007 by Saunders, an imprint of Elsevier Inc. All rights reserved.

1. According to the Progress Notes, what were Mr. Metcalf's drinking habits at the time of his visit on 1/4/07?

2. How much coffee did Mr. Metcalf admit to drinking in a day?

→ • Scroll down in the Progress Notes and read the documentation for the chief complaint for Mr. Metcalf's visit on 5/1/07.

3. What are Mr. Metcalf's drinking habits now?

4. How much coffee does he currently admit to drinking in a day?

5. What was the diagnosis documented by Dr. Meyer on 1/4/07?

6. What is Mr. Metcalf's diagnosis on 5/1/07?

→ • Click on the **Patient Medical Information** tab and select **5-General Health History Questionnaire**.
• Click on the arrow at the top right corner of the screen to turn to page 2 and read Wilson Metcalf's Health History form that was completed on 1/4/07.

Copyright © 2014, 2011, 2007 by Saunders, an imprint of Elsevier Inc. All rights reserved.

7. Who do you think filled out the Health History form?

8. Under Section IV, General Health Attitude and Habits, what was Mr. Metcalf's response to the question about how much alcohol he drinks, if any?

9. According to the form, did Mr. Metcalf believe he had a problem with alcohol?

10. On this form, how much coffee did Mr. Metcalf say he drank?

11. Are Wilson Metcalf's answers on the form consistent with the documentation in his Progress Notes? Explain. If the answers are not consistent, why do you think this may have happened?

12. Why would it have been important for the medical assistant to review this history with Wilson Metcalf?

Copyright © 2014, 2011, 2007 by Saunders, an imprint of Elsevier Inc. All rights reserved.

13. Assume that you interviewed Wilson Metcalf on 1/4/07 and wrote the Progress Notes on that date. Complete the blank page of the General Health History Questionnaire below by answering the questions correctly for Mr. Metcalf based on the information he provided during the interview.

ANDRUS/CLINI-REC ® **HEALTH HISTORY QUESTIONNAIRE**

Chart No. ______

Identification Information

Today's Date ______

Name ______ Date of Birth ______

Occupation ______ Marital Status ______

PART A – PRESENT HEALTH HISTORY

I. CURRENT MEDICAL PROBLEMS

Please list the medical problems for which you came to see the doctor. About when did they begin?

Problems	Date Began

What concerns you most about these problems?

______

If you are being treated for any other illness or medical problems by another physician, please describe the problems and write the name of the physician or medical facility treating you.

Illness or Medical Problem	Physician or Medical Facility	City

II. MEDICATIONS

Please list all medications you are now taking, including those you buy without a doctor's prescription (such as aspirin, cold tablets or vitamin supplements).

______

III. ALLERGIES AND SENSITIVITIES

List anything that you are allergic to such as certain foods, medications, dust, chemicals or soaps, household items, pollens, bee stings, etc., and indicate how each affects you.

Allergic To:	Effect	Allergic To:	Effect
nuts			

IV. GENERAL HEALTH, ATTITUDE AND HABITS

How is your overall health now? Health now: Poor ___ Fair ___ Good ___ Excellent ___
How has it been most of your life? Health has been: Poor ___ Fair ___ Good ___ Excellent ___
In the past year:
Has your appetite changed? Appetite: Decreased ___ Increased ___ Stayed same ___
Has your weight changed? Weight: Lost ___ lbs. Gained ___ lbs. No change ___
Are you thirsty much of the time? Thirsty: No ___ Yes ___
Has your overall 'pep' changed? Pep: Decreased ___ Increased ___ Stayed same ___
Do you usually have trouble sleeping? Trouble sleeping: No ___ Yes ___
How much do you exercise? Exercise: Little or none ___ Less than I need ___ All I need ___
Do you smoke? Smokes: No ___ Yes ___ If yes, how many years? ___
How many each day? ___ Cigarettes ___ Cigars ___ Pipesfull
Have you ever smoked? Smoked: No ___ Yes ___ If yes, how many years? ___
How many each day? ___ Cigarettes ___ Cigars ___ Pipesfull
Do you drink alcoholic beverages? Alcohol: No ___ Yes ___ I drink ___ Beers ___ Glasses of wine
"Couple of Shots" Drinks of hard liquor - per day
Have you ever had a problem with alcohol? Prior problem: No ___ Yes ___
How much coffee or tea do you usually drink? Coffee/Tea: ___ cups of coffee or tea a day
Do you regularly wear seatbelts? Seatbelts: No ___ Yes ___

DO YOU:	Rarely/ Never	Occasionally	Frequently
Feel nervous?			
Feel depressed?			
Find it hard to make decisions?			
Lose your temper?			
Worry a lot?			
Tire easily?			
Have trouble relaxing?			
Have any sexual problems?			

DO YOU:	Rarely/ Never	Occasionally	Frequently
Ever feel like committing suicide?			
Feel bored with your life?			
Use marijuana?			
Use "hard drugs"?			

Do you want to talk to the doctor about a personal matter? No ___ Yes ___

C O N F I D E N T I A L

Created and Developed by "Medical Economics" Professional Systems
Copyright © 1979, 1983 Bibbero Systems International, Inc.

STOCK NO. 19-742-4 8/95 Page 1

Copyright © 2014, 2011, 2007 by Saunders, an imprint of Elsevier Inc. All rights reserved.

14. Suppose that Mac Wallace (born 10/23/1980) comes to the office stating he has a fever and sore throat. He has had difficulty swallowing and has had pain in his right ear. All of these symptoms have lasted for about 4 days and have become progressively worse each day. He has also run out of blood pressure medicine and wants the prescription to be refilled. Before his throat became sore, his child had strep throat. Document Mac Wallace's chief complaint on the Progress Notes below.

PATIENT'S NAME ______________________ ☐FEMALE ☐MALE Date of Birth: __/__/__

DATE	PATIENT VISITS AND FINDINGS

15. What subjective symptoms does Mac Wallace report?

16. Which of these subjective symptoms could become objective symptoms following physical examination?

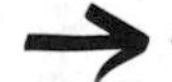

- Click **Close Chart** to return to the Check Out area.
- Click the exit arrow.
- Click **Return to Map** and select **Yes** at the pop-up menu to return to the office map or click **Exit the Program**.

Copyright © 2014, 2011, 2007 by Saunders, an imprint of Elsevier Inc. All rights reserved.

LESSON 15

Obtaining Vital Signs

Reading Assignment: Chapter 31—Vital Signs

- Factors That May Influence Vital Signs
- Temperature
- Pulse
- Respiration
- Blood Pressure

Patients: All

Learning Objectives:

- State the normal range for body temperature, based on the site used to measure the reading.
- Identify conditions or factors that alter body temperature.
- Identify the three terms used to describe the characteristics of the patient's pulse.
- Describe conditions or factors that alter the pulse rate and rhythm.
- Identify terms related to respiration.
- State the normal respiratory rate ranges, depth, and rhythm.
- Describe conditions that alter respiratory function.
- State the normal ranges for blood pressure.
- Describe conditions or factors that alter blood pressure, including age-related factors.
- Discuss what is meant by hypertension, prehypertension, and normal blood pressure.

Overview:

This lesson is intended to provide an understanding of the importance of correctly obtaining vital signs. Dr. John R. Simmons is a college professor who has a history of hypertension. Teresa Hernandez is a teenage patient. You will be using the Policy Manual to decide what steps you need to include in patient care to be in compliance with the physician's standing orders for these patients. After reviewing the information and answering questions about normal ranges for vital signs, you will be asked to check the vital signs of the patients in the Virtual Medical Office (VMO) and recognize which patients do not have normal vital sign results.

Copyright © 2014, 2011, 2007 by Saunders, an imprint of Elsevier Inc. All rights reserved.

Exercise 1

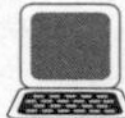

Online Activity—Obtaining Temperature, Pulse, and Respiration

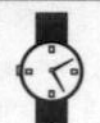

30 minutes

- Sign in to Mountain View Clinic.
- Select **Teresa Hernandez** from the patient list.
- Click on **Exam Room**.
- Click on **Policy** to open the office Policy Manual.
- Type "standing orders" in the search bar and click on the magnifying glass.

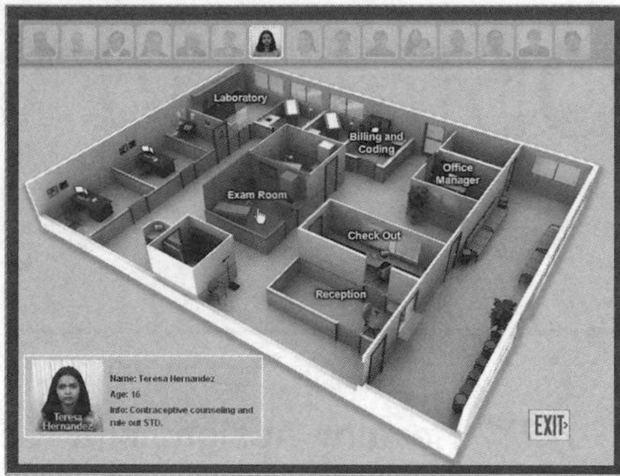

1. What are the standing order instructions regarding vital signs and physical examinations?

2. List five factors that can affect body temperature.

   (1)

   (2)

   (3)

   (4)

   (5)

3. If you were to check the temperature of a 6-year-old child who was playing outside in the sun during summer, would you expect the child's temperature to be slightly elevated?

Copyright © 2014, 2011, 2007 by Saunders, an imprint of Elsevier Inc. All rights reserved.

4. What course of action could you take to double-check and ensure that the body temperature was higher as a result of activity rather than illness?

5. A person with fever is described as ___________________, whereas a person without fever is considered ___________________.

6. Which of the following temperature readings would be considered normal in an adult patient?
   a. Oral 98.6
   b. Axillary 97.6
   c. Tympanic 98.6
   d. Options a, b, and c

7. Below, match each normal temperature with the age group to which it applies.

	Age Group	**Temperature**
_____	Newborn	a. 98.6 oral
_____	1 year	b. 96.8 oral
_____	6 years to adult	c. 98.2 axillary
_____	Elderly, over age 70 years	d. 99.7

8. What is specifically being measured when a person's pulse rate is obtained?

9. Consider all the patients at Mountain View Clinic. Which patient would you expect to have the highest pulse rate, as determined by age only?

Copyright © 2014, 2011, 2007 by Saunders, an imprint of Elsevier Inc. All rights reserved.

10. List the most common pulse sites.

11. Match each of the following age groups with the average pulse rate that applies.

	Average Pulse Rate	Age Group
_____	75-120	a. Newborns
_____	60-100	b. 1-2 years
_____	80-140	c. 3-6 years
_____	120-160	d. 7-11 years
_____	75-110	e. Adolescence to adulthood

12. Three characteristics of the patient's pulse are described by ____________________, ____________________, and ____________________.

13. What is meant by the term *arrhythmia*?

14. When discussing pulse volume, ________________________ indicates a fast, weak pulse, whereas ________________________ indicates an extremely full strong pulse.

15. The number of breaths (full inspiration and full expiration) that a patient takes during a 60-second interval should be documented as the patient's respiratory __________________.

Copyright © 2014, 2011, 2007 by Saunders, an imprint of Elsevier Inc. All rights reserved.

16. Which of the following factors affect respirations? Select all that apply.

_____ Age

_____ Physical activity

_____ Color of eyes

_____ Disease processes

_____ Emotional states

_____ Gender

_____ Medications

_____ Fever

17. Match each of the following respiratory terms to its definition.

	Term	Definition
_____	Rhonchi	a. A condition marked by rapid shallow respiration
_____	Wheezes	b. Abnormally prolonged and deep breathing associated with acute anxiety or emotional tension
_____	Hyperventilation	c. Abnormal rumbling sounds on expiration that indicate airway obstruction by thick secretions or spasms
_____	Tachypnea	d. High-pitched sound heard on expiration that indicates an obstruction or narrowing of the respiratory passages

18. Match each of the following average respiratory rate ranges with the age group to which it applies.

	Average Respiratory Rate Range	Age Group
_____	12-20	a. Newborns
_____	20-30	b. 1-3 years
_____	30-50	c. 4-6 years
_____	16-22	d. 7-11 years
_____	18-26	e. Adolescents/adults

Copyright © 2014, 2011, 2007 by Saunders, an imprint of Elsevier Inc. All rights reserved.

19. The taking in of oxygen is called ____________________, whereas the breathing out of carbon dioxide is called ____________________. Together, these two mechanisms are considered one ____________________.

20. Match each of the following terms with its definition.

	Definition	Term
_____	Individual must stand or sit to breathe comfortably	a. Apnea
_____	Bluish discoloration of the skin	b. Sleep apnea
_____	Difficult breathing	c. Stertorous
_____	Absence or cessation of breathing	d. Orthopnea
_____	Strenuous respiratory effort marked by a snoring sound	e. Dyspnea
_____	Absence of respirations during periods of rest	f. Cyanosis

21. Indicate whether each of the following statements is true or false.

a. _________ When an aural temperature is taken on a toddler, the auricle should be pulled down and back.

b. _________ When an aural temperature is taken on an adult, the auricle should be pulled up and back to expose the tympanic membrane.

c. _________ The patient should be told what procedures will be done when obtaining all vital signs.

d. _________ If a pulse rate is being taken before counting the respiratory rate, you should count the respiratory rate after releasing the pressure from the patient's wrist.

e. _________ Measuring a rectal temperature is a safe procedure for all patients.

f. _________ All patients can have the pulse taken at the radial site.

g. _________ When pulse rates are being recorded, any deviation of rhythm or volume should be documented.

h. _________ When respirations are being recorded, any deviation in rhythm or volume should be documented.

Copyright © 2014, 2011, 2007 by Saunders, an imprint of Elsevier Inc. All rights reserved.

Now that you have reviewed information regarding taking vital signs, continue with Teresa Hernandez as your patient.

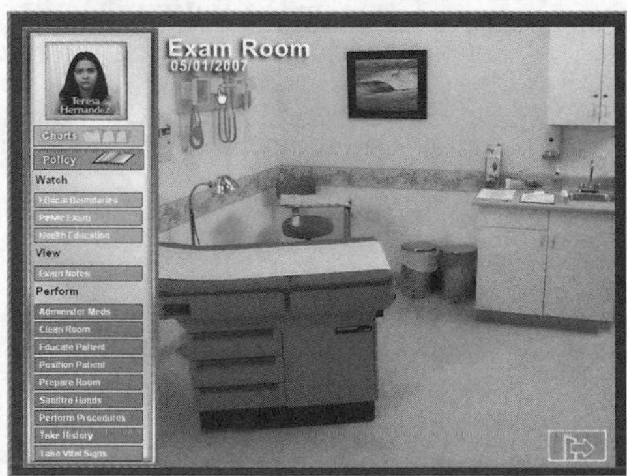

- Click **Close Manual** to return to the Exam Room.
- Click on the **Vital Signs Wall Unit**.
- Click **Take Blood Pressure**.
- Record the readings in the appropriate box at the bottom of the screen.
- Repeat this for all vital signs.
- If any of the patient's results are abnormal check the box next to "Check if Physician needs to be notified of Abnormality."
- Click **Finish** to return to the Exam Room.
- Click the exit arrow.
- On the Summary Menu, click on **Look at Your Performance Summary**.
- Scroll down the Performance Summary to the Take Vital Signs section and compare your answers with those chosen by the experts. The summary can be printed or saved for your instructor.
- Click **Close** to return to the Summary Menu.
- Click **Return to Map** and select **Yes** at the pop-up menu to return to the office map.

22. Which, if any, of Teresa Hernandez's vital signs are not within normal limits?

Critical Thinking Question

23. Suppose Teresa just arrived at the office and finished signing in when you were ready to move her into the examination room. Then you measured her pulse and it was 148 bpm, with her respirations at 36 breaths/min. While recording her chief complaint, she told you that she was out of breath because of walking up 16 flights of stairs to make it to the appointment and that a sign was posted on the elevator stating it was "out of order." Would these circumstances have any bearing on the readings you obtained? What would be the appropriate procedure to follow in this instance?

Copyright © 2014, 2011, 2007 by Saunders, an imprint of Elsevier Inc. All rights reserved.

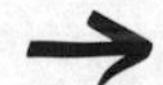

- Click on **Check Out**.
- Click on **Charts**.
- Click on the **Patient Medical Information** tab and select **1-Progress Notes** and read the final documentation of Teresa Hernandez's visit.

24. Did the medical assistant obtain the necessary vital signs? Explain your answer.

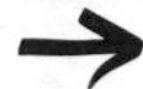

- Click **Close Chart** to return to the Check Out area.
- Click the exit arrow.
- Click **Return to Map** and select **Yes** at the pop-up menu to return to the office map.

Exercise 2

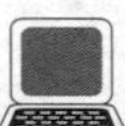

Online Activity—Obtaining Blood Pressure Readings

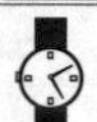

45 minutes

1. What is specifically assessed by blood pressure measurements?

2. The top number of the blood pressure reading is referred to as the ____________________ reading, and the bottom number is referred to as the ____________________ reading.

3. Match each of the following terms with its definition.

Term	Definition
_____ Hypertension	a. Pressure on the walls of the arteries when the heart is at rest
_____ Pulse pressure	b. Blood pressure over 140/90
_____ Systolic pressure	c. Blood pressure below 90/60
_____ Hypotension	d. Highest pressure that occurs when the heart is contracting and the first pulse beat is heard
_____ Diastolic pressure	e. The difference between systolic and diastolic pressure

Copyright © 2014, 2011, 2007 by Saunders, an imprint of Elsevier Inc. All rights reserved.

4. Which of the following factors affect blood pressure? Select all that apply.

_____ Time of day

_____ Age

_____ Environment

_____ Exercise

_____ Gender

_____ Emotions

_____ Body position

_____ Amount of sleep

_____ Medications

5. List the numerical categories for defining normal blood pressure, prehypertensive state, and hypertension, as published by the American Heart Association.

6. The equipment needed for obtaining blood pressure includes a ____________________ and ____________________.

7. If John R. Simmons were the patient, which size blood pressure cuff would you need to choose to check his blood pressure?

8. If Tristan Tsosie were the patient, which size blood pressure cuff would you need to choose to check his blood pressure?

Copyright © 2014, 2011, 2007 by Saunders, an imprint of Elsevier Inc. All rights reserved.

9. The sounds heard through the stethoscope as the blood pressure is being taken are called

_____________________.

- Select **John R. Simmons** from the patient list.
- Click on **Reception**.
- Under the Watch heading, click on **Patient Check-In** and watch the video.

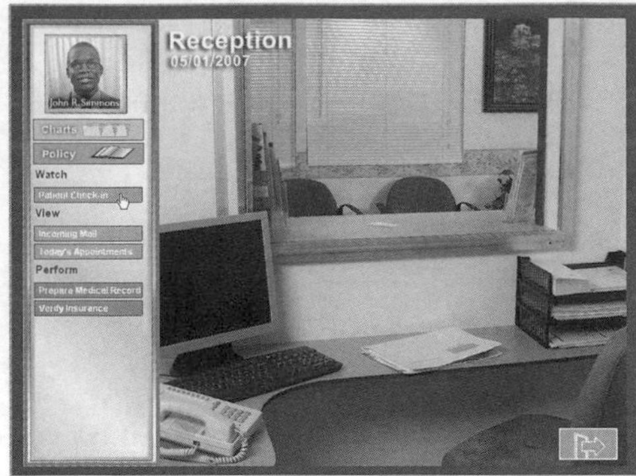

Critical Thinking Question

10. How should the office staff address John Simmons?

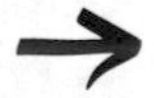

- Click the **X** on the video screen to close the video.
- Click the exit arrow.
- Click **Return to Map** and select **Yes** at the pop-up menu to return to the office map.
- Click on **Check Out**.
- Click on **Charts**.
- Click on the **Patient Medical Information** tab and select **1-Progress Notes**.
- Read the entire documentation of Dr. Simmons' visit.

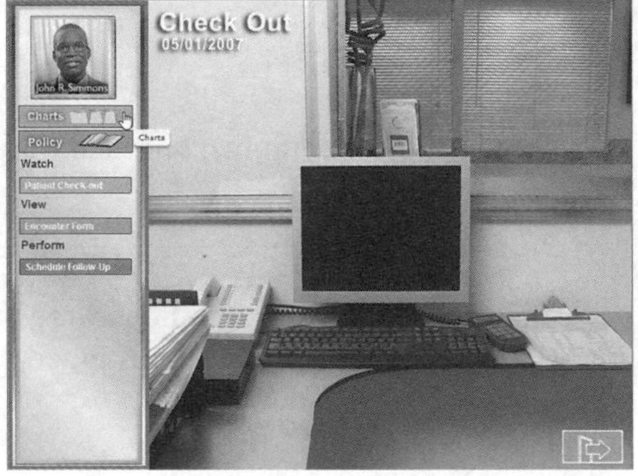

11. Dr. Simmons had his blood pressure monitored throughout his visit. Which, if any, of the vital signs for Dr. Simmons are not within normal limits?

Copyright © 2014, 2011, 2007 by Saunders, an imprint of Elsevier Inc. All rights reserved.

12. The blood pressure readings for Dr. Simmons are higher when taken the second time. What is a logical explanation for the difference?

13. Why do you think that Dr. Meyer wants Dr. Simmons to take blood pressure readings at home and record them?

14. Notice that Dr. Simmons' blood pressure reading taken from the left arm is more elevated than the reading from the right arm. What is an explanation for this?

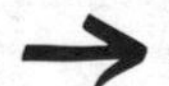

- Click **Close Chart** to return to the Check Out area.
- Click the exit arrow.
- Click **Return to Map** and select **Yes** at the pop-up menu to return to the office map.

Copyright © 2014, 2011, 2007 by Saunders, an imprint of Elsevier Inc. All rights reserved.

Exercise 3

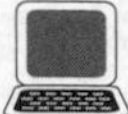

Online Activity—Documentation of Vital Signs

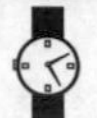

10 minutes

1. Using today's date and time, accurately document the following scenario on the form below:

   Judy Marks, age 69 (born 4/27/1938), is taking medication for hypertensive disease and is seen at the office on a regular basis. Today she has come in to have her vital signs checked by the medical assistant. Her pulse is 104, weak, and difficult to obtain, with a skipped beat every six beats. Her rate of breathing is 24 times a minute but shallow. Her temperature is 97.6 degrees. Blood pressure is 176/104 in the left arm and 170/102 in the right arm.

PATIENT'S NAME ______ ☐FEMALE ☐MALE Date of Birth: __/__/__

DATE	PATIENT VISITS AND FINDINGS

2. Which, if any, of the findings on the form in the previous question need to be reported to the physician before Judy Marks leaves the office? Which are abnormal?

Copyright © 2014, 2011, 2007 by Saunders, an imprint of Elsevier Inc. All rights reserved.

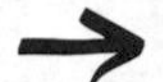

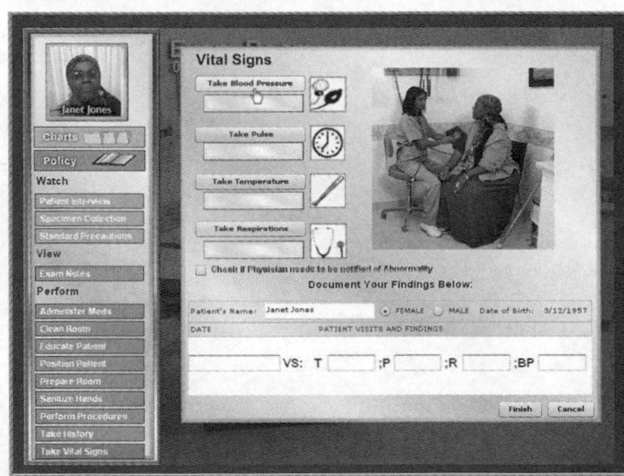

- Select **Janet Jones** from the patient list.
- Click on **Exam Room**.
- Click on the **Vital Signs Wall Unit**.
- Click **Take Blood Pressure**.
- Record the readings in the appropriate box at the bottom of the screen.
- Repeat this for all vital signs.
- If any of the patient's results are abnormal, check the box next to "Check if Physician needs to be notified of Abnormality."
- Click **Finish** to return to the Exam Room.
- Click the exit arrow.
- On the Summary Menu, click on **Look at Your Performance Summary**.
- Scroll down the Performance Summary to the Take Vital Signs section and compare your answers with those chosen by the experts. The summary can be printed or saved for your instructor.
- Complete question 3 (below) for your first patient.
- Click **Close** to return to the Summary Menu.
- Click **Return to Map** and select **Yes** at the pop-up menu to return to the office map.
- Repeat the previous steps for all the remaining patients at Mountain View Clinic, comparing your answer with the experts and documenting any errors in question 3.

3. Use this space to document any errors you made in transferring vital signs information or any failure to notify the physician of abnormalities in normal readings for any patients.

Copyright © 2014, 2011, 2007 by Saunders, an imprint of Elsevier Inc. All rights reserved.

LESSON 16

Measuring Height and Weight

Reading Assignment: Chapter 31—Vital Signs
- Anthropometric Measurement

Patients: Shaunti Begay, Jean Deere

Learning Objectives:

- Describe the correct methodology for measuring height on an adult.
- Describe the correct methodology for measuring weight on an adult.
- Convert height from inches to feet and inches.
- Convert height and weight from metric to English measurements.
- Convert height and weight from English to metric measurements.
- State the importance of measuring height and weight on each office visit.

Overview:

In this lesson you will view the videos to understand the correct methodology for measuring height and weight on a teenager and an adult. You will demonstrate how to convert a patient's height from inches to feet and inches for documentation. You will also perform conversions between metric and English measurements. One of these patients, Jean Deere, is confused. You will observe the handling of this patient and critique the actions of the medical assistant, as well as observe the medical assistant who handles a parent's negative remarks regarding her daughter's weight.

Copyright © 2014, 2011, 2007 by Saunders, an imprint of Elsevier Inc. All rights reserved.

Exercise 1

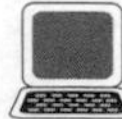

Online Activity—Measuring Height

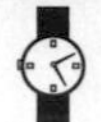

30 minutes

- Sign in to Mountain View Clinic.
- Select **Shaunti Begay** from the patient list.
- Click on **Exam Room**.
- Under the Watch heading, select **Health Promotion** and watch the video.
- Pause the video at the first fade-out by clicking the pause button.

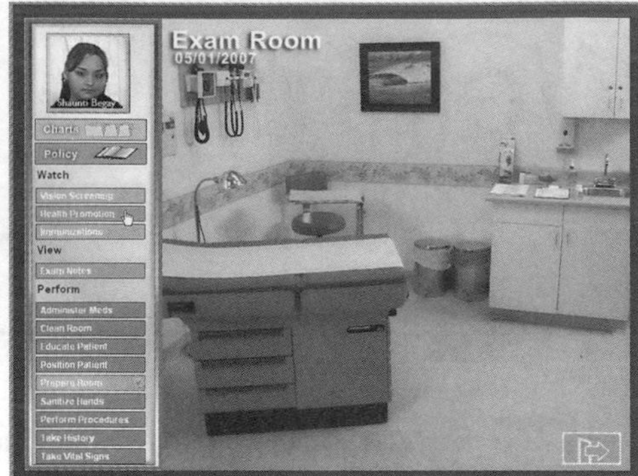

1. Why should Shaunti remove her shoes before her height and weight are measured?

2. Why is it important to measure a child's height at each office visit through adolescence?

3. What may occur in regard to height as an adult person ages?

4. Shaunti is wearing socks. If she were not wearing socks, what would have been the appropriate action by the medical assistant before having her stand on the scale?

Copyright © 2014, 2011, 2007 by Saunders, an imprint of Elsevier Inc. All rights reserved.

5. What is the correct angle of the head bar when measuring height?

6. The height measurements on medical scales are marked in _____-inch increments.

7. The medical assistant stated that Shaunti is 5 feet 2 inches tall, which would be __________ inches.

8. How do you think Shaunti felt about her mother's comment in regard to her weight?

→ • Click the **X** on the video screen to close the video.
• Click the exit arrow.
• Click **Return to Map** and select **Yes** at the pop-up menu to return to the office map.

Exercise 2

Online Activity—Measuring Weight

30 minutes

1. How is quality control performed on scales?

2. What safety steps does the medical assistant need to take with all patients when measuring weight?

Copyright © 2014, 2011, 2007 by Saunders, an imprint of Elsevier Inc. All rights reserved.

3. What weight calibration marking is used on most standing scales found in medical offices?

- Select **Jean Deere** from the patient list.
- Click on **Exam Room**.
- Under the Watch heading, select **Patient Assessment** and watch the video.

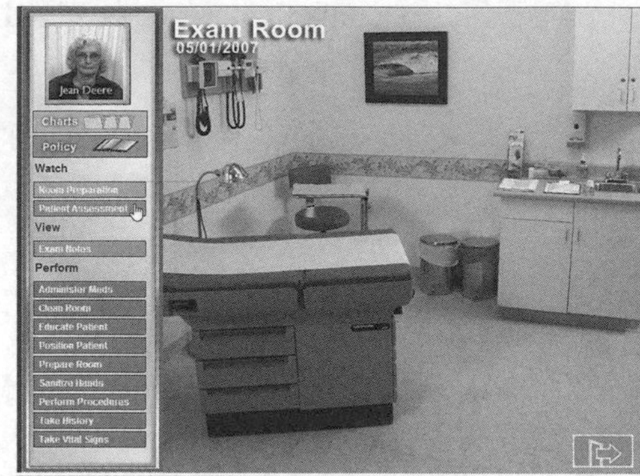

4. Did the medical assistant handle Ms. Deere appropriately to obtain an accurate measurement of the patient's weight?

5. The medical assistant offered to help Ms. Deere to the scales. Why would this be so important with this patient?

6. Notice the placement of the walker over the scales. Why is this important to help in supporting Ms. Deere? When a walker is used in this way, what observations must the medical assistant make to ensure an accurate reading?

Copyright © 2014, 2011, 2007 by Saunders, an imprint of Elsevier Inc. All rights reserved.

7. Ms. Deere is confused, and her son thinks she might have early Alzheimer's disease. Do you think that the medical assistant was professional and appropriate in her handling of the patient? Explain your answer. Was it appropriate for Ms. Deere's son to be with her during the weight measurement? Why or why not?

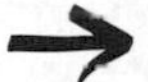

- Click the **X** on the video screen to close the video.
- Click on **Charts**.
- Click on the **Patient Medical Information** tab and select **1-Progress Notes**.

8. Based on the Progress Notes, what was Jean Deere's weight on her last visit on 9/21/06?

- Click **Close Chart** to return to the Exam Room.
- Click the exit arrow.
- Click **Return to Map** and select **Yes** at the pop-up menu to return to the office map.
- Click on **Check Out**.
- Click on **Charts**.
- Click on the **Patient Medical Information** tab and select **1-Progress Notes**.

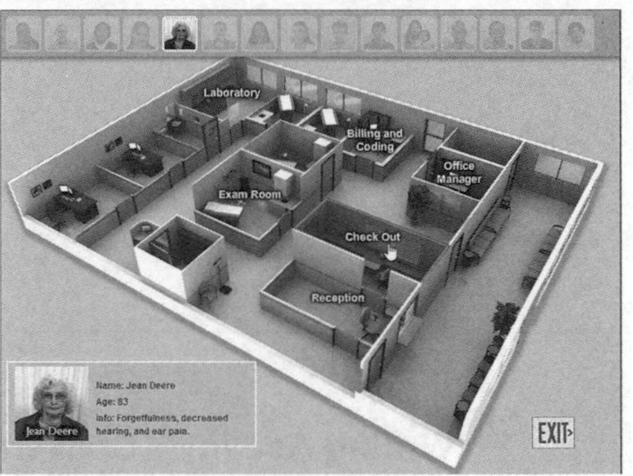

9. What is Ms. Deere's weight on today's visit, 05/01/07? Do you see a valid reason for the medical assistant to ask questions about her eating habits while taking the health history? Explain.

- Click **Close Chart** to return to the Check Out area.
- Click on **Policy** to open the office Policy Manual.
- Type "standing orders" in the search bar and click on the magnifying glass.
- Read the section of the Policy Manual on standing orders.

Copyright © 2014, 2011, 2007 by Saunders, an imprint of Elsevier Inc. All rights reserved.

10. Did the medical assistants follow the correct protocol for Shaunti Begay and Jean Deere, according to what you read in the Policy Manual? Explain your answer.

Critical Thinking Question

11. If a patient tells the medical assistant that he or she prefers not to be weighed, but it is the protocol of the office that all patients be weighed, what would be the best way for the medical assistant to proceed?

Exercise 3

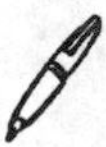

Writing Activity—Conversions for Mensuration

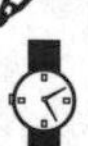

15 minutes

Use the formulas provided below to calculate answers to the questions in this exercise.

- Weight conversion of kilograms to pounds: Multiply kilograms by 2.2 (1 kg = 2.2 lb).
- Weight conversion of pounds to kilograms: Divide pounds by 2.2 (2.2 lb = 1 kg).
- Height conversion of inches to feet and inches: Divide the total number of inches by 12; then express the remainder as inches (12 in = 1 ft).
- Height conversion of inches to centimeters: Multiply inches by 2.5 (1 in = 2.5 cm).
- Height conversion of centimeters to inches: Divide centimeters by 2.5 (2.5 cm = 1 in).

Copyright © 2014, 2011, 2007 by Saunders, an imprint of Elsevier Inc. All rights reserved.

1. Joan Neiman weighs 64 kilograms. What is her weight in pounds?

2. Shaunti Begay is 5 feet 2 inches tall. What is her height in centimeters?

3. Jean Deere weighs 120 pounds. What is her weight in kilograms?

4. Sara McHugh is 68 inches tall. What is her height in feet and inches?

5. Isaiah Franklin is 185 centimeters tall. What is his height in inches? In feet and inches?

Copyright © 2014, 2011, 2007 by Saunders, an imprint of Elsevier Inc. All rights reserved.

LESSON 17

Preparing and Maintaining Examination and Treatment Areas

Reading Assignment: Chapter 32—Assisting with the Primary Physical Examination
- Physical Examination
- Preparing for the Physical Examination
- Supplies and Instruments Needed for the Physical Examination

Patients: Jean Deere, Louise Parlet, Rhea Davison, Jesus Santo

Learning Objectives:

- Describe the steps necessary in preparing an examination room for patient care.
- List supplies needed for a complete physical examination.
- Describe the steps necessary in cleaning the examination or treatment room following patient care.
- Document patient vital signs and history into the medical record.

Overview:

In this lesson you will list the supplies that are necessary in preparing an examination or treatment room for Jean Deere. After Ms. Deere has been examined by the physician, the examination or treatment room must be prepared for the next patient, Louise Parlet. A review of the necessary steps in infection control and disposal of biohazardous waste is presented, including questions addressing hand hygiene. You will also practice documenting in the patients health record.

Copyright © 2014, 2011, 2007 by Saunders, an imprint of Elsevier Inc. All rights reserved.

Exercise 1

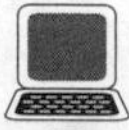
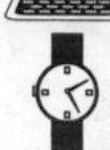

Online Activity—Preparing Examination or Treatment Room for Patient Care

30 minutes

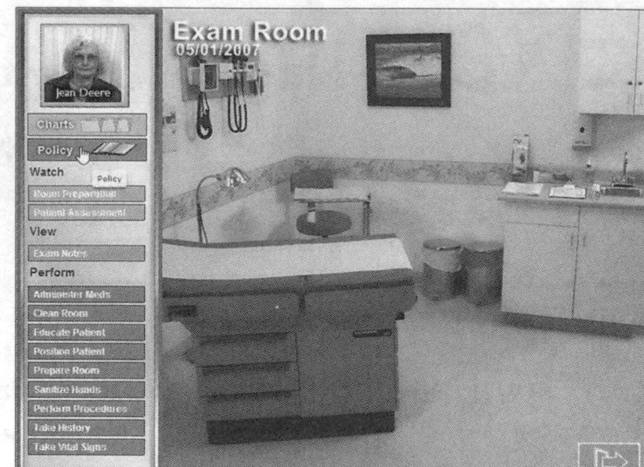

- Sign in to Mountain View Clinic.
- Select **Jean Deere** from the patient list.
- Click on **Exam Room**.
- Click on **Policy** to open the office Policy Manual.
- Type "room maintenance" in the search bar and click on the magnifying glass.
- Read the office policy on the preparation of examination/treatment rooms.
- Click **Close Manual** to return to the Exam Room.
- Under the Watch heading, select **Room Preparation** and watch the video.

1. The medical assisting extern washed her hands before setting up the examination/treatment room. Why is this an important step in room preparation?

2. The medical assistant extern asked Ameeta about Ms. Deere's symptoms. Why is this information important when preparing a room for the patient?

Copyright © 2014, 2011, 2007 by Saunders, an imprint of Elsevier Inc. All rights reserved.

3. Indicate whether each of the following statements is true or false.

a. _________ Infection control is important when preparing a room for a patient.

b. _________ When preparing the room for a physical examination, all equipment must be in good working order, properly disinfected, and readily available for the physician's use during the examination.

c. _________ The general cleanliness of the room has nothing to do with the patient's feelings about the entire medical office.

d. _________ Waste receptacles in the examination/treatment room should be emptied frequently.

e. _________ Biohazardous receptacles should be changed after any patient care that involves gross biohazard waste.

f. _________ Sharps biohazard containers should be emptied daily.

g. _________ Equipment for the examination should be placed at easy access for the physician and, if possible, in the order of use.

h. _________ The medical assistant should know how to operate and care for the equipment found in examination and treatment rooms.

i. _________ The appropriate room temperature should be determined by what is comfortable for the physician.

j. _________ All equipment in the examination room should be disposable.

k. _________ Proper disposal of equipment following use is an important factor in infection control.

l. _________ Improperly checked equipment and supplies may cause injury to a patient.

Copyright © 2014, 2011, 2007 by Saunders, an imprint of Elsevier Inc. All rights reserved.

4. Match each of the following pieces of equipment to its description or purpose.

Equipment

_____ Sphygmomanometer

_____ Drape

_____ Patient gown

_____ Thermometer

_____ Cotton-tipped applicator

_____ Tongue depressor

_____ Lubricant

_____ Tape measure

_____ Tuning fork

_____ Percussion hammer

_____ Speculum

_____ Ophthalmoscope

_____ Otoscope

_____ Stethoscope

_____ Penlight

_____ Gooseneck lamp

_____ Disposable gloves

Description or Purpose

a. Light on movable stand

b. Covering to reduce patient exposure

c. Used to test neurological reflexes

d. Long stick with cotton cover used to obtain specimens or to cleanse an area when dampened

e. Small flashlight used to check pupils

f. Instrument used to check auditory acuity

g. Instrument used to measure blood pressure

h. Instrument used to measure temperature

i. Instrument used to auscultate sounds

j. A device used to measure parts of the body

k. A covering for hands for good infection control practices

l. A covering with sleeves to provide modesty and warmth for the patient

m. Smooth wooden blade used to examine mouth and throat

n. Instrument used to examine eyes

o. Instrument used to open a body orifice

p. Instrument used to examine ear canal

q. Agent used to reduce friction

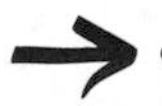

- Click the **X** on the video screen to close the video.
- Click on the **Exam Notes** file folder and read the documentation for Jean Deere's visit.

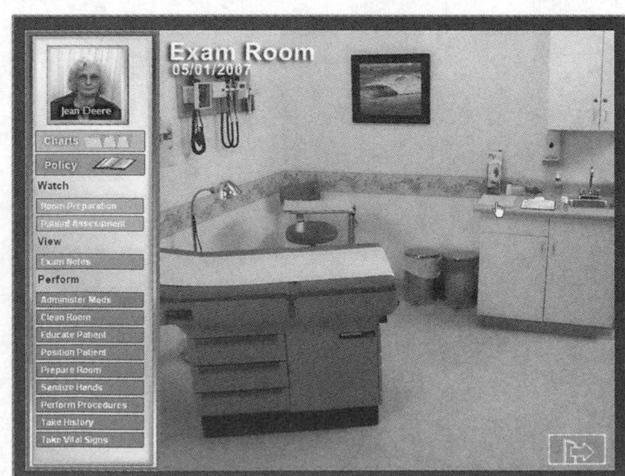

Copyright © 2014, 2011, 2007 by Saunders, an imprint of Elsevier Inc. All rights reserved.

5. Ameeta was correct in assuming Dr. Meyer would want to do an ear lavage and a pulse oximeter reading. What additional test did Dr. Meyer want done at this visit?

6. Why does the patient have to return tomorrow too?

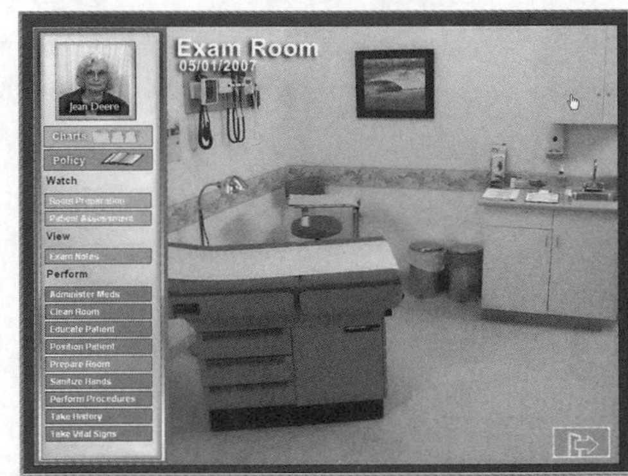

- Click **Finish** to return to the Exam Room.
- Click on the **Supply Cabinet**.
- Add the supplies needed for the patient's exam by clicking on the supply from the Available Supplies list and clicking **Add Item** to confirm your choice.
- If you wish to remove a chosen supply, highlight the supply in the Selected Supplies box and click **Remove**.
- Repeat this step until you are satisfied you have everything you need from the list.
- Click **Finish** to return to the Exam Room.

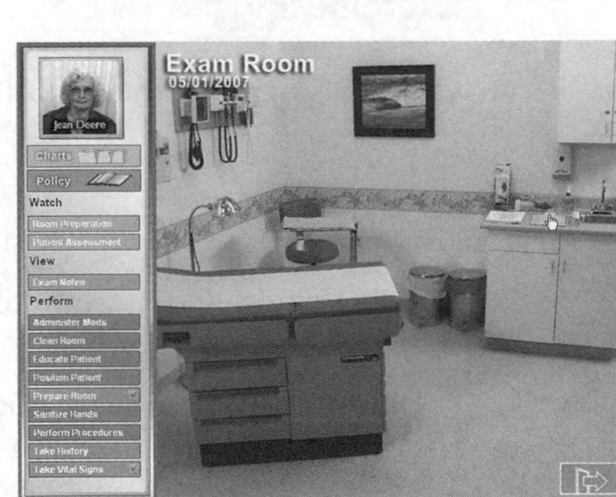

- Click on the **Vital Signs Wall Unit**.
- Click **Take Blood Pressure**.
- Record the readings in the appropriate box at the bottom of the screen.
- Repeat this for all vital signs.
- If any of the patient's results are abnormal, check the box next to "Check if Physician needs to be notified of Abnormality."
- Click **Finish** to return to the Exam Room.
- Click on the **Medical Record** clipboard.
- Click on the **Ask** buttons to view the patient's answers to the questions regarding her medical history.

Copyright © 2014, 2011, 2007 by Saunders, an imprint of Elsevier Inc. All rights reserved.

- Record the information in the patient's medical record in the box under "Document all findings below." Enter your name after your documentation as instructed by your instructor.
- At the bottom of the page, click **Next** to view additional questions and responses related to the patient's history.
- Use the checkboxes to select any other information you would need to ask the patient.
- If requested by your instructor, print the information by clicking on **Print** at the bottom of the screen.
- Click **Finish** to close the History Taking window and answer **Yes** at the pop-up window to return to the Exam Room.
- Click the exit arrow.
- On the Summary Menu, click on **Look at Your Performance Summary**.
- Scroll down the Performance Summary to the Prepare Room, Take History, and Take Vital Signs sections and compare your answers with those chosen by the experts. The summary can be printed or saved for your instructor.
- Click **Close** to return to the Summary Menu.
- Click **Return to Map** and select **Yes** at the pop-up menu to return to the office map.

7. After reviewing the Performance Summary, were there any items you selected that did not agree with the experts? What impact would these discrepancies have on patient care?

Exercise 2

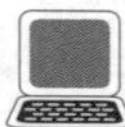

Online Activity—Maintaining the Examination or Treatment Room Following Patient Care

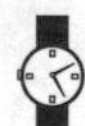

30 minutes

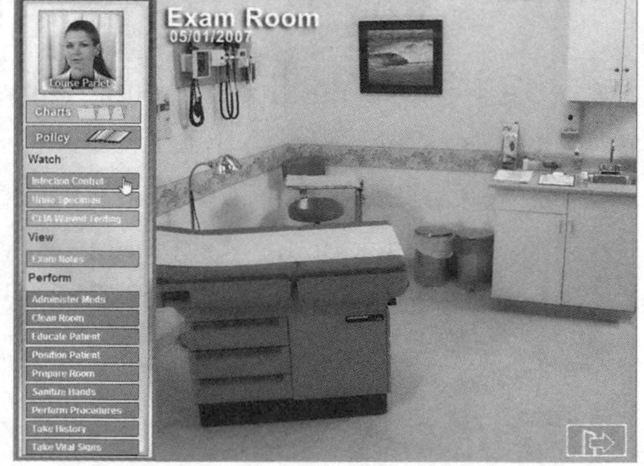

- Select **Louise Parlet** from the patient list.
- Click on the **Exam Room**.
- Under the Watch heading, click on **Infection Control** and watch the video. Pay close attention to the extern's actions throughout the entire video.
- Click the **X** on the video screen to close the video.
- Click on **Policy** to open the Policy Manual.
- Type "room maintenance" in the search bar and click on the magnifying glass.
- Read the section of the Policy Manual on room maintenance.

Copyright © 2014, 2011, 2007 by Saunders, an imprint of Elsevier Inc. All rights reserved.

1. What does the Policy Manual indicate should be performed after each patient has been seen?

2. During the video, did the medical assistant follow the Policy Manual while cleaning the room? Explain your answer.

3. During the video, did you see a break in infection control by the medical assisting extern? Explain.

4. Would it have been acceptable for the medical assisting extern to clean the table without gloves if she had sanitized her hands before and immediately after disposing of the table paper and gown? Why or why not?

Copyright © 2014, 2011, 2007 by Saunders, an imprint of Elsevier Inc. All rights reserved.

5. Indicate whether each of the following statements is true or false.

   a. _________ The medical assistant should use gloves, gown, and face shield when cleaning the examination room after a patient.

   b. _________ The medical assistant should disinfect the table, supply tray, and counter/table tops after each patient.

   c. _________ The nondisposable supplies and equipment should be disinfected and properly stored when cleaning the room.

   d. _________ Nondisposable equipment should be sanitized and sterilized as necessary before storage.

   e. _________ The office Policy Manual contains all information needed for the correct cleaning of a room following a patient examination.

   f. _________ The physician will inform the medical assistant of the items that must be discarded and those that should be sanitized and used again.

   g. _________ Items such as ophthalmoscopes, otoscopes, and tuning forks do not require sanitization following use in patient care.

   h. _________ Standard precautions should be followed when preparing and cleaning the examination/treatment room.

   i. _________ If the medical assistant does not have time between patients to completely clean the room, it is more important to keep the appointment schedule on time than to clean the room.

   j. _________ It is permissible for the medical assistant to clean a room after the following patient has been placed in the examination/treatment room.

   k. _________ Teamwork is essential in keeping the office neat, clean, and ready for patients.

6. What do you think would be the best action to take if you entered a room with a patient and discovered that the room had not been prepared as it should have been?

→ • Click **Close Manual** to return to the Exam Room.

• Click on the **Supply Cabinet**.

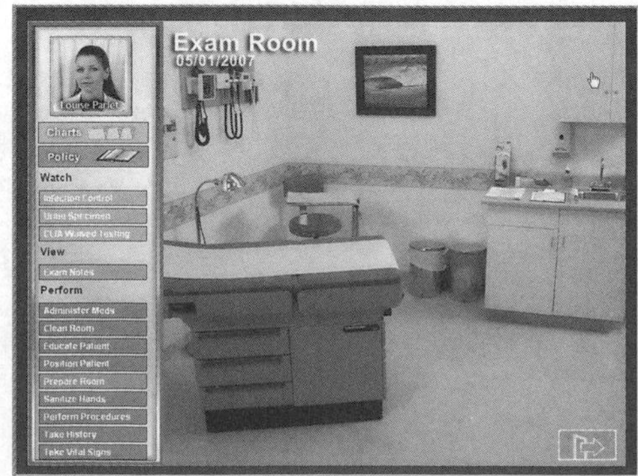

Copyright © 2014, 2011, 2007 by Saunders, an imprint of Elsevier Inc. All rights reserved.

- Add the supplies needed for the patient's exam by clicking on the supply from the Available Supplies list and clicking **Add Item** to confirm your choice.
- If you wish to remove a chosen supply, highlight the supply in the Selected Supplies box and click **Remove**.
- Repeat this step until you are satisfied you have everything you need from the list.
- Click **Finish** to return to the Exam Room.
- Click on the **Vital Signs Wall Unit**.
- Click **Take Blood Pressure**.
- Record the readings in the appropriate box at the bottom of the screen.
- Repeat this for all vital signs.
- If any of the patient's results are abnormal, check the box next to "Check if Physician needs to be notified of Abnormality."
- Click **Finish** to return to the Exam Room.
- Click on the **Medical Record** clipboard.
- Click on the **Ask** buttons to view the patient's answers to the questions regarding her medical history.
- Record the information in the patient's medical record in the box under "Document all findings below." Enter your name after your documentation as instructed by your instructor.
- At the bottom of the page, click **Next** to view additional questions and responses related to the patient's history.
- Use the checkboxes to select any other information you would need to ask the patient.
- If requested by your instructor, print the information by clicking on **Print** at the bottom of the screen.
- Click **Finish** to close the History Taking window and answer **Yes** at the pop-up window to return to the Exam Room.
- Click the exit arrow.
- On the Summary Menu, click on **Look at Your Performance Summary**.
- Scroll down the Performance Summary to the Prepare Room, Take History, and Take Vital Signs sections and compare your answers with those chosen by the experts. The summary can be printed or saved for your instructor.
- Click **Close** to return to the Summary Menu.
- Click **Return to Map** and select **Yes** at the pop-up menu to return to the office map.

Exercise 3

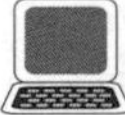

Online Activity—Maintaining and Cleaning the Treatment Room Following Patient Care

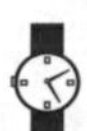

10 minutes

In this activity you will choose the correct way to clean the examination room after the physician provides care to a patient.

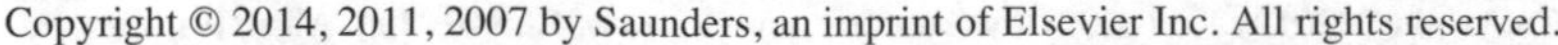
Copyright © 2014, 2011, 2007 by Saunders, an imprint of Elsevier Inc. All rights reserved.

- Select **Rhea Davison** from the patient list.
- Click on **Exam Room**.
- Click on the **Exam Notes** file folder and read the documentation regarding Rhea Davison's visit.
- Click **Finish** to return to the Exam Room.

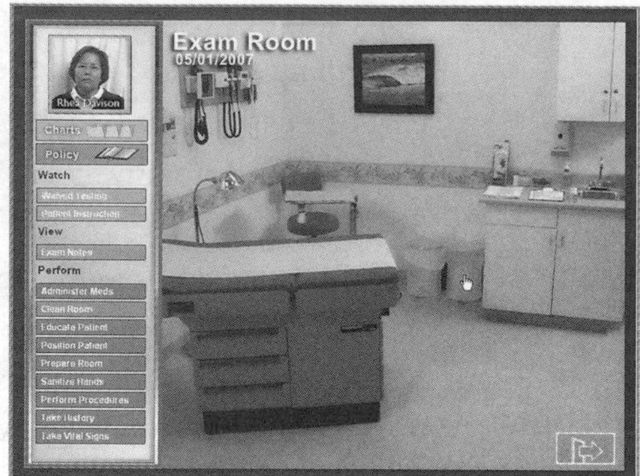

- Click on the **Waste Receptacles**.
- Use the checkboxes to select the appropriate steps necessary to clean the Exam Room after Rhea Davison's exam.
- Click **Finish** to return to the Exam Room.
- Click the exit arrow.
- On the Summary Menu, click on **Look at Your Performance Summary**.
- Scroll down the Performance Summary to the Clean Room section and compare your answers with those chosen by the experts. The summary can be printed or saved for your instructor.
- Click **Close** to return to the Summary Menu.
- Click **Return to Map** and select **Yes** at the pop-up menu to return to the office map.
- Select **Jesus Santo** from the patient list.
- Click on **Exam Room**.
- Click on the **Exam Notes** file folder and read the documentation regarding Jesus Santo's visit.
- Click **Finish** to return to the Exam Room.

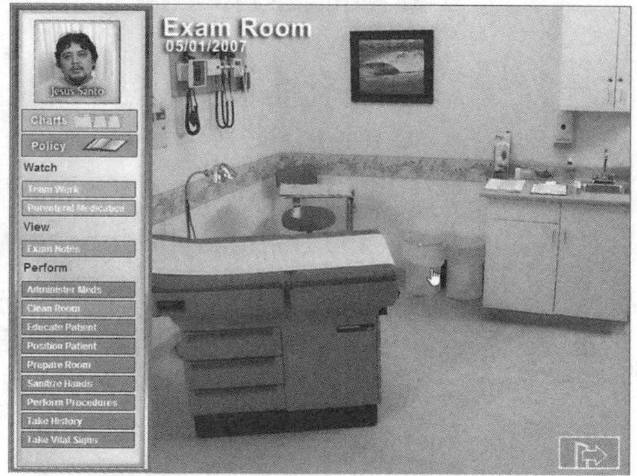

- Click on the **Waste Receptacles**.
- Use the checkboxes to select the appropriate steps necessary to clean the Exam Room after Jesus Santo's exam.
- Click **Finish** to return to the Exam Room.
- Click the exit arrow.
- On the Summary Menu, click on **Look at Your Performance Summary**.
- Scroll down the Performance Summary to the Clean Room section and compare your answers with those chosen by the experts.
- You may save and print the Performance Summary for your records or turn it in to your instructor. The icons for saving and printing the Performance Summary are located at the top right corner of the screen.
- Click **Close** to return to the Summary Menu.
- Click **Return to Map** and select **Yes** at the pop-up menu to return to the office map or click Exit the Program.

Copyright © 2014, 2011, 2007 by Saunders, an imprint of Elsevier Inc. All rights reserved.

LESSON 18

Preparing the Patient and Assisting with a Routine Physical Examination

Reading Assignment: Chapter 32—Assisting with the Primary Physical Examination
- Physical Examination
- Assisting with the Physical Examination
- Principles of Body Mechanics
- Examination Sequence
- Role of the Medical Assistant

Patients: Teresa Hernandez, Jean Deere

Learning Objectives:

- Identify the information needed to prepare the patient for a physical examination.
- Prepare the patient for a physical examination following office policy and procedures.
- Understand legal and ethical boundaries when preparing a patient for a physical examination.
- Choose the correct patient positioning for the physical examination.
- Recognize the ethical role of the medical assistant when assisting with physical examinations.
- Discuss patient safety measures during a physical examination.
- Describe the importance of efficiency when assisting the examiner.
- Understand the importance of using correct body mechanics while assisting with physical examinations.
- Recognize what instruments are needed when assisting with the physical examination.

Overview:

In this lesson you will study the necessary steps in patient preparation for a routine physical examination. Teresa Hernandez is a new teenage patient, whereas Jean Deere is an established geriatric patient. Ms. Deere wants her son James to assist in getting her ready for a physical exam. With each patient, ethical and legal issues are of concern.

Copyright © 2014, 2011, 2007 by Saunders, an imprint of Elsevier Inc. All rights reserved.

Exercise 1

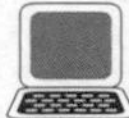

Online Activity—Preparing an Established Patient for Physical Examination

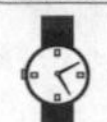

20 minutes

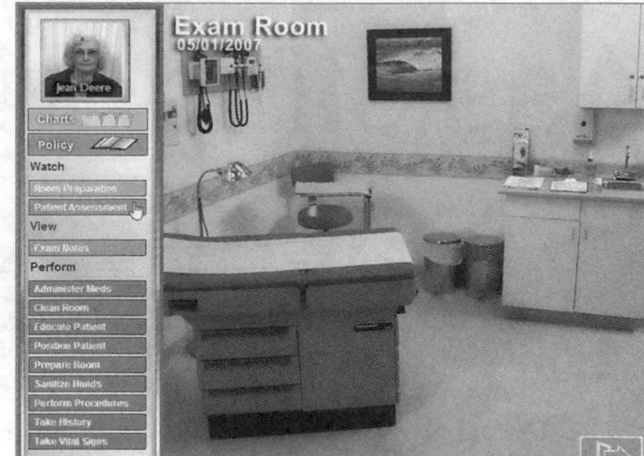

- Sign in to Mountain View Clinic.
- Select **Jean Deere** from the patient list.
- Click on **Exam Room**.
- Under the Watch heading, select **Patient Assessment** to view the video.
- At the end of the video, click **Close** to return to the Exam Room.
- Click the **X** on the video screen to close the video.
- Click on **Policy** to open the office Policy Manual.
- Type "standing orders" in the search bar and click on the magnifying glass.

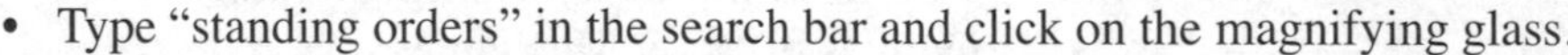

- Read the section of the Policy Manual on standing orders.

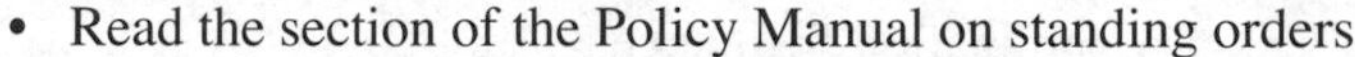

1. What clothing should be removed for Ms. Deere's physical examination?

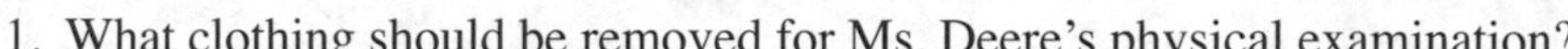

2. What supplies should Ameeta be sure are available on the table to assist Ms. Deere's son James in preparing his mother for the examination?

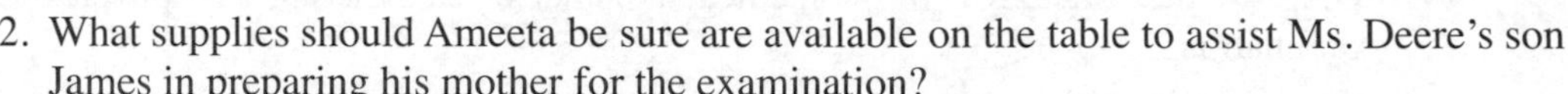

3. Ameeta has allowed Ms. Deere's son to assist with disrobing. Is that appropriate? Why or why not?

Copyright © 2014, 2011, 2007 by Saunders, an imprint of Elsevier Inc. All rights reserved.

4. When would it not be appropriate to allow a family member to help disrobe a patient?

5. Why is it important for Ameeta to offer to help Ms. Deere onto the table?

6. If Ameeta had to assist with lifting Ms. Deere, which of her muscle groups should she use—those of the back or the large muscles of the arms and legs?

7. If Ms. Deere seemed to be weak on her left side, to which side would Ameeta provide support, while using the correct body mechanics?

8. For safety reasons, when should Ms. Deere be positioned on the exam table?

9. Is it acceptable to leave the room when a confused, debilitated, or geriatric patient is on the exam table? Why or why not?

Copyright © 2014, 2011, 2007 by Saunders, an imprint of Elsevier Inc. All rights reserved.

- Click **Close Manual** to return to the Exam Room.
- Click on the **Exam Table**.
- Use the checkboxes to select all positions in which the patient will be placed during her exam.
- Click **Finish** to return to the Exam Room.
- Click the exit arrow.
- On the Summary Menu, click on **Look at Your Performance Summary**.
- Scroll down the Performance Summary to the section and compare your answers with those chosen by the experts. The summary can be printed or saved for your instructor.
- Click **Close** to return to the Summary Menu.
- Click **Return to Map** and select **Yes** at the pop-up menu to return to the office map.

Exercise 2

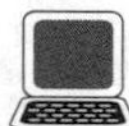

Online Activity—Preparing a Young Adult and Assisting with a Routine Physical Examination

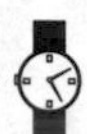

25 minutes

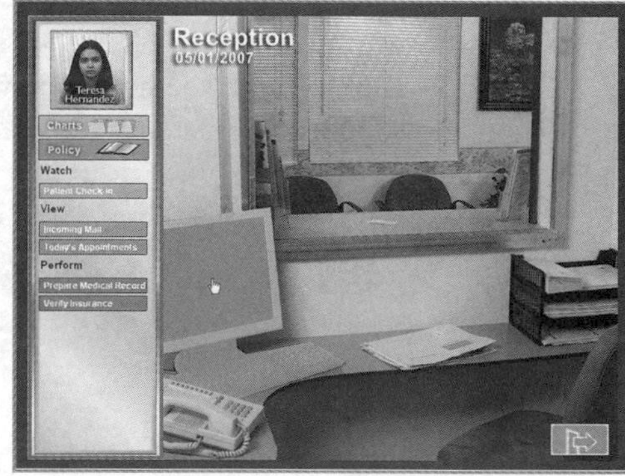

- Select **Teresa Hernandez** from the patient list.
- Click on **Reception**.
- Click on the **Computer**.
- Find the reason for Teresa's visit on the schedule
- Click **Finish** to return to the Reception area.
- Under the Watch heading, click on **Patient Check-In** and watch the video.
- You may also review the Policy Manual section on Standing Orders once more before answering the following questions.

1. What is the reason for Teresa Hernandez's appointment, and what is her status in the medical office that will affect preparations for the physical examination?

Copyright © 2014, 2011, 2007 by Saunders, an imprint of Elsevier Inc. All rights reserved.

2. Did you feel that Kristin was professional in speaking with Teresa about correcting the forms she was asked to fill out, even though the patient was concerned about her parents finding out she had an appointment at the office?

Critical Thinking Question

3. Someone else came to stand behind Teresa while she was talking with Kristin. Why do you think he was shaking his head at the end of the video?

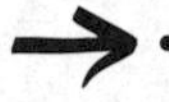

- Click the **X** on the video screen to close the video.
- Click the exit arrow.
- Click **Return to Map** and select **Yes** at the pop-up menu to return to the office map.
- Click on **Exam Room**.
- Under the Watch heading, click on **Ethical Boundaries** and watch the video.

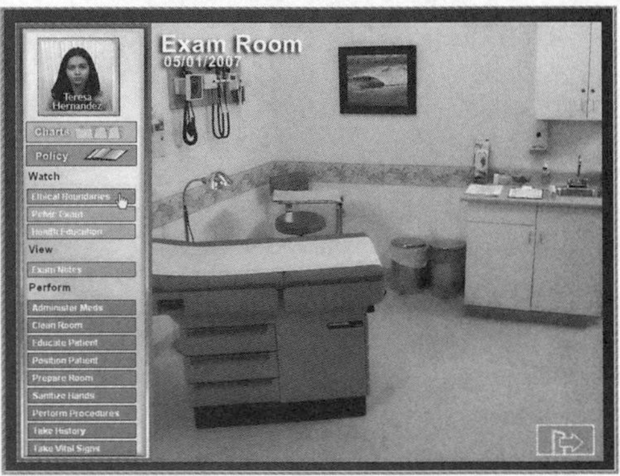

4. What preliminary steps must the clinical medical assistant complete before a physical examination?

5. What clothing should Teresa remove for her physical examination?

Copyright © 2014, 2011, 2007 by Saunders, an imprint of Elsevier Inc. All rights reserved.

6. Teresa appears to be very nervous and uneasy about discussing her chief complaint. What do you think of the way that Ameeta, the medical assistant, handled the situation?

7. Because of the privacy issues surrounding contraception, especially with a teenage patient, Ameeta was faced with ethical and confidentiality boundaries in preparing Teresa to talk with the physician. Do you think that Ameeta provided the guidance needed to place Teresa more at ease? Explain your answer.

8. Would it have been appropriate for Ameeta to tell Teresa that what is said in the office is confidential? Why or why not?

9. Ameeta instructed Teresa to completely disrobe and to put on the gown, but can you identify any important information that she did not include in her instructions?

Copyright © 2014, 2011, 2007 by Saunders, an imprint of Elsevier Inc. All rights reserved.

- Click the **X** on the video screen to close the video.
- Click on the **Exam Table**.
- Use the checkboxes to select all positions in which the patient will be placed during her exam.
- Click **Finish** to return to the Exam Room.
- Under the Watch heading, click on **Pelvic Exam** and watch the video.

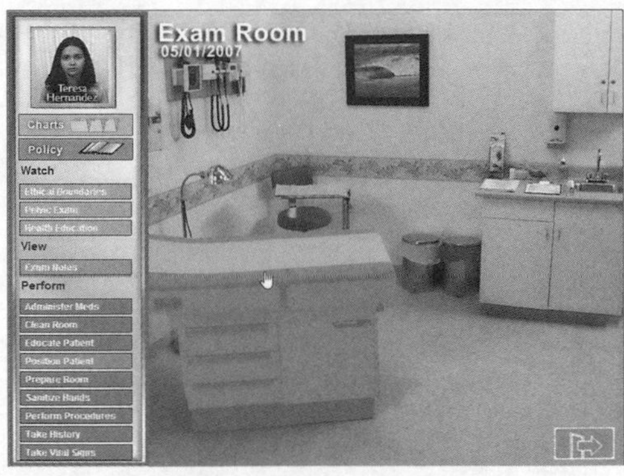

10. In the video, what are the ways that Ameeta assists Dr. Hayler? Select all that apply.

_____ Passes instruments

_____ Takes instruments after use

_____ Waits for Dr. Hayler to ask for instruments

_____ Is prepared to give Dr. Hayler needed supplies promptly

_____ Explains the procedure and the need for infection control

_____ Disposes of Dr. Hayler's disposable equipment

_____ Asks Dr. Hayler to dispose of equipment

_____ Has prepared tray and passes all supplies on the tray for use

_____ Has supplies prepared that might be used for a pelvic exam

_____ Accepts specimen for laboratory testing

_____ Prepares label for specimen transport

_____ Has gooseneck lamp adjusted for proper lighting of area being examined

_____ Has the patient in proper position for a pelvic examination

11. How did Ameeta provide safety measures for Teresa?

12. What was one thing Ameeta could have asked Teresa to do before helping her sit up.

Copyright © 2014, 2011, 2007 by Saunders, an imprint of Elsevier Inc. All rights reserved.

13. Why is it important for Ameeta to have all the supplies and equipment available for the physician and to efficiently hand these to the physician without his asking?

14. Teresa was placed in the ____________________ position.

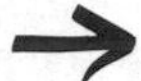

- Click the **X** on the video screen to close the video.
- Click the exit arrow.
- On the Summary Menu, click on **Look at Your Performance Summary**.
- Scroll down the Performance Summary to the Position Patient section and compare your answers with those chosen by the experts. The summary can be printed or saved for your instructor.
- Click **Close** to return to the Summary Menu.
- Click **Return to Map**, then click **Yes** at the pop-up menu to return to the office map or click **Exit the Program**.

Exercise 3

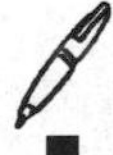

Writing Activity—Appropriate Body Mechanics

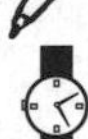

10 minutes

Answer the following questions regarding using proper body mechanics while assisting with patient examinations.

1. If you are reaching for an object, you should avoid twisting and turning and instead move your feet to face the object. What is the purpose of doing this?

Copyright © 2014, 2011, 2007 by Saunders, an imprint of Elsevier Inc. All rights reserved.

2. What is the risk involved with placing the popliteal area of your legs behind the knees next to the edge of the chair?

3. It is advisable to not cross your legs while sitting. What is the reason for this recommendation?

4. What precautions should be taken when lifting heavy objects?

5. If possible, slide, roll, or push a heavy item rather than _______________ or _______________ it.

6. When standing, how should your weight be distributed?

Copyright © 2014, 2011, 2007 by Saunders, an imprint of Elsevier Inc. All rights reserved.

LESSON 19

Administering Parenteral Medications and Immunizations

Reading Assignment: Chapter 33—Principles of Pharmacology
- Drug Names
- Factors That Affect Drug Action

Chapter 34—Pharmacology Math

Chapter 35—Administering Medications (including IV Therapy)
- Safety in Drug Administration
- Drug Forms and Administration

Patients: Shaunti Begay, Jesus Santo, Jade Wong

Learning Objectives:

- Describe preparation of medications according to physician's orders.
- Discuss the steps necessary to administer a parenteral injection according to physician's orders.
- Choose appropriate supplies for assisting with the administration of medication (based on volume ordered).
- Identify the correct supplies for assisting with an examination.
- List the Seven Rights of patient medication administration.
- Identify the necessary steps for patient safety with the administration of medications.
- Identify local resources for immunizations and for patient education.
- Correlate the importance of timing the collection of laboratory specimens with the administration of medication.
- Choose the appropriate biohazard container for disposal of supplies utilized in the administration of medication.
- Understand documentation and recordkeeping procedures for the administration of medication and immunizations.
- Correctly document the administration of medication.

Overview:

In this lesson the administration of medication based on the physician's order is presented. You will choose syringes and the volume of medication to help prepare patients for the administration of parenteral medications and immunizations. You will also complete documentation of these injections. The appropriate way to provide referrals to community resources for health maintenance and prevention will also be presented.

Copyright © 2014, 2011, 2007 by Saunders, an imprint of Elsevier Inc. All rights reserved.

Exercise 1

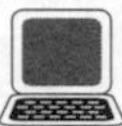

Online Activity—Administering Parenteral Medications

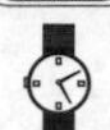

20 minutes

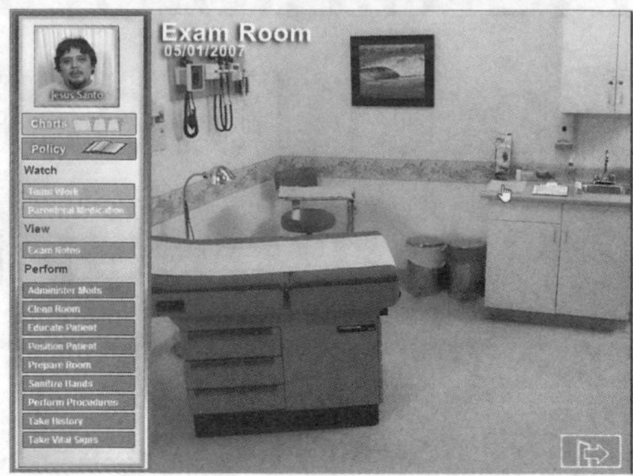

- Sign in to Mountain View Clinic.
- Select **Jesus Santo** from the patient list.
- Click on **Exam Room**.
- Click on the **Exam Notes** file folder and read the documentation on Jesus Santo's visit.
- Click **Finish** to return to the Exam Room.
- Click on the **Supply Cabinet**.
- Add the supplies needed for the patient's exam by clicking on the supply from the Available Supplies list and clicking **Add Item** to confirm your choice.
- If you wish to remove a chosen supply, highlight the supply in the Selected Supplies box and click **Remove**.
- Repeat this step until you are satisfied you have everything you need from the list.
- Do NOT close this window. Keep the Prepare Room wizard open as you continue with the lesson.

1. The medical assistant is asked to prepare Bicillin-LA 1,200,000 units for injection. If the medication is available as Bicillin-LA 600,000 units/mL, how many milliliters would Charlie prepare to give Mr. Santo?

2. What is the classification of the Bicillin-LA? (*Hint:* Use the Internet or a drug reference if you need help.)

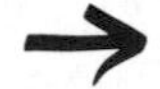

- From the list of Available Supplies, click on **Parenteral Injection** and review the contents on the tray as shown in the photo.

3. Four syringes, a tuberculin syringe, a 5-mL syringe, an insulin syringe, and a 3-mL syringe are on the parenteral injection tray. Which is the correct syringe for the administration of the medication ordered?

Copyright © 2014, 2011, 2007 by Saunders, an imprint of Elsevier Inc. All rights reserved.

4. Choose the correct syringe and indicate the amount of medication that should be given to Jesus Santo by shading in the appropriate area.

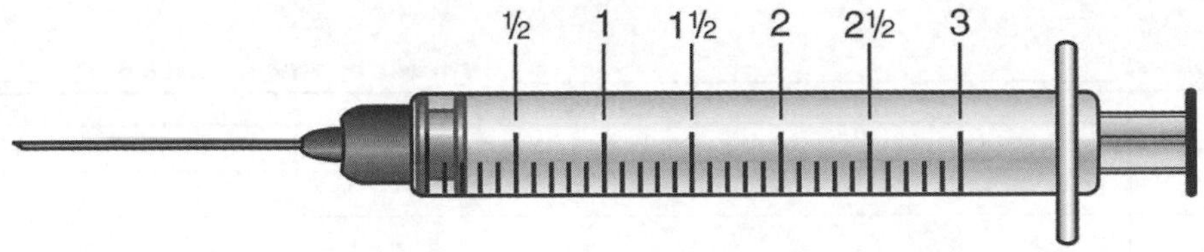

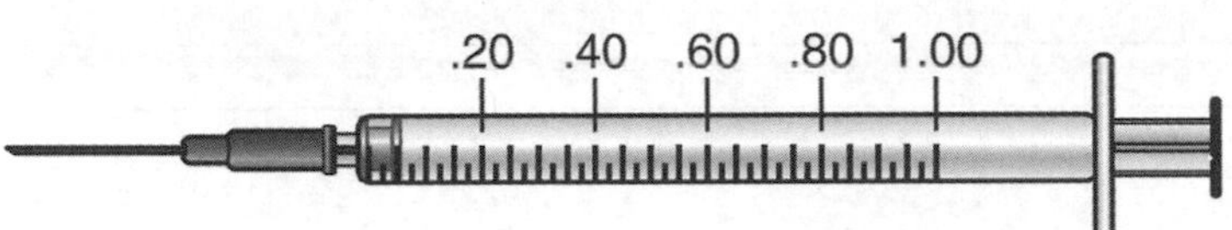

- Click **Finish** to return to the Exam Room.
- Click on the **Medication Cup**.
- Use the checkboxes to select the appropriate actions necessary to prepare medications for the patient.
- Click **Finish** to return to the Exam Room.
- Click on the **Waste Receptacles**.
- Use the checkboxes to select the appropriate steps necessary to clean the Exam Room after the patient's exam.
- Click **Finish** to return to the Exam Room.

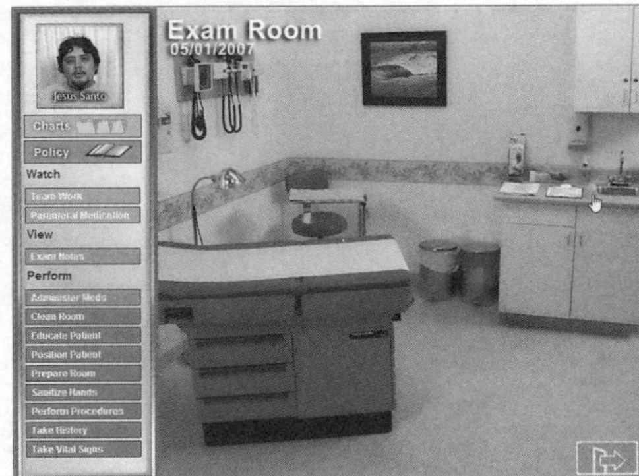

5. What is the correct disposal of the syringe following the administration of the Bicillin-LA?
   a. In a regular waste container
   b. In a biohazard waste container
   c. In a puncture-proof biohazard waste container

6. What is the proper disposal of the used supplies, other than the syringe, following the administration of Bicillin-LA?
   a. In a regular waste container
   b. In a biohazard waste container
   c. In a puncture-proof biohazard waste container

Copyright © 2014, 2011, 2007 by Saunders, an imprint of Elsevier Inc. All rights reserved.

7. Properly document the injection given to Mr. Santo, using the date and time at present.

PATIENT'S NAME ______ ☐FEMALE ☐MALE Date of Birth: __/__/__

DATE	PATIENT VISITS AND FINDINGS

Critical Thinking Question

8. The Exam Notes state that the complete blood count (CBC) should be drawn before administration of the Bicillin LA. Why should the CBC be drawn first and then the medication administered?

9. Why is it important for Mr. Santo to stay in the office for 15 to 20 minutes following the injection of Bicillin-LA?

10. The physician has stated in the Exam Notes that the patient should wait for 15 to 20 minutes before leaving the office. Mr. Santo was brought to the medical office by his employer, Mr. Freeman. If Mr. Freeman does not want to wait, what should the medical assistant at the check-out desk do? Apply your critical thinking skills while answering this question.

Copyright © 2014, 2011, 2007 by Saunders, an imprint of Elsevier Inc. All rights reserved.

11. The Exam Notes state that Mr. Santo should receive two written prescriptions. Fill out the following blank prescription forms for the physician's signature. Use 33344888 for the Drug Enforcement Administration (DEA) number.

Mountain View Clinic
4412 Broadway Ave
London XY 55555
Phone 555-555-1234 FAX 555-555-1239

Patient Name ____________________ Age ________
Address ____________________ Date ________

℞ } Superscription
Inscription {
Subscription {
Signatura {

☐ Dispense as Written
Refill NR 1 2 3 4

Signature ____________________
DEA # ____________________

Mountain View Clinic
4412 Broadway Ave
London XY 55555
Phone 555-555-1234 FAX 555-555-1239

Patient Name ____________________ Age ________
Address ____________________ Date ________

℞ } Superscription
Inscription {
Subscription {
Signatura {

☐ Dispense as Written
Refill NR 1 2 3 4

Signature ____________________
DEA # ____________________

Copyright © 2014, 2011, 2007 by Saunders, an imprint of Elsevier Inc. All rights reserved.

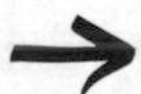

- Click the exit arrow.
- On the Summary Menu, click on **Look at Your Performance Summary**.
- Scroll down the Performance Summary to the Administer Meds, Clean Room, and Prepare Room sections and compare your answers with those chosen by the experts. The summary can be printed or saved for your instructor.
- Click **Close** to return to the Summary Menu.
- Click **Return to Map** and select **Yes** at the pop-up menu to return to the office map.

Exercise 2

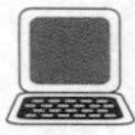

Online Activity—Administering and Documenting Immunizations

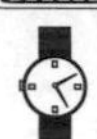

30 minutes

- Select **Shaunti Begay** from the patient list.
- Click on the **Exam Room**.
- Under the Watch heading, click on **Immunizations** and watch the video.

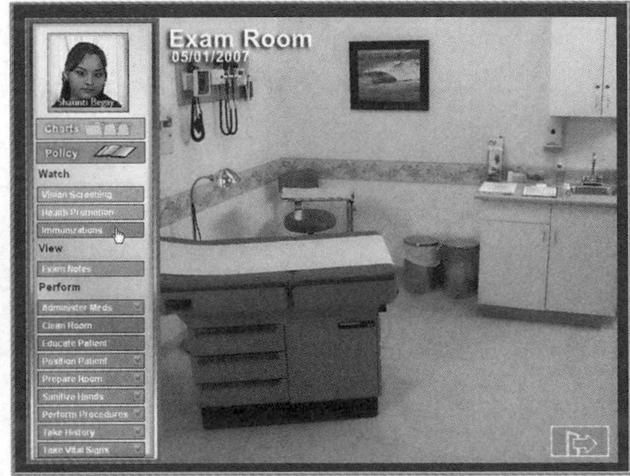

1. What is the site of the hepatitis B immunization?

2. When is the next dose of hepatitis B due?

3. When the hepatitis B vaccine is being prepared for administration, when should the medical assistant check the medication against the physician's order before administering it?

Copyright © 2014, 2011, 2007 by Saunders, an imprint of Elsevier Inc. All rights reserved.

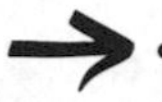

- Click the **X** on the video screen to close the video.
- Click the exit arrow.
- Click on **Return to Map** and select **Yes** at the pop-up menu to return to the office map.
- Click on **Check Out**.
- Click on **Charts**.

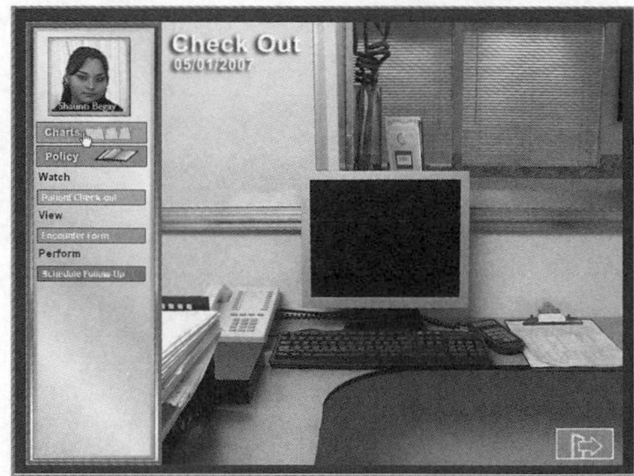

4. What volume of hepatitis B vaccine is being given to Shaunti?

5. Mark the diagram below to indicate the amount of vaccine that should be administered to Shaunti for the hepatitis B immunization.

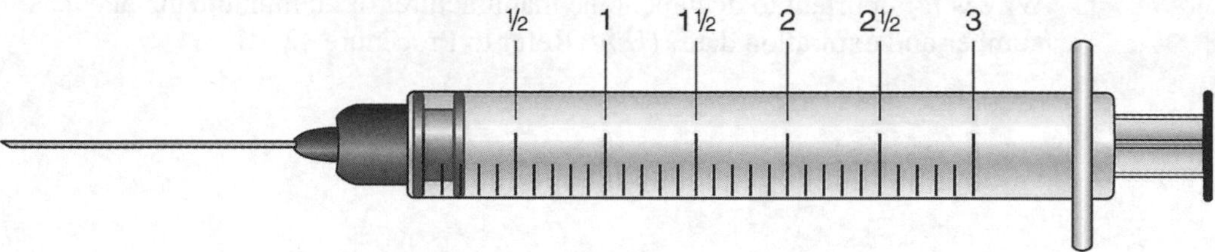

6. What is the expiration date of the hepatitis B vaccine?

7. What is most important about this expiration date?

Critical Thinking Question

8. What steps should the medical assistant take when noticing the expiration date was before the date given? What do you think went wrong with the administration of this injection?

Copyright © 2014, 2011, 2007 by Saunders, an imprint of Elsevier Inc. All rights reserved.

9. What is a VIS statement? Why is this required for an immunization?

10. What are the Seven Rights of medication administration?

11. Why is it important to document the manufacturer of an immunizing agent as well as the lot number and expiration date? (*Hint:* Refer to Procedure 42-1.)

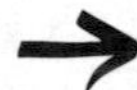

- Click **Close Chart** to return to the Check Out area.
- Click the exit arrow.
- Click on **Return to Map** and select **Yes** at the pop-up menu to return to the office map.

Exercise 3

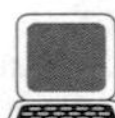

Online Activity—Immunizations as Indicated in Well-Child Visits

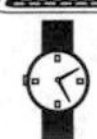

25 minutes

- Select **Jade Wong** from the patient list.
- Click on **Exam Room**.
- Under the Watch heading, click on **Immunizations** and watch the video.
- Click the **X** on the video screen to close the video.
- Click on the **Exam Notes** file folder and read the documentation of Jade's visit.

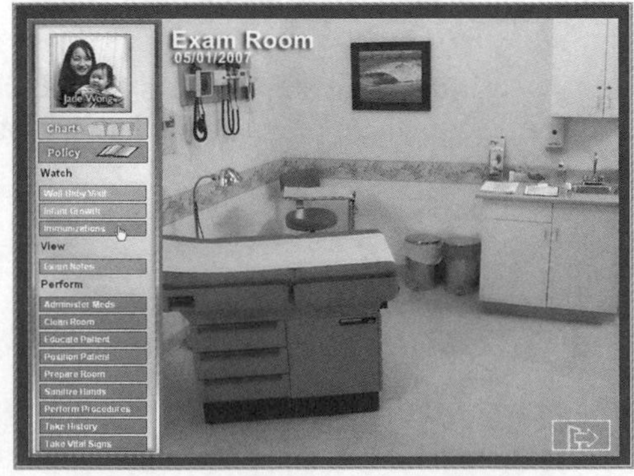

Copyright © 2014, 2011, 2007 by Saunders, an imprint of Elsevier Inc. All rights reserved.

1. Why is it important to provide the parents with information, including the VIS, concerning the immunizations that the child will receive?

2. The medical assistant asked whether Jade had any problems with previous immunizations. Why is this information important before administering the immunizations at this visit?

3. What immunizations will be given to Jade? Be sure to include the diseases that these immunizations protect against (not just the abbreviations of the immunizations).

4. The Exam Notes indicate that Jade's mother has not received the polio vaccine. Why is the injectable polio vaccine safer for the mother?

5. What resources are available in your community for the mother to obtain the polio vaccine if she wants to get it some place other than the physician's office?

Copyright © 2014, 2011, 2007 by Saunders, an imprint of Elsevier Inc. All rights reserved.

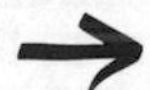

- Click on **Finish** to return to the Exam Room.
- Click the exit arrow.
- Click on **Return to Map** and select **Yes** at the pop-up menu to return to the office map.
- Click on **Check Out**.
- Click on **Charts**.
- Click on the **Patient Medical Information** tab and select **1-Progress Notes**.

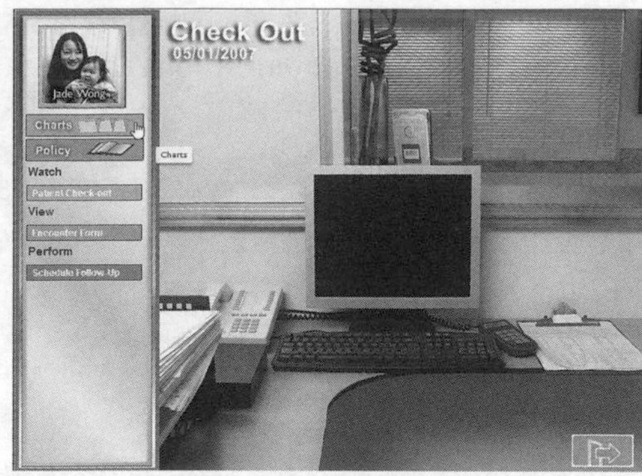

6. In the Progress Notes, the medical assistant states that Jade seemed to tolerate the immunizations with no problems. Why is this documentation important?

7. What volume of Pediarix will be administered to Jade?

8. Indicate on the syringe below the volume of Pediarix that Jade should receive.

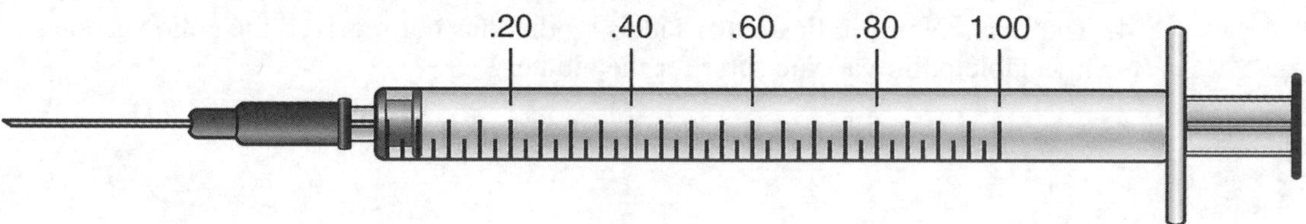

Copyright © 2014, 2011, 2007 by Saunders, an imprint of Elsevier Inc. All rights reserved.

9. Below, document the immunizations that have been given to Jade today. Be sure to follow CDC guidelines.

Vaccine Administration Record for Children and Teens

Patient name: ____________________

Birthdate: ____________________

Chart number: ____________________

Before administering any vaccines, give copies of all pertinent Vaccine Information Statements (VISs) to the child's parent or legal representative and make sure he/she understands the risks and benefits of the vaccine(s). Always provide or update the patient's personal record card.

Vaccine	Type of Vaccine[1]	Date given (mo/day/yr)	Funding Source (F,S,P)[2]	Site[3]	Vaccine		Vaccine Information Statement (VIS)		Vaccinator[6] (signature or initials & title)
					Lot #	Mfr.	Date on VIS[4]	Date given[4]	
Hepatitis B[6] (e.g., HepB, Hib-HepB, DTaP-HepB-IPV) Give IM.[7]									
Diphtheria, Tetanus, Pertussis[6] (e.g., DTaP, DTaP/Hib, DTaP-HepB-IPV, DT, DTaP-IPV/Hib, Tdap, DTaP-IPV, Td) Give IM.[7]									
***Haemophilus influenzae* type b[6]** (e.g., Hib, Hib-HepB, DTaP-IPV/Hib, DTaP/Hib) Give IM.[7]									
Polio[6] (e.g., IPV, DTaP-HepB-IPV, DTaP-IPV/Hib, DTaP-IPV) Give IPV SC or IM.[7] Give all others IM.[7]									
Pneumococcal (e.g., PCV7, PCV13, conjugate; PPSV23, polysaccharide) Give PCV IM.[7] Give PPSV SC or IM.[7]									
Rotavirus (RV1, RV5) Give orally (po).									
Measles, Mumps, Rubella[6] (e.g., MMR, MMRV) Give SC.[7]									
Varicella[6] (e.g., VAR, MMRV) Give SC.[7]									
Hepatitis A (HepA) Give IM.[7]									
Meningococcal (e.g., MCV4; MPSV4) Give MCV4 IM[7] and MPSV4 SC.[7]									
Human papillomavirus (e.g., HPV2, HPV4) Give IM.[7]									
Influenza (e.g., TIV, inactivated; LAIV, live attenuated) Give TIV IM.[7] Give LAIV IN.[7]									
Other									

How to Complete this Record

1. Record the generic abbreviation (e.g., Tdap) or the trade name for each vaccine (see table at right).
2. Record the funding source of the vaccine given as either F (federal), S (state), or P (private).
3. Record the site where vaccine was administered as either RA (right arm), LA (left arm), RT (right thigh), LT (left thigh), or IN (intranasal).
4. Record the publication date of each VIS as well as the date the VIS is given to the patient.
5. To meet the space constraints of this form and federal requirements for documentation, a healthcare setting may want to keep a reference list of vaccinators that includes their initials and titles.
6. For combination vaccines, fill in a row for each antigen in the combination.
7. IM is the abbreviation for intramuscular; SC is the abbreviation for subcutaneous; IN is the abbreviation for intranasal.

Abbreviation	Trade Name & Manufacturer
MMR	MMRII (Merck)
VAR	Varivax (Merck)
MMRV	ProQuad (Merck)
HepA	Havrix (GlaxoSmithKline [GSK]), Vaqta (Merck)
HepA-HepB	Twinrix (GSK)
HPV2	Cervarix (GSK)
HPV4	Gardasil (Merck)
LAIV (Live attenuated influenza vaccine]	FluMist (MedImmune)
TIV (Trivalent inactivated influenza vaccine)	Afluria (CSL Biotherapies); Agriflu (Novartis); Fluarix (GSK), FluLaval (GSK); Fluvirin (Novartis); Fluzone (sanofi)
MCV4	Menactra (sanofi pasteur); Menveo (Novartis)
MPSV4	Menomune (sanofi pasteur)

Technical content reviewed by the Centers for Disease Control and Prevention, August 2010.

www.immunize.org/catg.d/p2022.pdf • Item #P2022 (8/10)

Distributed by the Immunization Action Coalition • (651) 647-9009 • www.immunize.org • www.vaccineinformation.org

Copyright © 2014, 2011, 2007 by Saunders, an imprint of Elsevier Inc. All rights reserved.

10. Why is the use of a 1-mL syringe more appropriate when administering the medication to Jade?

- Click **Close Chart** to return to the Check Out area.
- Under the Watch heading, click on **Patient Check-Out** and watch the video.

11. The medical assistant provides Jade's father, Mr. Wong, with information concerning child nutrition and community resources. She indicates that Mr. Wong and his wife are open to this help. Why is it important that the implied permission is provided, either verbally or nonverbally, before giving information?

12. The Progress Notes also state that Jade's mother has been referred to ESL classes. What does ESL mean?

13. Using the Internet or a local resource guide, list the resources for ESL education in your area.

- Click the **X** on the video screen to close the video.
- Click **Close** and return to the Check Out area.
- Click the exit arrow.
- Click on **Return to Map** and select **Yes** at the pop-up menu to return to the office map or click **Exit the Program**.

Copyright © 2014, 2011, 2007 by Saunders, an imprint of Elsevier Inc. All rights reserved.

LESSON 20

Fecal Specimen Collection

Reading Assignment: Chapter 39—Assisting in Gastroenterology
- The Medical Assistant's Role in the Gastrointestinal Examination

Patient: John R. Simmons

Learning Objectives:

- Understand the reasons for collecting fecal specimens.
- Using the package insert of the fecal occult test, identify the correct steps to give the patient when providing patient education for preparing and collecting the specimen.
- Describe the development of the fecal occult test and the visual appearance of the controls.
- Identify the possible indications of a positive fecal occult test.
- Understand the need for quality control when obtaining and testing a fecal specimen.

Overview:

In this lesson Dr. John R. Simmons, a college professor, will be asked to provide the medical office with fecal specimens to be tested for occult blood. The medical assistant has the responsibility of providing Dr. Simmons with the necessary preparation to ensure that a quality test will be obtained. Dr. Simmons has not been asked to do this test previously, so specific instructions must be provided. Discussing fecal specimens tends to embarrass most patients, so it is important that the medical assistant respond with dignity and professionalism. Furthermore, it is imperative that the correct instructions be given; otherwise, the patient may provide a specimen that cannot be tested.

Copyright © 2014, 2011, 2007 by Saunders, an imprint of Elsevier Inc. All rights reserved.

Exercise 1

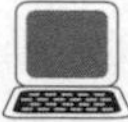

Online Activity—Patient Instruction for Collecting Fecal Specimens

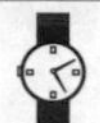

40 minutes

- Sign in to Mountain View Clinic.
- Select **John R. Simmons** from the patient list.
- Click on **Exam Room**.
- Under the **Watch** heading, select **Patient Instruction** and watch the video.

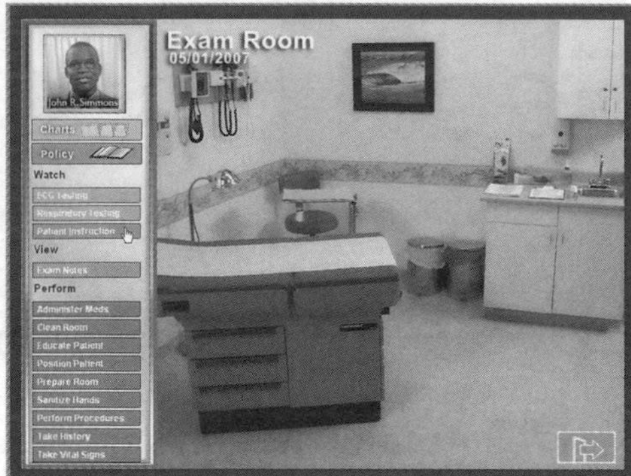

1. Dr. Simmons seems embarrassed by the need to collect stool specimens. How did the medical assistant attempt to put him at ease?

2. What is a guaiac test? How is this test related to fecal specimens?

3. Which supplies do patients need to obtain fecal specimens at home? Select all that apply.

_____ Gloves

_____ Wooden applicator sticks

_____ Test kits (the number is based on the physician's policy)

_____ Plastic wrap

_____ Written instructions

_____ Addressed envelope

Copyright © 2014, 2011, 2007 by Saunders, an imprint of Elsevier Inc. All rights reserved.

- Go to your Evolve account and enter the course area for this textbook. Under the Course Documents heading, access the document "Fecal Occult Testing Kit Package Insert." This is one type of fecal occult testing kit. Answer the following questions using the package insert.

  Note that in the physician's office, you may have a variation of instructions, depending on which test kit is being used. For this question, however, use the package insert provided.

4. Which information should the medical assistant give the patient when providing instructions for preparing to obtain a fecal specimen? Select all that apply.

   _____ Avoid all vegetables for 3 days.

   _____ Eat a high-fiber diet for 3 days.

   _____ Do not eat red meat, including processed meats and cold cuts, for 3 days.

   _____ Take all medications ordered by the physician.

   _____ Avoid taking aspirin, corticosteroids, and NSAIDs for a week before collecting the specimen.

   _____ Do not collect stool specimens during a menstrual period or for 3 days afterward.

   _____ Eat foods that will cause softening of stools to make the specimen easier to obtain.

   _____ Eat small amounts of food that contain vitamin C.

   _____ Do not eat raw fruits and vegetables, especially melons, radishes, turnips, and horseradish.

   _____ Eat cooked vegetables.

   _____ Drink at least three glasses of milk per day.

   _____ Do not take iron or vitamin C for 3 days.

   _____ Eat moderate amounts of bran cereal, popcorn, and other roughage.

5. When test kits are taken home, how should the patient store the kits until the specimens are collected?

6. What directions should be given to the patient about the timing of specimens?

Copyright © 2014, 2011, 2007 by Saunders, an imprint of Elsevier Inc. All rights reserved.

7. Which of the following are correct instructions to give to the patient about obtaining the stool specimen? Select all that apply.

_____ Using the wooden applicator stick, collect a sample of stool either from a container or from toilet paper.

_____ If the stool falls in the commode, collect the sample as you would from the container or the toilet paper.

_____ Open the flap of the first kit on the left (be sure there are two square boxes inside, labeled A and B); then smear a small amount of stool on the filter paper labeled A, making sure to spread it until thin.

_____ Using the same wooden stick, collect a second sample of stool from another area of the stool.

_____ Place this sample on top of the sample already collected.

_____ Place the second sample in the filter paper box labeled B.

_____ Close the front flap.

_____ Tear this test kit from the other two and place in the envelope provided.

_____ Add the date and time of collection on the flap.

_____ Repeat the same procedure with the next two stools (if three test kits were provided).

_____ Allow the specimens to air-dry before returning to the office.

_____ Place the specimens in a standard letter-sized envelope and mail.

_____ Place the specimens in an aluminum-lined envelope designed for sending to the medical office.

8. Why is it important that the smears be taken from two different areas of the stool?

9. Why is it important that the patient add roughage to the diet?

Copyright © 2014, 2011, 2007 by Saunders, an imprint of Elsevier Inc. All rights reserved.

10. On the form below, document the procedure for instructing the patient in the collection of a fecal specimen.

PATIENT'S NAME ____________ ☐FEMALE ☐MALE Date of Birth: __/__/__

DATE	PATIENT VISITS AND FINDINGS

- Click the **X** on the video screen to close the video.
- Click the exit arrow.
- Click **Return to Map** and select **Yes** at the pop-up menu to return to the office map or click **Exit the Program**.

Exercise 2

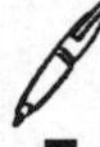

Writing Activity—Developing a Hemoccult Slide Test

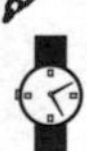

20 minutes

A week after his visit, Dr. John R. Simmons has returned the Hemoccult slides to the medical office for development. In this exercise, you will describe the steps necessary to develop the test and provide documentation to the physician.

1. Which of the following are the proper supplies needed for developing the Hemoccult test? Select all that apply.

_____ Sterile gloves

_____ Gloves

_____ Gown and goggles

_____ Developer solution

_____ Wooden sticks

_____ Watch

_____ Reference card

_____ Biohazard waste container

Copyright © 2014, 2011, 2007 by Saunders, an imprint of Elsevier Inc. All rights reserved.

2. Now that you have chosen the proper supplies for developing the Hemoccult, match the following columns to show the correct order of the steps.

	Order	Action
_____	Step 1	a. Ensure quality control by checking the expiration date on slides and developer.
_____	Step 2	b. Don the correct personal protective equipment.
_____	Step 3	c. Dispose of the used Hemoccult slides in proper waste container.
_____	Step 4	d. Read the results in 60 seconds.
_____	Step 5	e. Open the back flap of the slides.
_____	Step 6	f. Document the results in the medical record.
_____	Step 7	g. Sanitize hands following the procedure.
_____	Step 8	h. Sanitize hands before the procedure.
_____	Step 9	i. Compare the results with the reference card.
_____	Step 10	j. Apply two drops of developing solution to the guaiac test paper and the quality control area.

3. Why is it important to read the Hemoccult slide results at the end of 60 seconds?

4. The result of the first specimen obtained by Dr. Simmons was negative, but slides 2 and 3 were positive. Document these results on the Progress Notes below.

PATIENT'S NAME ______________________ ☐FEMALE ☐MALE Date of Birth: ___/___/___

DATE	PATIENT VISITS AND FINDINGS

Copyright © 2014, 2011, 2007 by Saunders, an imprint of Elsevier Inc. All rights reserved.

5. What does a positive Hemoccult test indicate?

6. What are the indications if the positive quality control area does not change to a blue color?

7. What are two possible causes of invalid tests?

Copyright © 2014, 2011, 2007 by Saunders, an imprint of Elsevier Inc. All rights reserved.

LESSON 21

Assisting with a Prenatal/ Gynecological Examination

Reading Assignment: Chapter 41—Assisting in Obstetrics and Gynecology
- Pregnancy
- The Medical Assistant's Role in Gynecological and Obstetric Procedures

Patients: Renee Anderson, Louise Parlet

Learning Objectives:

- Choose the necessary questions to ask the patient to obtain information for a thorough health history and gynecological and prenatal examinations.
- Understand the appropriate positions in which the patient will be placed for the gynecological examination
- Discuss the legal and ethical boundaries of preparing a patient for a gynecological/prenatal examination.
- Discuss the legal and ethical issues associated with assault/domestic abuse.
- Document the patient information into the medical record.
- Understand how a medical assistant should handle domestic abuse concerns ethically and professionally.
- Assess how verbal and nonverbal communications are important to assess with victims of domestic abuse.
- Read a health history form to obtain information that may indicate the patient has been abused.

Overview:

This lesson is designed around two patients: Louise Parlet, an established patient who is having a routine prenatal examination, and Renee Anderson, a new patient coming in for a routine gynecological examination. Ms. Anderson is also a victim of domestic abuse.

Copyright © 2014, 2011, 2007 by Saunders, an imprint of Elsevier Inc. All rights reserved.

Exercise 1

Online Activity—Assisting with a Routine Prenatal Examination

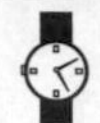

45 minutes

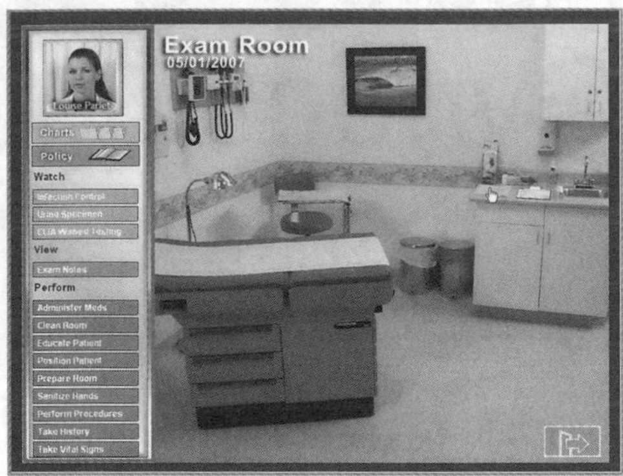

- Sign in to Mountain View Clinic.
- Select **Louise Parlet** from the patient list.
- Click on **Exam Room**.
- Click on the **Exam Notes** file folder and read the documentation for Louise Parlet's visit.
- Click on **Finish** to return to the Exam Room.
- Click on the **Supply Cabinet**.
- Add the supplies needed for the patient's exam by clicking on the supply from the Available Supplies list and clicking **Add Item** to confirm your choice.
- If you wish to remove a chosen supply, highlight the supply in the Selected Supplies box and click **Remove**.
- Repeat this step until you are satisfied you have everything you need from the list.
- Do NOT close this window. Keep the Prepare Room wizard open as you continue with the lesson.

1. Match the columns below to indicate the order in which you will use the items needed for a gynecological examination.

	Order of Use	**Item**
_____	First	a. Water-soluble lubricant
_____	Second	b. Cytobrush/spatula
_____	Third	c. Laboratory requisition form
_____	Fourth	d. Gloves for physician
_____	Fifth	e. Speculum
_____	Sixth	f. Gloves for the medical assistant
_____	Seventh	g. Culture transport, if applicable

Copyright © 2014, 2011, 2007 by Saunders, an imprint of Elsevier Inc. All rights reserved.

- Confirm that you have chosen the necessary supplies for Ms. Parlet's Pap smear.
- Click **Finish** to return to the Exam Room.
- Click on the **Exam Table**.
- Use the checkboxes to select all positions in which the patient will be placed during her exam.
- Click **Finish** to return to the Exam Room.

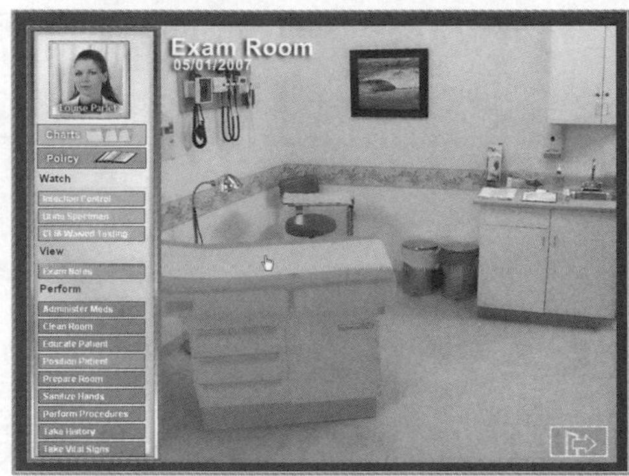

2. Practice documenting in the patient's medical record by following these steps.

- Click on the **Medical Record** clipboard.
- Click on the **Ask** buttons to view the patient's answers to the questions regarding her medical history.
- Record the information into the patient's medical record in the box under "Document all findings below." Enter your name after your documentation as instructed by your instructor.
- At the bottom of the page, click **Next** to view additional questions and responses related to the patient's history.

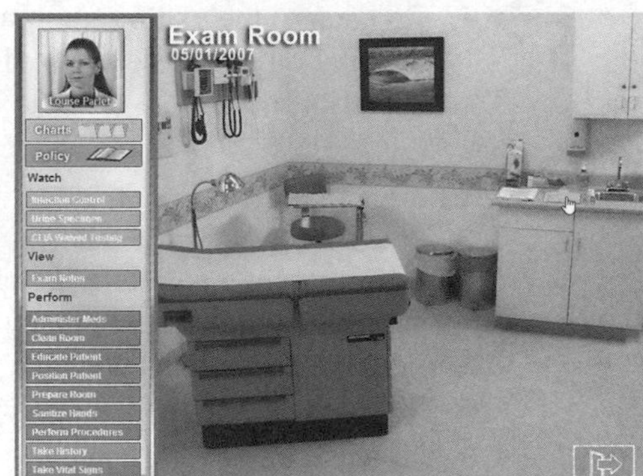

- Use the checkboxes to select any other information you would need to ask the patient.
- If requested by your instructor, print the information by clicking on Print at the bottom of the screen.
- Click **Finish** to close the History Taking window and answer **Yes** at the pop-up window to return to the Exam Room.

3. What information is important to obtain before a prenatal examination?

Copyright © 2014, 2011, 2007 by Saunders, an imprint of Elsevier Inc. All rights reserved.

4. What information did Ms. Parlet provide that might indicate that she is pregnant?

5. How many times has Ms. Parlet conceived? What was the outcome?

→ • Go back to the examination notes if needed. You may also open Ms. Parlet's chart by clicking on the **Patient Medical information** tab and select **5-General Health History Questionnaire**.

Thought Questions

6. Why might a patient who has previously had a spontaneous abortion be "afraid" of complications of pregnancy and therefore phone the office more frequently with questions than other patients who are pregnant?

7. What are ways the medical assistant can alleviate apprehension and provide emotional support to these patients?

Copyright © 2014, 2011, 2007 by Saunders, an imprint of Elsevier Inc. All rights reserved.

8. List the positions used for Ms. Parlet's examination in the order they will be used.

   (1)

   (2)

   (3)

9. Explain the use of each of the positions chosen.

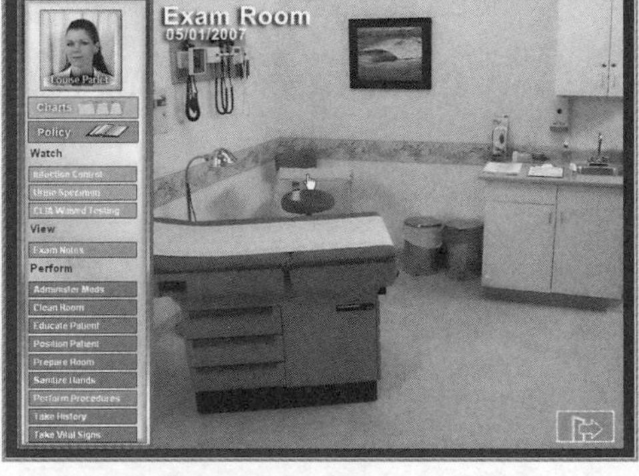

- Click on the **Mayo Stand**.
- Click on **Exam Notes**.
- Click on **Finish** to return to the Perform Procedures window.
- Use the checkboxes to select the procedures that should be performed on the patient during her visit.
- Click **Finish** to return to the Exam Room.
- Click the exit arrow.
- On the Summary Menu, click on **Look at Your Performance Summary**.
- Use the scroll bar to review the areas you performed. The summary can be printed or saved for your instructor.
- Click **Close** to return to the Summary Menu.
- Click **Return to Map** and select **Yes** at the pop-up menu to return to the office map.

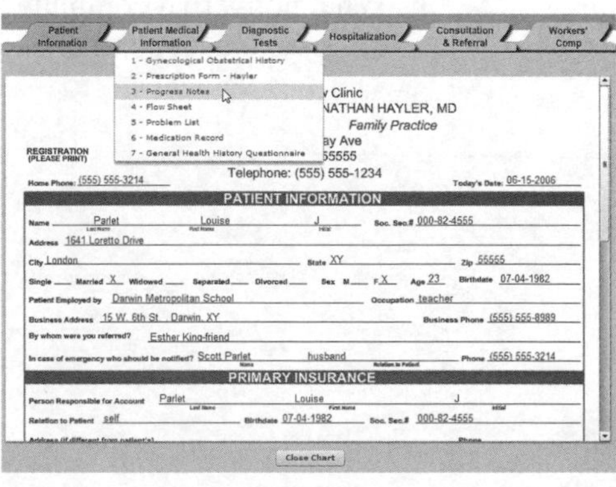

- Click on **Check Out**.
- Click on **Charts**.
- Click on the **Patient Medical Information** tab and select **3-Progress Notes**.

Copyright © 2014, 2011, 2007 by Saunders, an imprint of Elsevier Inc. All rights reserved.

10. Which procedures were accomplished? Why were these needed for the prenatal examination?

11. According to Dr. Hayler's documentation, Ms. Parlet is __________ weeks pregnant.

- Click **Close Chart** to return to the Check Out area.
- Click the exit arrow.
- Click **Return to Map** and select **Yes** at the pop-up menu to return to the office map.

Exercise 2

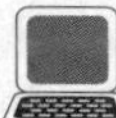

Online Activity—Assisting with a Gynecological Examination

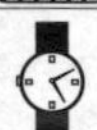

30 minutes

- Select **Renee Anderson** from the patient list.
- Click on **Reception**.
- Under the watch heading, click on **Patient Check-In** and watch the video.

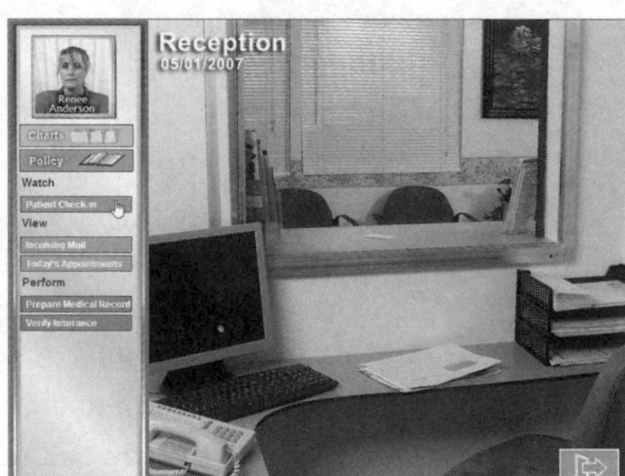

1. What nonverbal communication is most important in this video for the medical assistant to observe and respond to?

Copyright © 2014, 2011, 2007 by Saunders, an imprint of Elsevier Inc. All rights reserved.

2. Did the medical assistant at check-in handle the confidentiality question correctly and accurately? Explain your answer.

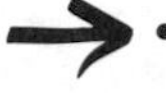

- Click the **X** on the video screen to close the video.
- Click on the **Medical Record**.
- Click on the **Perform** button next to Assemble Medical Record.
- Add forms needed in the Patient Information tab by clicking on the forms from the Forms Available list and clicking **Add** to confirm your choice.
- Continue adding forms to the appropriate tabs in the patient's medical record. To select a new tab, either click on the tab on the medical record or use the drop-down menu on the right.

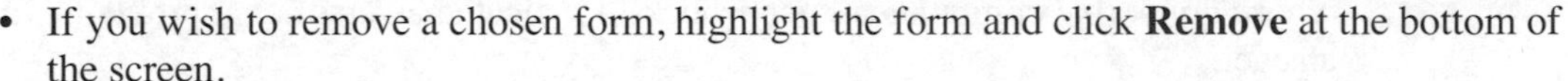

- If you wish to remove a chosen form, highlight the form and click **Remove** at the bottom of the screen.
- Click **Finish** to close the chart and return to the Reception area.

- Click the exit arrow.
- On the Summary Menu, click on **Look at Your Performance Summary**.
- Scroll down the Performance Summary to the Assemble Medical Record sections and compare your answers with those chosen by the experts. The summary can be printed or saved for your instructor.

- Click **Close** to return to the Summary Menu.
- Click **Return to Map**, then click **Yes** at the pop-up menu to return to the office map.
- Click on **Exam Room**.
- Under the Watch heading, click on **Patient Care** and watch the video.

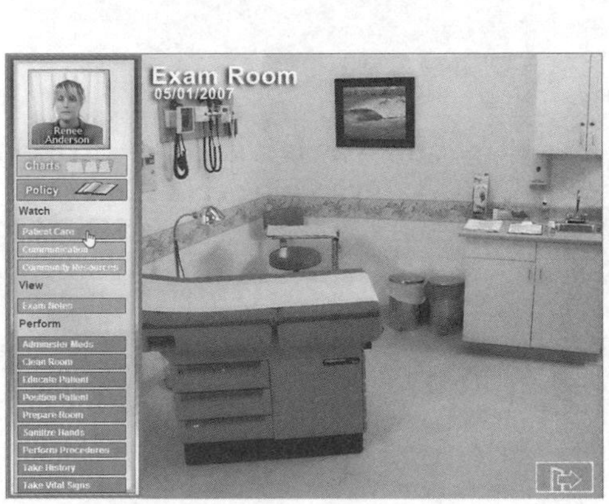

Copyright © 2014, 2011, 2007 by Saunders, an imprint of Elsevier Inc. All rights reserved.

3. In the video, Susan states that she missed a question on the lab request form concerning previously abnormal Pap smears. Why is this important?

4. During the examination, what nonverbal communication did the patient provide to the medical assistant and physician that might have led to an examination for spousal abuse by the physician?

5. Do you think that Susan provided the appropriate verbal and nonverbal support for a patient whose nonverbal communication at check-in indicated an emotional problem? Explain your answer.

6. Why is it important to include the instructions for breast self-examination with each gynecological patient?

Copyright © 2014, 2011, 2007 by Saunders, an imprint of Elsevier Inc. All rights reserved.

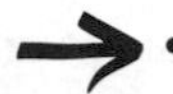

- Click the **X** on the video screen to close the video.
- Click on **Charts**.
- Click on the **Patient Medical Information** tab and select **1-General Health History Questionnaire**.

7. Dr. Hayler suggests that Ms. Anderson have a mammogram. Other than finding a breast lump, what reason would be appropriate for suggesting this mammogram? (*Hint:* Check the Patient Information Form in her chart for age and health history.)

8. Along with the physical findings documented on page 6 of the health history form, what additional information on the form provides a hint of spousal abuse?

- Click on **Close Chart** to return to the Exam Room.
- Under the Watch heading, click on **Communication** and watch the video.

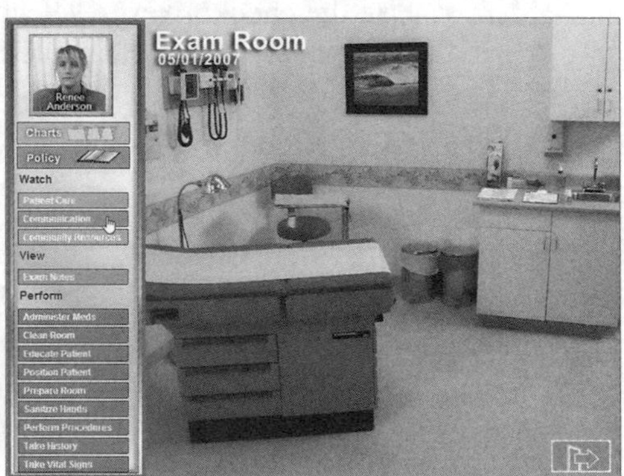

9. When Ms. Anderson arrived for her appointment, ethical and confidential matters were discussed. What did Dr. Hayler and the medical assistant do to continue the ethical and confidential manner of the examination?

Copyright © 2014, 2011, 2007 by Saunders, an imprint of Elsevier Inc. All rights reserved.

10. How do you feel about the manner that Dr. Hayler used when talking with Ms. Anderson, as well as the response of the medical assistant, Susan, to the patient's nonverbal communication?

11. What responsibilities did the medical assistant have concerning the cleaning of the room before Dr. Hayler returned to discuss treatment with Ms. Anderson?

- Click the **X** on the video screen to close the video.
- Click on the **Waste Receptacles**.
- Use the checkboxes to select the appropriate steps necessary to clean the Exam Room after the patient's exam.
- Click **Finish** to return to the Exam Room.

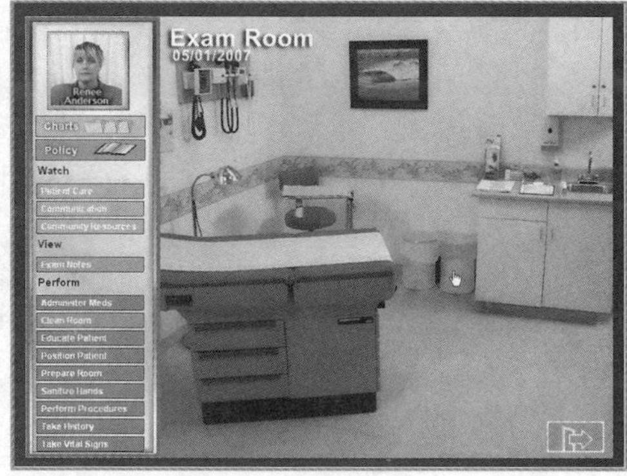

12. Indicate whether each of the following statements is true or false.

   a. _________ The date of the last menstrual period is not important on the lab requisition form for a Pap smear.

   b. _________ The medical assistant is responsible for asking the site of specimen collection during a Pap smear if this information is not provided by the physician.

   c. _________ When assisting with a pelvic examination, the medical assistant should be near the supply tray to pass needed supplies to the physician but should also be at the side of the patient to provide support and to observe nonverbal communication.

   d. _________ With a female patient and a male examiner, the medical assistant has a legal and ethical responsibility to remain in the room at all times.

Copyright © 2014, 2011, 2007 by Saunders, an imprint of Elsevier Inc. All rights reserved.

13. Why is it important that a Pap smear not be collected during the menstrual period or for several days following?

Critical Thinking Question

14. In the video, Dr. Hayler's assistant, who was present during the examination of his patient, is a woman. Why is it recommended that a female assistant, rather than having Charlie, the male medical assistant, assist with the prenatal examination?

Critical Thinking Question

15. Why is it important to keep the patient covered with the gown and drape as much as possible rather than removing the entire drape during the pelvic examination?

Critical Thinking Question

16. What legal problems could arise if the patient and physician are alone during the time the patient is disrobed during a gynecological examination?

Copyright © 2014, 2011, 2007 by Saunders, an imprint of Elsevier Inc. All rights reserved.

Critical Thinking Question

17. What should the next step be in caring for a patient who may be the victim of domestic abuse?

- Under the Watch heading, click on **Community Resources** and watch the video.

18. In your opinion, did Susan give the community resource information to Ms. Anderson in a professional manner? Would you have done anything differently?

- Click the **X** on the video screen to close the video.
- Click the exit arrow.
- Scroll down the Performance Summary to the Clean Room section and compare your answers with those chosen by the experts. The summary can be printed or saved for your instructor.
- Click **Close** to return to the Summary Menu.
- Click **Return to Map**, then click **Yes** at the pop-up menu to return to the office map or click **Exit the Program**.

Copyright © 2014, 2011, 2007 by Saunders, an imprint of Elsevier Inc. All rights reserved.

LESSON 22

Assisting with a Pediatric Examination

Reading Assignment: Chapter 5—Interpersonal Skills and Human Behavior
- Multicultural Issues

Chapter 42—Assisting in Pediatrics
- Normal Growth and Development
- Immunizations
- The Pediatric Patient
- The Medical Assistant's Role in Pediatric Procedures

Patient: Jade Wong

Learning Objectives:

- Describe the steps necessary in preparing a child for a pediatric examination.
- Identify similarities and differences when obtaining mensurations in children and in adults.
- Plot height and weight on a growth chart for children, and identify trends in percentile ranking.
- Describe the role of the medical assistant in a pediatric examination.
- Understand the importance of effective verbal and nonverbal communication with persons of different cultures.
- Understand methods of parental involvement while preparing infants for a physical examination.
- Read the Progress Notes to obtain information about the patient's visit.

Overview:

In this lesson students will be introduced to the pediatric examination and will be expected to identify the differences in examining a pediatric patient versus an adult patient. Jade Wong's parents are of Asian descent and speak little English. During Jade's pediatric visit, the medical assistant explains the needs to the father, who acts as a interpreter. The mother is also provided with information concerning immunizations for health promotion and disease prevention.

Copyright © 2014, 2011, 2007 by Saunders, an imprint of Elsevier Inc. All rights reserved.

Exercise 1

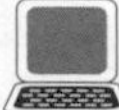

Online Activity—Assisting with a Pediatric Examination

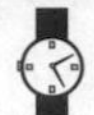

45 minutes

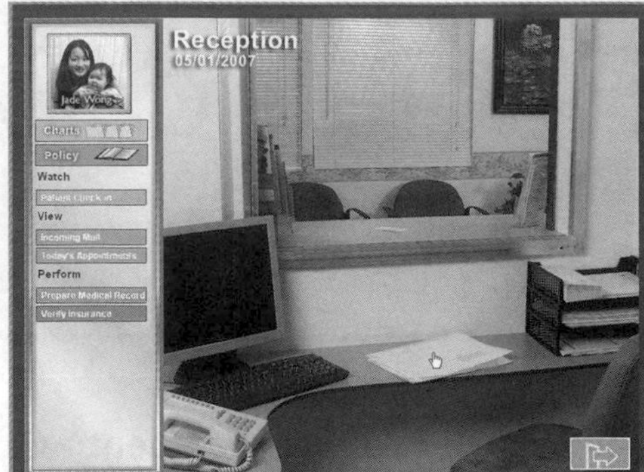

- Sign in to Mountain View Clinic.
- Select **Jade Wong** from the patient list.
- Click on **Reception**.
- Click on the **Medical Record**.
- Click on the **Perform** button next to Assemble Medical Record.
- Add forms needed in the Patient Information tab by clicking on the forms from the Forms Available list and clicking Add to confirm your choice.
- Continue adding forms to the appropriate tabs in the patient's medical record. To select a new tab, either click on the tab on the medical record or use the drop-down menu on the right.

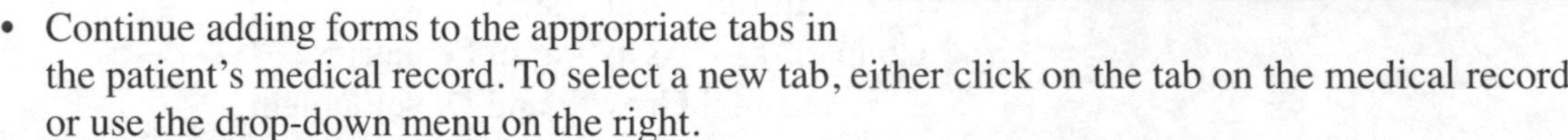

- If you wish to remove a chosen form, highlight the form and click **Remove** at the bottom of the screen.
- Click **Finish** to close the chart and return to the Reception area.

- Click the exit arrow.
- On the Summary Menu, click on **Look at Your Performance Summary**.
- Scroll down the Performance Summary to the Assemble Medical Record section and compare your answers with those chosen by the experts. The summary can be printed or
- Click **Close** to return to the Summary Menu.
- Click **Return to Map** and select **Yes** at the pop-up menu to return to the office map.

- Click on **Exam Room**.
- Under the Watch heading, select **Well-Baby Visit** and watch the video.

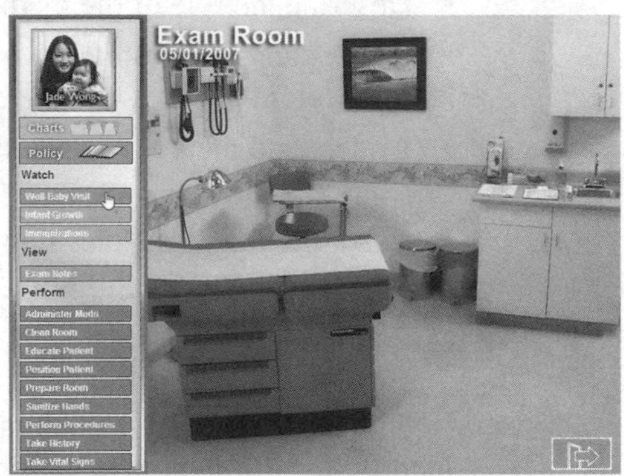

1. What measurements would you expect the medical assistant to obtain on Jade for a well-baby visit? How does this differ from an adult measurement?

Copyright © 2014, 2011, 2007 by Saunders, an imprint of Elsevier Inc. All rights reserved.

2. Why is it important for the medical assistant to develop rapport with a child and with parents when assisting with a well-child office visit?

3. As the medical assistant works with Jade, she is using the father as an interpreter and is allowing the mother to have an active part in the medical care through this means. Do you feel this is an important part of the care, or do you believe the medical assistant should provide care and speak only with the father? Explain your answer.

4. Why is it important to remove the clothing before weighing the infant? Why should the diaper be removed?

Critical Thinking Question

5. What are some of the differences between the preparation of a 4-year-old child for an examination versus the preparation of an adult for an examination?

Copyright © 2014, 2011, 2007 by Saunders, an imprint of Elsevier Inc. All rights reserved.

6. What tactics may be used with older children to gain their confidence?

7. What roles do verbal communication and nonverbal communication play in a pediatric examination?

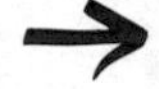

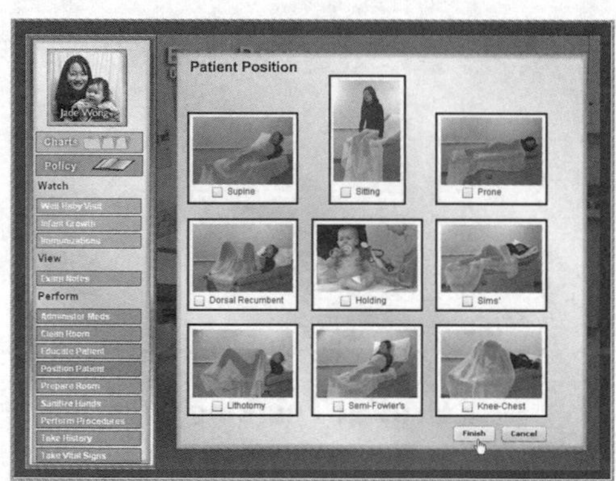

- Click the **X** on the video screen to close the video.
- Click on the **Exam Table**.
- Use the checkboxes to select all positions in which the patient will be placed during her exam.
- Click **Finish** to return to the Exam Room.
- Under the Watch heading, click on **Infant Growth** and watch the video.
- Click the **X** on the video screen to close the video.
- Under the Watch heading, click on **Immunizations** and watch the video.
- Click the **X** on the video screen to close the video.
- Click the exit arrow.
- On the Summary Menu, click on **Look at Your Performance Summary**.
- Scroll down the Performance Summary to the Position Patient section and compare your answers with those of the experts. The summary can be printed or saved for your instructor.
- Click **Close** to return to the Summary Menu.
- Click **Return to Map** and select **Yes** at the pop-up menu to return to the office map.

Copyright © 2014, 2011, 2007 by Saunders, an imprint of Elsevier Inc. All rights reserved.

- Click on **Billing and Coding**.
- Click on **Charts**.
- Click on the **Patient Medical Information** tab and select **6-Newborn Health Summary**.

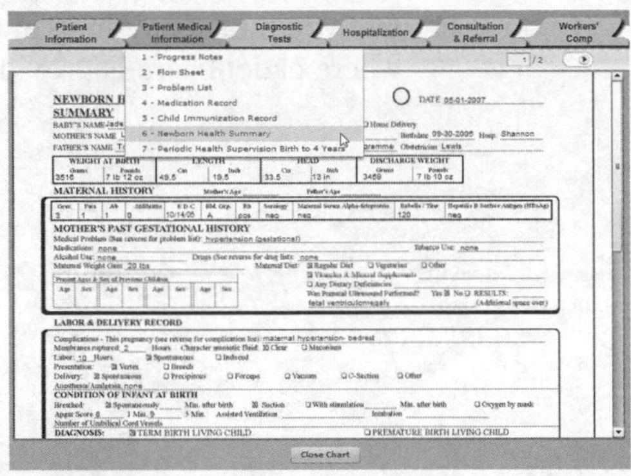

8. Record Jade's birth weight and length from the medical history in the Newborn Health Summary.

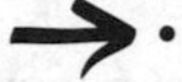

- Click again on the **Patient Medical Information** tab and select **1-Progress Notes**.

9. What measurements were recorded from today's visit?

- Look again at the Progress Notes and read the chief complaint documented for today's visit.

10. As you watched the videos of Jade's visit to the medical office, what role did the clinical medical assistant play throughout the visit?

Copyright © 2014, 2011, 2007 by Saunders, an imprint of Elsevier Inc. All rights reserved.

11. Did you notice anything in the examination room that should not have been in the room where patient care is provided?

12. Why is the chief complaint in quotation marks?

13. Indicate whether each of the following statements is true or false.

a. ________ The growth charts are the same for both genders and for all ages.

b. ________ A well-baby visit is usually scheduled every 2 months for the first 6 months so that the child can receive the needed immunizations on schedule.

c. ________ After the age of 6 months, well-baby visits are scheduled every 3 months until age 18 months.

d. ________ After 2 years of age, well-child visits are scheduled every 2 years.

e. ________ The medical assistant should obtain information about the motor and cognitive development of the child at each visit.

f. ________ If a child is seen for a sick-child visit between well-baby visits, the child does not need to have weight and length obtained.

g. ________ When measuring the circumference of the head and chest, the measurement should be taken at the greatest circumference.

h. ________ Infant scales measure weight in pounds and ounces rather than in pounds and fractions of pounds as with adult.

i. ________ When measuring the height of an infant, the measurement should be from the heel to the crown of the head.

j. ________ When a child becomes old enough to stand on a scale, he or she will sometimes be difficult to weigh and may be afraid or have difficulty balancing without holding onto something.

k. ________ When weighing a young child who is afraid of the balance beam scales or who weighs more than the infant scale can accommodate, an alternative is to weigh the mother and child together on an adult scale and then weigh the mother alone. After obtaining the two weights, you can determine the weight of the child by subtracting the mother's weight from the combined weight of the two.

Copyright © 2014, 2011, 2007 by Saunders, an imprint of Elsevier Inc. All rights reserved.

- Click **Close Chart** to return to the Billing and Coding area.
- Click the exit arrow.
- Click **Return to Map**, then click **Yes** at the pop-up menu to return to the office map or click **Exit the Program**.

Exercise 2

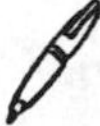

Writing Activity—Plotting a Growth Chart and Recognizing Trends in Percentiles

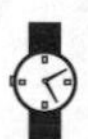

20 minutes

1. On the next page, plot the growth chart for Kaitlynn Griffin using these measurements.

   3 months 22 3/4 inches 11 pounds

   6 months 26 inches 14 pounds, 8 ounces

   9 months 27 1/2 inches 16 pounds, 4 ounces

   13 months 30 1/2 inches 19 pounds

   16 months 31 1/2 inches 20 pounds, 8 ounces

   24 months 34 3/4 inches 27 pounds

2. Compare Kaitlynn's percentiles. What trend do you see on her length?

3. What trend did you see in her weight gain?

Copyright © 2014, 2011, 2007 by Saunders, an imprint of Elsevier Inc. All rights reserved.

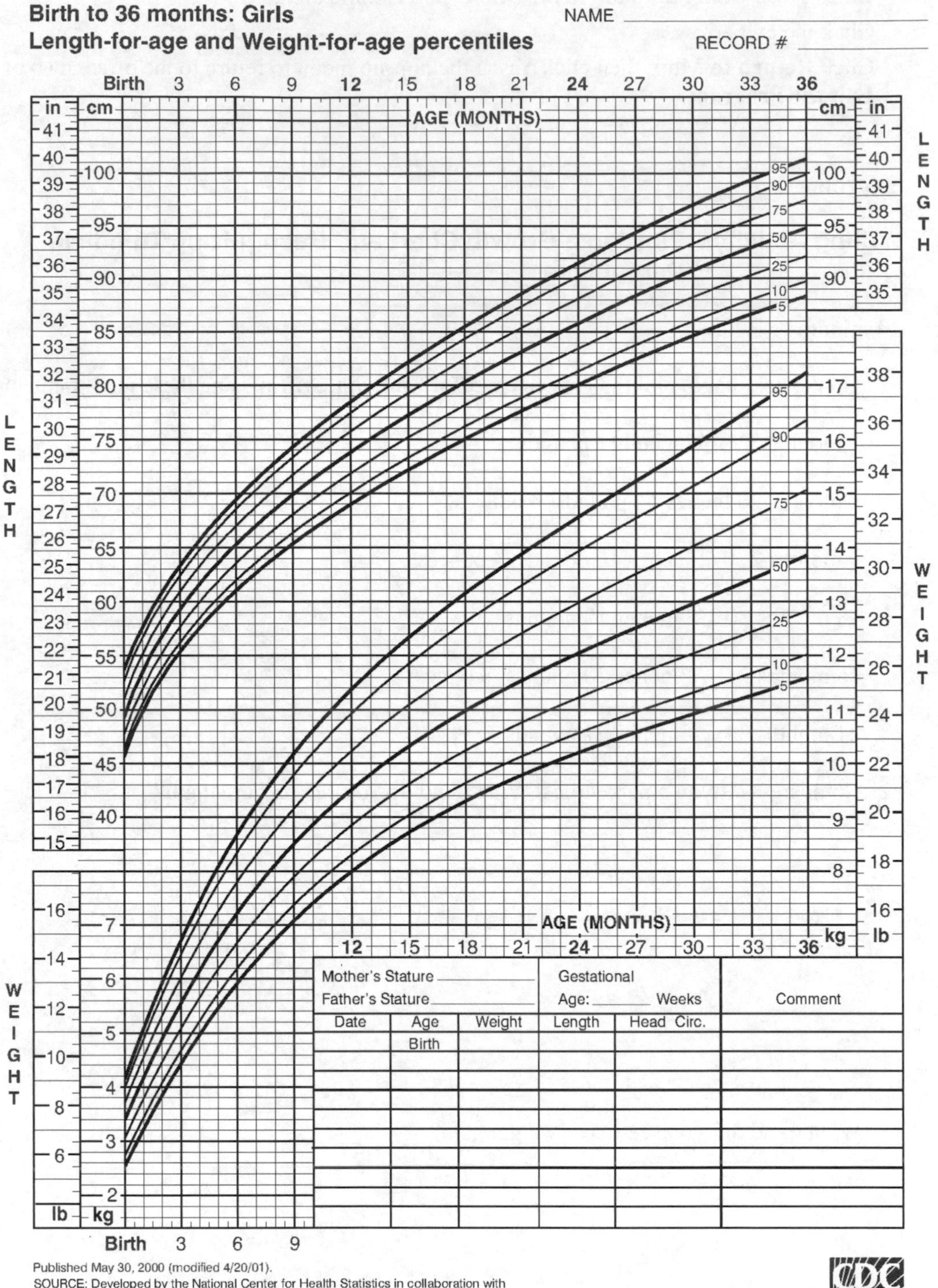

Copyright © 2014, 2011, 2007 by Saunders, an imprint of Elsevier Inc. All rights reserved.

LESSON 23

Respiratory Testing

Reading Assignment: Chapter 46—Assisting in Pulmonary Medicine
- Major Diseases of the Respiratory System
- The Medical Assistant's Role in Pulmonary Procedures
- Table 46-3
- Legal and Ethical Issues

Patients: John R. Simmons, Hu Huang

Learning Objectives:

- Understand the purpose of pulmonary function tests.
- Be familiar with abbreviations associated with pulmonary function tests and their definitions.
- Identify pulmonary function tests performed in the physician's office.
- Identify indications for spirometry testing.
- Distinguish between lung function tests.
- Identify the necessary steps in patient preparation for respiratory testing.
- Understand the unique role of the medical assistant in spirometry testing.
- Identify possible reasons for obtaining a sputum specimen.
- Correctly document the spirometry results into the patient's Progress Notes of the health record.
- Explain the benefits of peak flow measurements in monitoring patients who have asthma.
- Give examples of patients who may need home oxygen therapy.

Overview:

This lesson is designed to provide instruction in respiratory testing and the proper documentation of the procedure. Dr. John R. Simmons, a college professor, will have respiratory testing as a part of his complete medical examination. Another patient, Hu Huang, has a suspected diagnosis of avian flu that he may have acquired during a trip to Asia. He will be providing sputum specimens for a differential diagnosis. Standard precautions will be necessary while performing the test and when discarding supplies following the testing and sputum collection.

You will be asked to explain the role of peak flow monitoring in controlling asthma symptoms and give examples of patients who may need to have oxygen therapy administered at their homes.

Copyright © 2014, 2011, 2007 by Saunders, an imprint of Elsevier Inc. All rights reserved.

Exercise 1

Writing Activity—Elements in Respiratory Testing

15 minutes

1. What are the purposes of pulmonary function tests?

2. Identify the method of testing pulmonary function in the physician's office setting?

3. List at least three indications for spirometry testing.

4. Match each spirometry testing term with its correct definition.

	Term	Definition
_____	Maximum volume ventilation (MVV)	a. Amount of air that can be forcefully exhaled from a maximum inhalation
_____	Functional residual volume (FRV)	b. Volume of air left in the lungs after a forced expiration
_____	Expiratory reserve volume (ERV)	c. Maximum amount of air that can be expired after a maximum inspiration
_____	Residual volume (RV)	d. Maximum volume the patient can breathe in and out in 1 minute
_____	Forced vital capacity (FVC)	e. Volume of air inspired and expired during a normal respiration
_____	Vital capacity (VC)	f. Maximum amount of air that can be expired after a normal inspiration
_____	Inspiratory capacity (IC)	g. Amount of air left in the lungs after a normal expiration
_____	Tidal volume (TV)	h. Maximum volume of air that can be exhaled after a normal inspiration

Copyright © 2014, 2011, 2007 by Saunders, an imprint of Elsevier Inc. All rights reserved.

Exercise 2

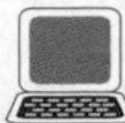

Online Activity—Preparing the Patient and Performing Spirometry Testing

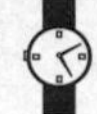

30 minutes

- Sign in to Mountain View Clinic.
- Select **John R. Simmons** from the patient list.
- Click on **Exam Room**.
- Under the Watch heading, click on **Respiratory Testing** and watch the video.

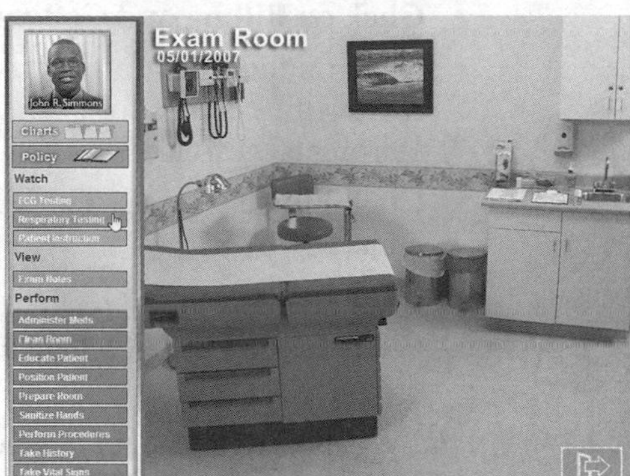

1. What preparation of the patient was provided during the video?

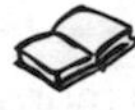

2. During the video, Dr. Simmons asks the medical assistant what the "contraption" is. How would you answer this question? (*Hint:* First, clarify what Dr. Simmons is being asked to perform during the video—spirometry testing or peak flow monitoring? Refer to Procedure 46-1, Figure 1, and Figure 46-13 in your textbook to see the devices used for each of these procedures.)

3. What was the physician's order regarding respiratory testing?

Copyright © 2014, 2011, 2007 by Saunders, an imprint of Elsevier Inc. All rights reserved.

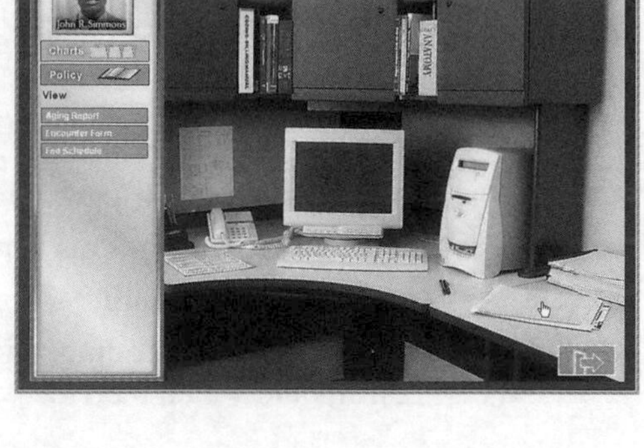

- Click the **X** on the video screen to close the video.
- Click the exit arrow.
- Click **Return to Map** and select **Yes** at the pop-up menu to return to the office map.
- Click on **Billing and Coding**.
- Click on the **Encounter Form** clipboard to review the charges for peak flow monitoring or spirometry testing.
- Click **Finish** to return to the Billing and Coding area.
- Click on **Charts**.
- Click on the **Patient Medical Information** tab and select **1-Progress Notes**.

4. What was the patient charged for? Is a specific place provided for peak flow testing on the Encounter Form?

Critical Thinking Question

5. Since spirometry and peak flow testing both fall under respiratory testing, could the physician be more specific when writing the order? Should the Encounter Form be more specific by having respiratory testing as a heading that includes both peak flow monitoring and spirometry testing?

6. What other instructions should be given to patients who are coming to the medical office for spirometry testing?

Copyright © 2014, 2011, 2007 by Saunders, an imprint of Elsevier Inc. All rights reserved.

7. How many attempts should the patient be given to obtain quality testing?

8. During the testing, what should the medical assistant do to encourage an acceptable test?

→ • Click on the **Exam Notes** file folder and read the documentation for this visit.

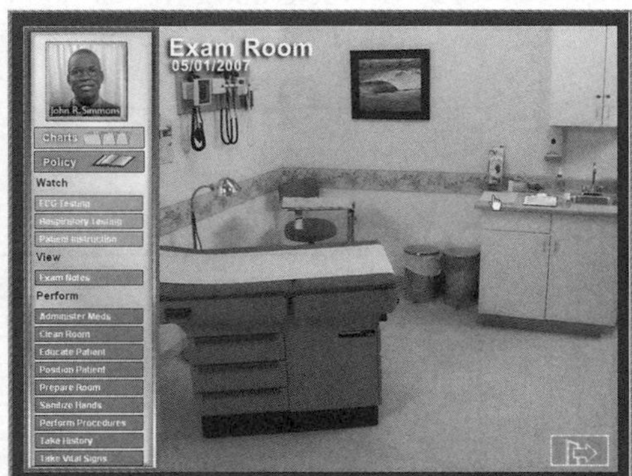

9. What vital signs should the medical assistant record prior to spirometry testing?

Critical Thinking Question

10. As a medical assistant, if you read the order as written by the Mountain View Clinic physician, would you need to clarify what test the physician wanted performed? Explain your answer.

Copyright © 2014, 2011, 2007 by Saunders, an imprint of Elsevier Inc. All rights reserved.

11. Indicate whether each of the following statements is true or false.

   a. ________ During the video, the medical assistant provided the needed information for Dr. Simmons to obtain an acceptable test.

   b. ________ The patient's lips may be loosely pursed around the mouthpiece without affecting the results of the test.

   c. ________ The medical assistant should obtain the patient's height and weight before performing the test for computerized spirometers to make the correct calculations.

   d. ________ When the test is completed, the mouthpiece may be reused.

   e. ________ The medical assistant should provide coaching only while the patient is exhaling air into the mouthpiece.

12. On the blank Progress Notes below, document Dr. Simmons' spirometry testing, including his results of 250, 290, and 330 on peak flow testing.

PATIENT'S NAME ____________ ☐FEMALE ☐MALE Date of Birth: __/__/__

DATE	PATIENT VISITS AND FINDINGS

13. Continue reviewing the written documentation of Dr. Simmons' testing in the Exam Notes. Which documentation would be more helpful to the physician—the notes with the readings of the spirometry testing or the Exam Notes?

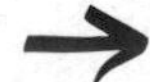

- Click **Finish** to return to the Exam Room.
- Click the exit arrow.
- On the Summary Menu, click **Return to Map** and select **Yes** at the pop-up menu to return to the office map.

Copyright © 2014, 2011, 2007 by Saunders, an imprint of Elsevier Inc. All rights reserved.

Exercise 3

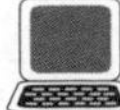

Online Activity—Collecting Sputum Specimens

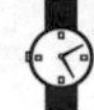

15 minutes

- Select **Hu Huang** from the patient list.
- Click on **Exam Room**.
- Under the Watch heading, click on **Sputum Collection** and watch the video.

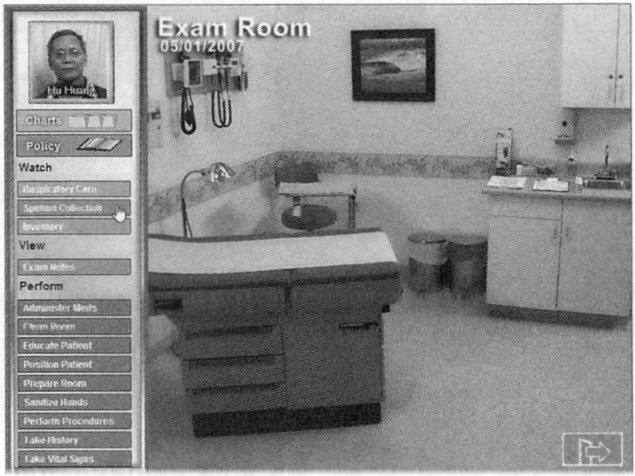

1. What directions should be provided to the patient before obtaining a sputum specimen?

2. Why are sputum specimens usually collected?

3. What types of testing are usually performed on sputum tests?

Copyright © 2014, 2011, 2007 by Saunders, an imprint of Elsevier Inc. All rights reserved.

4. Which of the following PPE and other supplies are essential for preventing cross contamination when obtaining a sputum specimen? Select all that apply.

_____ Sterile gloves

_____ Gloves

_____ Gown

_____ Goggles/face shield

_____ Shoe covers

_____ Mask

_____ Table covering

_____ Puncture-proof biohazard container

_____ Biohazard waste bag

5. On the blank form below, document the collection of Hu Huang's sputum specimen using today's date, time, and your name.

PATIENT'S NAME ________________ ☐FEMALE ☐MALE Date of Birth: ___/___/___

DATE	PATIENT VISITS AND FINDINGS

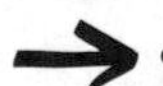

- Click the **X** on the video screen to close the video.
- Click the exit arrow.
- Click **Return to Map**, then click **Yes** at the pop-up menu to return to the office map or click **Exit the Program**.

Copyright © 2014, 2011, 2007 by Saunders, an imprint of Elsevier Inc. All rights reserved.

Exercise 4

Writing Activity—Peak Flow Measurement and Oxygen Therapy

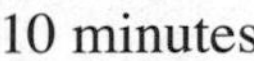

10 minutes

1. Define *asthma*.

2. List some of the symptoms that a person with asthma experiences.

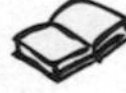

3. Identify some of the things that may trigger an asthma attack. (*Hint:* Refer to Chapter 42 in your textbook if needed.)

Critical Thinking Question

4. Ethan Griffin is a patient at your clinic. He has chronic asthma and takes several medications to help control his asthma attacks. The physician has recommended that Ethan's parents use a peak flow meter at home. How would you explain to Ethan's parents the importance of performing the peak flow meter measurement and documenting his results for the medical office?

Copyright © 2014, 2011, 2007 by Saunders, an imprint of Elsevier Inc. All rights reserved.

5. Give examples of when a patient might need home oxygen therapy.

Critical Thinking Question

6. After home oxygen therapy is initiated, how will the physician know if the patient is responding?

7. What are safety guidelines that should be followed when a patient is prescribed at home oxygen therapy? (*Hint:* Use the Internet to locate this information, if needed.)

Copyright © 2014, 2011, 2007 by Saunders, an imprint of Elsevier Inc. All rights reserved.

LESSON 24

Electrocardiogram

Reading Assignment: Chapter 47—Assisting in Cardiology
- Anatomy and Physiology of the Heart
- Diagnostic Procedures and Treatments
- Diseases and Disorders of the Heart

Chapter 49—Principles of Electrocardiography
- The Electrical Conduction System of the Heart
- The Electrocardiograph
- Performing Electrocardiography
- Interpreting an ECG Strip

Patients: John R. Simmons, Shaunti Begay

Learning Objectives:

- Discuss the purpose of electrocardiography (ECG).
- Explain when Holter monitoring would be indicated.
- Identify the correct placement of leads for ECG.
- Identify the waves, segments, and intervals that show up on an ECG that are representative of the cardiac cycle.
- State the need for quality control and the use of standardization marks when performing ECGs.
- Discuss the proper way to handle ECG paper.
- Describe patient preparation for an ECG.
- Identify the 12 leads found on an electrocardiogram.
- Understand what an artifact is and what causes it.
- Discuss ways of maintaining professionalism and ethical behavior to make a patient more comfortable when performing electrocardiography.
- Identify what modifications in lead placement should be made if the patient has amputations, wounds, or injuries.
- Document correctly that an ECG was performed on a patient.
- Prepare written information to give to a patient as it applied to the Holter monitor and event recording.

Copyright © 2014, 2011, 2007 by Saunders, an imprint of Elsevier Inc. All rights reserved.

Overview:

In this lesson Dr. John R. Simmons, a college professor, will have a routine electrocardiogram. You will be asked to show your knowledge of the heart and to discuss the means of testing the electrical activity of the heart. Shaunti Begay has questions about the event recording that the cardiology clinic will be performing. To alleviate her fears before she sees the cardiologists, you will prepare a general information pamphlet to give Shaunti and her parents regarding the purpose of Holter monitoring and event recording.

Exercise 1

Writing Activity—Basic Anatomy of the Heart and Risk Factors

15 minutes

1. The heart has _______ chambers. The top chambers are called ____________________, and the bottom chambers are called ____________________.

2. The heart is about the same size as an adult's ____________________.

3. The average adult heart pumps about _______ liters of blood every minute.

4. The sac that encloses the heart is called the ____________________.

5. ____________________ located between the chambers of the heart help ensure that blood flows from one chamber to another as it should.

6. List four risk factors for heart disease that cannot be changed.

   (1)

   (2)

   (3)

   (4)

7. List six risk factors for heart disease that can be modified or treated.

   (1)

   (2)

   (3)

   (4)

   (5)

   (6)

Copyright © 2014, 2011, 2007 by Saunders, an imprint of Elsevier Inc. All rights reserved.

8. What is the purpose of having a patient wear a Holter monitor?

9. What information must the patient record while wearing a Holter monitor?

Exercise 2

Writing Activity—Understanding the Purpose and Components of an Electrocardiogram

45 minutes

1. What is electrocardiography?

2. What does the electrocardiograph machine measure?

3. Define *cardiac cycle*.

4. In an adult, what is the average length of the cardiac cycle?

Copyright © 2014, 2011, 2007 by Saunders, an imprint of Elsevier Inc. All rights reserved.

5. Label the diagram below to show the main structures of the heart.

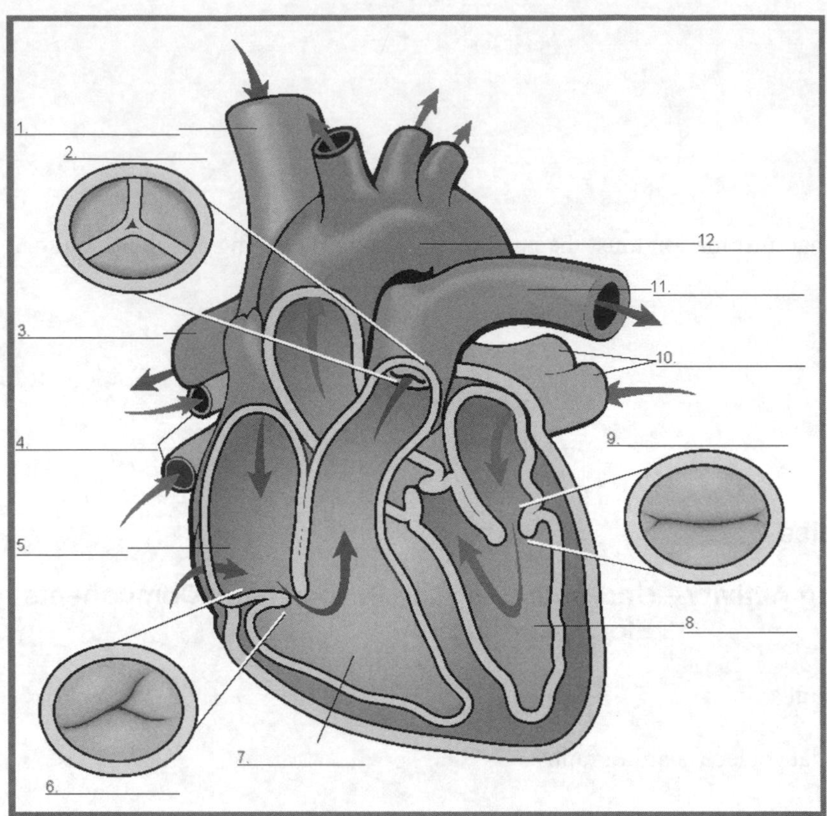

6. Label the waves, segments, and intervals on the ECG tracing below.

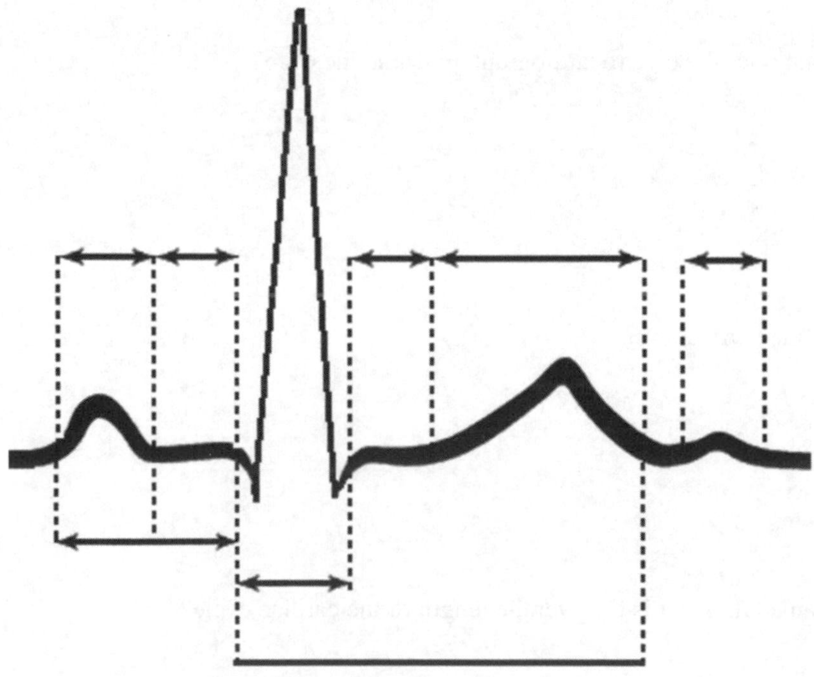

Copyright © 2014, 2011, 2007 by Saunders, an imprint of Elsevier Inc. All rights reserved.

7. What does a wave in an electrocardiogram tracing indicate?

8. What does the ST segment in an electrocardiogram tracing indicate?

9. What does the QT interval on an electrocardiogram tracing indicate?

10. What does the QRS complex indicate on an electrocardiogram tracing?

11. How does the physician use electrocardiograph paper to interpret the tracing?

12. Why is it important that the ECG tracing be handled carefully and not be allowed to smear or be folded in any way?

Copyright © 2014, 2011, 2007 by Saunders, an imprint of Elsevier Inc. All rights reserved.

13. What is the purpose of the standardization mark on an electrocardiogram? How is it used?

14. a. When the electrical impulse arrives and the heart muscle is ready to contract, this is called ________________________.

    b. When the electrical impulse is received and the heart muscle contracts, this is called ________________________.

    c. When the electrical impulse ends and the heart muscle is at rest, this is called ________________________.

15. What electrical activity of the heart is indicated by the P wave?

16. What electrical activity of the heart is indicated by the T wave?

17. Why would a physician order a Holter monitor test?

18. What are some of the conditions that a Doppler study can identify?

Copyright © 2014, 2011, 2007 by Saunders, an imprint of Elsevier Inc. All rights reserved.

Exercise 3

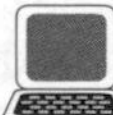

Online Activity—Preparing for the Electrocardiogram

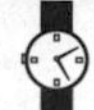

30 minutes

1. On the diagram below, show the locations and the markings of the leads to be placed for obtaining an electrocardiograph.

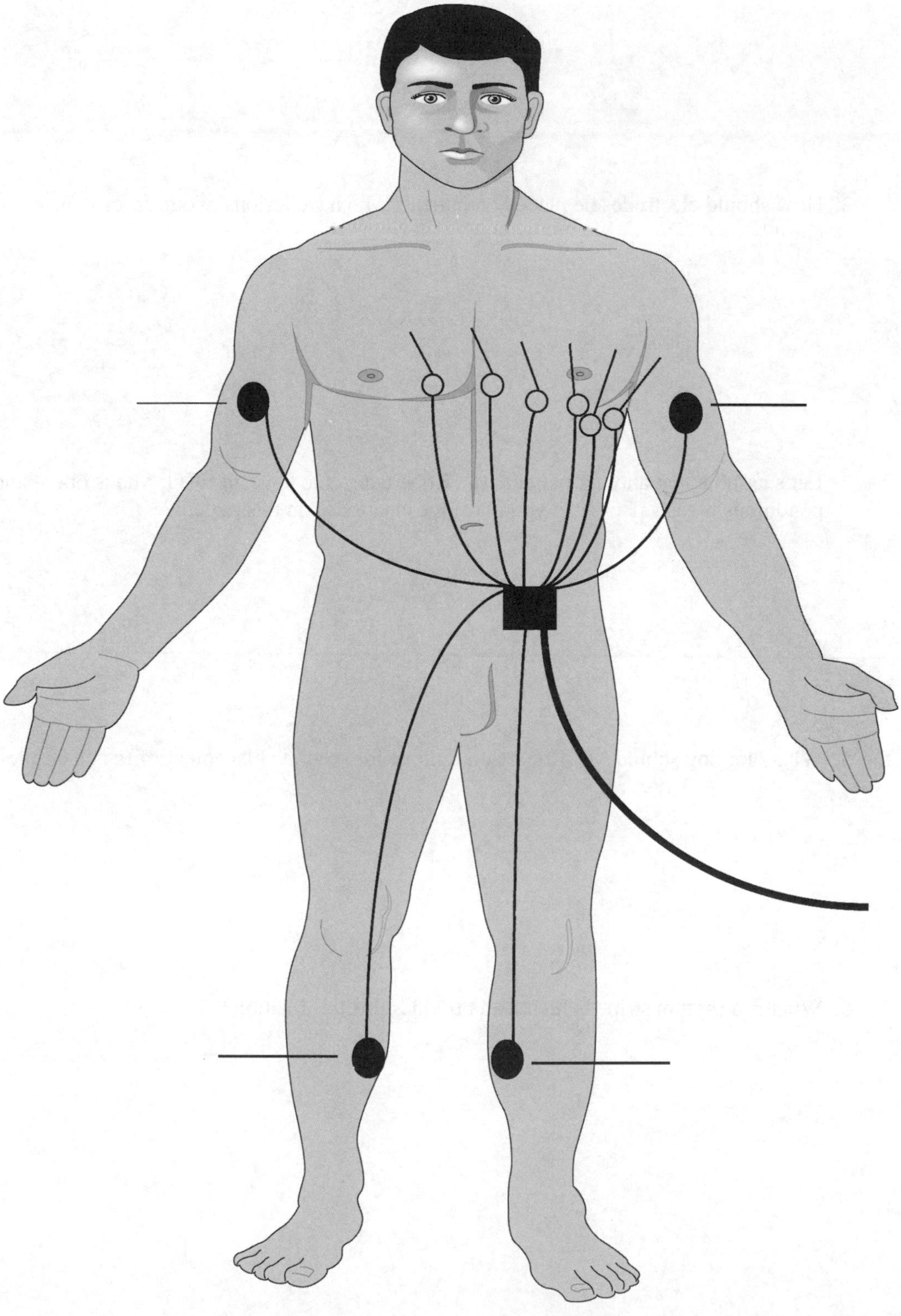

Copyright © 2014, 2011, 2007 by Saunders, an imprint of Elsevier Inc. All rights reserved.

Critical Thinking Questions

Questions 2 through 5 require critical thinking. In some cases, your textbook may not include all of the answers, but you may encounter similar circumstances as a medical assistant. If you need to refer to another source, please document the source you used.

2. If Dr. Simmons had a limb amputation or a bandage or cast on one of his extremities, how would the ECG lead be placed?

3. How should electrodes be placed on patients who have lesions, wounds, or incisions on the chest?

4. Let's assume that another patient, Ms. Robertson, is to have an ECG. She is obese and has pendulous breasts. How can you place the electrodes on this patient?

5. What clothing should Ms. Robertson remove for accurate placement of the electrodes?

6. What is a rhythm strip? Which lead provides this information?

Copyright © 2014, 2011, 2007 by Saunders, an imprint of Elsevier Inc. All rights reserved.

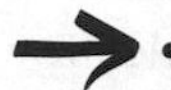

- Sign in to Mountain View Clinic.
- Select **John R. Simmons** from the patient list.
- Click on **Exam Room**.
- Under the Watch heading, click on **ECG Testing** and watch the video.

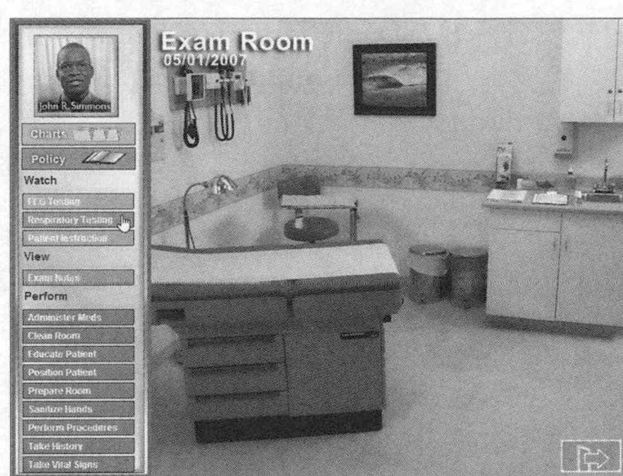

7. Describe Dr. Simmons' position on the table and how he is dressed. Based on this, do you think that he has been appropriately prepared for the ECG?

8. Is it always necessary to remove the patient's shoes and socks when performing an ECG? Why or why not?

9. Dr. Simmons asked Danielle, the medical assisting extern, whether everything was all right. He also stated that his hand was itching during the ECG. Why do you think Dr. Simmons tried to offer a reason for there being a problem with the ECG?

10. Imagine that you were the patient. What reaction do you think you would have if you saw such a perplexed look on the medical assisting extern's face?

Copyright © 2014, 2011, 2007 by Saunders, an imprint of Elsevier Inc. All rights reserved.

11. Danielle then stated that the recording was "fuzzy." What are fuzzy lines on the electrocardiograph called? What causes these lines?

12. What steps did Danielle take to correct this problem? What other steps could have been taken if her initial attempts had not corrected the problem?

13. Why is it important for Danielle to be sure the abnormal tracing is an artifact, rather than a dysrhythmia?

→ • Resume playing the video by clicking the play button.
• Pause the video at the next fade-out by clicking the pause button.

14. Do you think Danielle acted in a professional manner when discussing the ECG tracing with Dr. Simmons? Explain your answer.

Copyright © 2014, 2011, 2007 by Saunders, an imprint of Elsevier Inc. All rights reserved.

- Click the play button and watch the remainder of the video.

15. Do you feel that the medical assistant correctly handled the fact that Danielle had discussed the ECG tracing with Dr. Simmons? Explain your answer.

16. On the blank Progress Notes below, document the obtaining of the electrocardiograph on Dr. Simmons. Use today's date and time for the documentation.

PATIENT'S NAME ______________________ ☐FEMALE ☐MALE Date of Birth: __/__/__

DATE	PATIENT VISITS AND FINDINGS

- Click the **X** on the video screen to close the video.
- Click the exit arrow.
- Click **Return to Map**, then click **Yes** at the pop-up menu to return to the office map or click **Exit the Program**.

Copyright © 2014, 2011, 2007 by Saunders, an imprint of Elsevier Inc. All rights reserved.

LESSON 25

Collecting Urine Specimens

Reading Assignment: Chapter 52—Assisting in the Analysis of Urine
• Collecting a Urine Specimen

Patient: Louise Parlet

Learning Objectives:

- Discuss the reason for giving appropriate instructions to the patient before obtaining cleancatch midstream urine specimens.
- Identify the correct order of the steps needed to prepare a patient, either male or female, for obtaining a clean-catch midstream urine specimen.
- Discuss how breaks in proper technique can lead to possible errors in diagnoses.
- Distinguish between correct and incorrect instructions for collecting a urine specimen.
- Complete a laboratory requisition form for a urine specimen.
- Understand the time limit for allowing urine to sit at room temperature before specimen integrity is compromised.

Overview:

Clean-catch midstream urine specimens are routinely obtained from patients for analysis for chemicals and possible bacteria. Because urinary catheterization is an invasive procedure, contamination by bacteria can be a problem. The clean-catch midstream procedure is the most effective means of obtaining a specimen that is as free of bacteria as possible. However, for the specimen to be of acceptable quality for examination, the patient must be given clear and specific instructions for collection. This lesson will focus on the medical assistant's role in providing patient education and ensuring the necessary steps for quality collection of a clean-catch midstream urine sample.

Copyright © 2014, 2011, 2007 by Saunders, an imprint of Elsevier Inc. All rights reserved.

Exercise 1

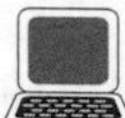

Online Activity—Patient Education for Clean-Catch Midstream Urine Collection

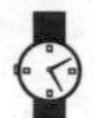

30 minutes

1. Why is it so important to provide proper patient education about the correct collection method for obtaining a clean-catch midstream urine specimen?

2. Indicate whether each of the following statements is true or false.

 a. ________ All urine specimens collected in the medical office must be clean-catch midstream samples.

 b. ________ The container used to obtain a clean-catch midstream urine sample must be aseptically clean.

 c. ________ The clean-catch midstream procedure requires the patient to follow specific instructions when obtaining the specimen.

 d. ________ A clean-catch midstream urine sample is used to check for urinary tract infections.

 e. ________ The patient has responsibility in the proper collection of the specimen.

 f. ________ Before collecting the specimen, a female patient should cleanse the perineum from back to front.

 g. ________ Before collecting the specimen, a male patient should cleanse the head of the penis in a circular motion from the urethral opening outward.

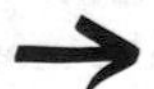

- Sign in to the Mountain View Clinic.
- Select **Louise Parlet** from the patient list.
- Click on **Exam Room**.
- Under the Watch heading, click on **Urine Specimen Collection** and watch the video.

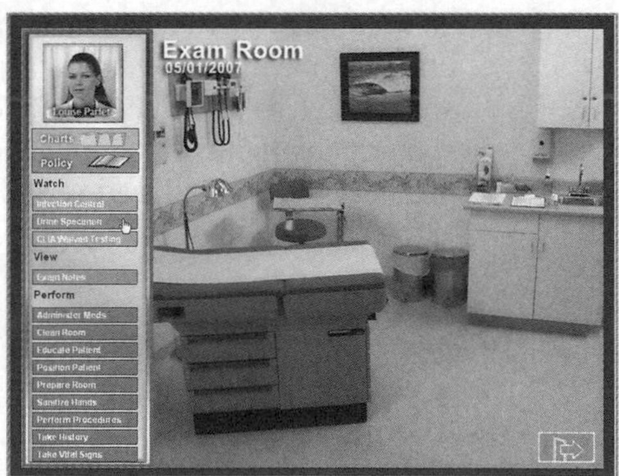

Copyright © 2014, 2011, 2007 by Saunders, an imprint of Elsevier Inc. All rights reserved.

3. In the video, the medical assistant provided information that is not correct. What incorrect information was given to the patient? What is the correct instruction?

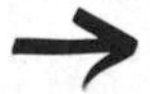

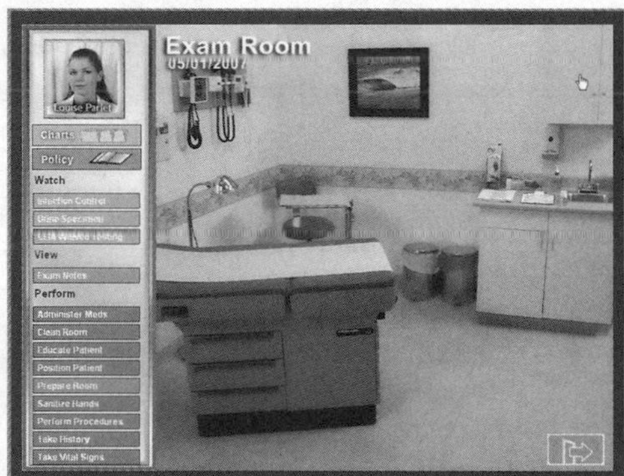

- Click the **X** on the video screen to close the video.
- Click on the **Supply Cabinet**.
- Add the supplies needed for the patient's exam by clicking on the supply from the Available Supplies list and clicking **Add Item** to confirm your choice.
- If you wish to remove a chosen supply, highlight the supply in the Selected Supplies box and click Remove.
- Repeat this step until you are satisfied you have everything you need from the list.
- Click **Finish** to return to the Exam Room.
- Click the exit arrow.
- On the Summary Menu, click on **Look at Your Performance Summary**.
- Scroll down the Performance Summary to the Prepare Room section and compare your answers with those chosen by the experts. The summary can be printed or saved for your instructor.
- Click **Close** to return to the Summary Menu.
- On the Summary Menu, click **Return to Map** and select **Yes** at the pop-up menu to return to the Office Map.

Copyright © 2014, 2011, 2007 by Saunders, an imprint of Elsevier Inc. All rights reserved.

4. Match the following columns to show the correct order of steps in the collection of a clean-catch midstream urine specimen.

Order		Action
_____	Step 1	a. Wipe, redress, wash your hands, and return urine to the place designated.
_____	Step 2	b. Wash your hands and open the towelette packages for easy access.
_____	Step 3	c. Cleanse each side of the urinary meatus with a front-to-back motion from the pubis to the anus, using a separate antiseptic wipe to clean each side. Clean directly across the urinary meatus with a third wipe.
_____	Step 4	d. Complete voiding into the toilet.
_____	Step 5	e. Void a small amount of urine, not catching the urine in the container.
_____	Step 6	f. Void into the container.
_____	Step 7	g. Move the container into position to catch the urine.
_____	Step 8	h. Remove undergarment, sit on the toilet swinging one leg to the side, and expose the urinary meatus by spreading apart the labia with one hand.
_____	Step 9	i. Open collection container without touching the rim or inside and place the lid facing up on a paper towel.
_____	Step 10	j. Close container, taking care to not touch rim or inside.

5. Why is it important that the patient be reminded to wash his or her hands before obtaining the specimen?

6. What are some of the possible problems that may be encountered if the patient is not properly prepared for obtaining the urine specimen?

Copyright © 2014, 2011, 2007 by Saunders, an imprint of Elsevier Inc. All rights reserved.

7. After the specimen has been collected, how long should it be allowed to stand before testing?

Critical Thinking Question

8. The physician asks you to have Joe Smith collect a clean-catch midstream urine specimen before he leaves the office after an 11:30 appointment. You instruct Mr. Smith to bring the urine specimen into the laboratory when he is finished collecting the specimen. After you get back from lunch, you check the examination rooms and the patient restroom and find a container with urine in it sitting on the shelf in the bathroom. The cup is labeled Joe Smith. It is now 1:00 in the afternoon. What should you do?

9. What data should be included in charting the collection a clean-catch midstream urine specimen? Select all that apply.

_____ Date of collection

_____ Time of collection

_____ Time that the specimen was provided to the laboratory

_____ Type of specimen collected

_____ Instructions provided to the patient

_____ Type of test ordered

_____ Signature of person responsible for giving the patient instructions and processing the specimen

Copyright © 2014, 2011, 2007 by Saunders, an imprint of Elsevier Inc. All rights reserved.

- Click on **Laboratory**.
- Click on the **Specimen Collection Tray**.
- Use the checkboxes to select the tests that need to be collected for the patient's visit. (*Hint:* If you wish to review the notes for this visit, click on **Charts** and select **3-Progress Notes** from the menu under the **Patient Medical Information** tab.)
- Click **Next**.
- Answer all the questions related to each test using the check boxes and radio buttons provided. (*Hint:* The Policy Manual can be opened at any time for reference as you answer the questions.)
- Click **Finish** to return to the Laboratory.

- Click on **Charts**.
- Click on the **Patient Medical Information** tab and select **3-Progress Notes**.

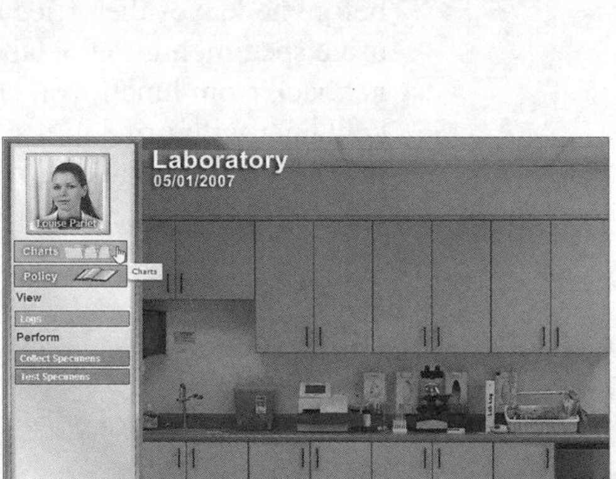

Copyright © 2014, 2011, 2007 by Saunders, an imprint of Elsevier Inc. All rights reserved.

10. Below, complete the laboratory requisition form as ordered in the Progress Notes by Dr. Hayler.

Lab Services

IMPORTANT
Patient instructions and map on back

PHYSICIAN ORDERS

Patient ______ (Last Name) ______ (First) ___ (M.I.) D.O.B. ______ M ☐ F ☐ Patient SS# ___ – ___ – ___

Address ______ City ______ Zip ______ Phone # ______

Physician ______

Date & Time of Collection: ______

ATTACH COPY OF INSURANCE CARD

Drawing Facility: ______

Diagnosis/ICD-9 Code ______
(Additional codes on reverse)

☐ 789.00 Abdominal Pain
☐ 285.9 Anemia (NOS)
☐ 414.9 Coronary Artery Disease (CAD)
☐ 250.0 DM (diabetes mellitus)
☐ 780.7 Fatigue/Malaise
☐ 272.0 Hypercholesterolemia
☐ 244.9 Hypothyroidism
☐ 272.4 Hyperlipidemia
☐ 401.9 Hypertension
☐ 465.9 URI (upper respiratory infection)

☐ ROUTINE ☐ PHONE RESULTS TO: # ______
☐ ASAP ☐ FAX RESULTS TO: # ______
☐ STAT ☐ COPY TO: ______

HEMATOLOGY

☐ 1021 CBC, Automated Diff (incl. Platelet Ct.)
☐ 1023 Hemoglobin/Hematocrit
☐ 1020 Hemogram
☐ 1025 Platelet Count
☐ 1150 Pro Time Diagnostic
☐ 1151 Pro Time, Therapeutic
☐ 1155 PTT
☐ 1315 Reticulocyte Count
☐ 1310 Sed Rate/Westergren

URINE

☐ 1059 Urinalysis
☐ 1082 Urinalysis w/Culture if indicated
Urine-24 Hr ______ Spot ______
Ht. ______ Wt. ______
☐ 3033 Creatinine
☐ 3036 Creatinine Clearance (also requires blood)
☐ 3398 Protein
☐ 3096 Sodium/Potassium
☐ Microalbumin 24 Hr ______ Spot ______

SEROLOGY

☐ 8020 ANA (Antinuclear Antibody)
☐ 8040 Mono Spot
☐ 3494 Rheumatoid Factor
☐ 8010 RPR
☐ 5365 Rubella

CHEMISTRY

☐ 5550 Alpha Fetoprotein, Prenatal
☐ 3000 Amylase
☐ 3153 B12/Folate
☐ 3156 Beta HCG, Quantitative
☐ 3321 Bilirubin, Total
☐ 3324 Bilirubin, Total/Direct
☐ 3009 BUN
☐ 3159 CEA
☐ 3348 Cholesterol
☐ 3030 Creatinine, Serum
☐ 3509 Digoxin (recommend 12 hrs., after dose)
☐ 3515 Dilantin
☐ 3168 Ferritin
☐ 3193 FSH
☐ 3066 ▼ Glucose, Fasting
☐ 3061 Glucose, 1° Post 50 g Glucola
☐ 3075 ▼ Glucose, 2° Post Glucola
☐ 3060 Glucose, 2° Post Prandial (meal)
☐ 3049 ▼ Glucose Tolerance Oral GTT
☐ 3047 ▼ Glucose Tolerance Gestational GTT
☐ 3650 Hemoglobin, A1C

CHEMISTRY

☐ 5232 HBsAg
☐ 3175 HIV (Consent required)
☐ 3581 Iron & Iron Binding Capacity
☐ 3195 LH
☐ 3590 Magnesium
☐ 3527 Phenobarbital
☐ 3095 Potassium
☐ 3689 Pregnancy Test, Serum (HCG, qual)
☐ 3653 Pregnancy Test, Urine
☐ 3197 Prolactin
☐ 3199 PSA
☐ 3339 SGOT/AST
☐ 3342 SGPT/ALT
☐ 3093 Sodium/Potassium, Serum
☐ 3510 Tegretol
☐ 3551 Theophylline
☐ 3333 Uric Acid

MICROBIOLOGY

Source ______
☐ 7240 Culture, AFB
☐ 7200 Culture, Blood x ______
☐ Draw Interval ______
☐ 7280 Culture, Fungus
☐ Culture, Routine
☐ 7005 Culture, Stool
☐ 7010 Culture, Throat
☐ 7000 Culture, Urine
☐ 7300 Gram Stain
☐ 7355 Occult Blood x ______
☐ 7365 Ova & Parasites x ______
☐ 7400 Smear & Suspension (includes Gram Stain/Wet Mount)
☐ 7060 Rapid Strep A Screen (Nega confirm by cult)
☐ 7065 Rapid Strep A Screen only
☐ 7030 Beta Strep Culture
☐ 5207 GC by DNA Probe
☐ 5130 Chlamydia by DNA Probe
☐ 5555 Chlamydia/GC by DNA Probe
☐ 7375 Wright Stain, Stool

Additional Tests ______

PANELS & PROFILES

☐ ✗ 3309 CHEM 12
Albumin, Alkaline Phosphatase, BUN, Calcium, Cholesterol, Glucose, LDH, Phosphorus, AST, Total Bilirubin, Total Protein, Uric Acid

☐ ▼ 3315 CHEM 20
Chem 12, Electrolyte Panel, Creatinine, Iron, Gamma GT, ALT, Triglycerides

☐ ▼ 3357 CARDIAC RISK PANEL
Cholesterol, HDL, LDL, Risk Factors, VLDL Triglycerides

☐ ✗ 3042 CRITICAL CARE PANEL
BUN, Chloride, CO2, Glucose, Potassium, Sodium

☐ 3046 ELECTROLYTE PANEL
Chloride, CO2, Potassium, Sodium

☐ ▼ 3399 EXECUTIVE PANEL
Chem 20, Iron, Cardiac Risk Panel, CBC, RPR, Thyroid Cascade

☐ 5242 HEPATITIS PANEL, ACUTE
HAVIgMAb, HBsAg, HBsAb, HBcAb, HCVAb

☐ ▼ 3355 LIPID MONITORING PANEL
Cholesterol, Triglycerides, HDL, LDL, VLDL, ALT, AST

☐ 3312 LIVER PANEL
Alkaline Phospatase, AST, Total Bilirubin, Gamma GT, Total Protein, Albumin, ALT

☐ ✗ 3083 METABOLIC STATUS PANEL
BUN, Osmolality (calculated), Chloride, CO2 Creatinine, Glucose, Potassium, Sodium, BUN/Creatinine, Ratio, Anion Gap

☐ ✗ 3376 PANEL B
Chem 12, CBC, Electrolyte Panel

☐ ▼ 3382 PANEL D
Chem 20, CBC, Thyroid Cascade

☐ ✗ 3388 PANEL F
Chem 12, CBC, Electrolyte Panel, Thyroid Cascade

☐ ▼ 3391 PANEL G
Chem 20, Cardiac Risk Panel, CBC, Thyroid Cascade

☐ ▼ 3393 PANEL H
Chem 20, CBC, Cardiac Risk Panel Rheumatoid Factor, Thyroid Cascade

☐ ▼ 3397 PANEL J
Chem 20, Cardiac Risk Panel

☐ 5351 PRENATAL PANEL
Antibody Screen ABO/Rh, CBC Rubella, HBsAg, RPR
☐ 1059 with Urinalysis, Routine
☐ 1082 with Urinalysis w/Culture if indicated

☐ ✗ 3102 RENAL PANEL
Metabolic Status Panel, Calcium, Phosphorus

☐ 3188 THYROID CASCADE
TSH, Reflex Testing

▼ - patient required to fast for 12-14 hours

✗ - patient recommended to fast 12-14 hours

LAB USE ONLY INIT ______
☐ SST ☐ PLASMA
☐ PURPLE ☐ SERUM
☐ YELLOW ☐ SWAB
☐ BLUE ☐ SLIDES
☐ GREEN ☐ DNA PROBE
☐ GREY ☐ B. CULT BTLS
☐ URINE
☐ BLACK
☐ OTHER ______
REC'V. SPECIMEN: ☐ FROZEN
☐ AMBIENT ☐ ON ICE

Special Instructions/Pertinent Clinical Information ______

Physician's Signature ______ **Date** ______

These orders may be FAXed to: 449-5288

7060-500 (7/96)

LAB

Copyright © 2014, 2011, 2007 by Saunders, an imprint of Elsevier Inc. All rights reserved.

11. Note that a urine culture can be ordered in two different places on the lab requisition. What is the difference between the two?

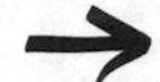

- Click **Close Chart** to return to the Laboratory.
- Click the exit arrow.
- On the Summary Menu, click on **Look at Your Performance Summary**.
- Scroll down the Performance Summary to the Collect Specimens section and compare your answers with those chosen by the experts. The summary can be printed or saved for your instructor.
- Click **Close** to return to the Summary Menu.
- Click **Return to Map**, then click **Yes** at the pop-up menu to return to the office map or click **Exit the Program**.

Copyright © 2014, 2011, 2007 by Saunders, an imprint of Elsevier Inc. All rights reserved.

LESSON 26

Urinalysis

Reading Assignment: Chapter 51—Assisting in the Clinical Laboratory
- Specimen Collection, Processing, and Storage
- Quality Assurance and Quality Control

Chapter 52—Assisting in the Analysis of Urine
- Collecting a Urine Specimen
- Routine Urinalysis
- Urine Toxicology

Patient: Janet Jones

Learning Objectives:

- Discuss the reasons for performing urinalysis.
- Identify the most common methods of collecting urine specimens in the physician's office.
- Understand the differences in testing results that can be expected with random and cleancatch midstream specimens.
- Identify the guidelines for using reagent strips in performing urinalysis.
- Identify the components of urine.
- Prepare a laboratory requisition for a dipstick urinalysis.
- Differentiate between reliability and accuracy of quality control.
- Identify examples of toxins that can be identified in urine.
- List instructions to be given to a patient who will be collecting a 24-hour urine specimen.
- Document urinalysis results correctly.
- Correlate urine characteristics of a patient with diabetes.

Overview:

This lesson is designed to reinforce the proper procedures for obtaining a clean-catch midstream urine specimen and then performing physical and chemical urinalyses. Janet Jones has a history of kidney disease and will need a urinalysis to provide a differential diagnosis for her back pain. As the medical assistant, you will be expected to understand the necessary information to perform a urinalysis, ensuring quality control.

Copyright © 2014, 2011, 2007 by Saunders, an imprint of Elsevier Inc. All rights reserved.

Exercise 1

Writing Activity—Urine Components and Collection

25 minutes

1. Match the organs of the urinary tract to the diagram below.

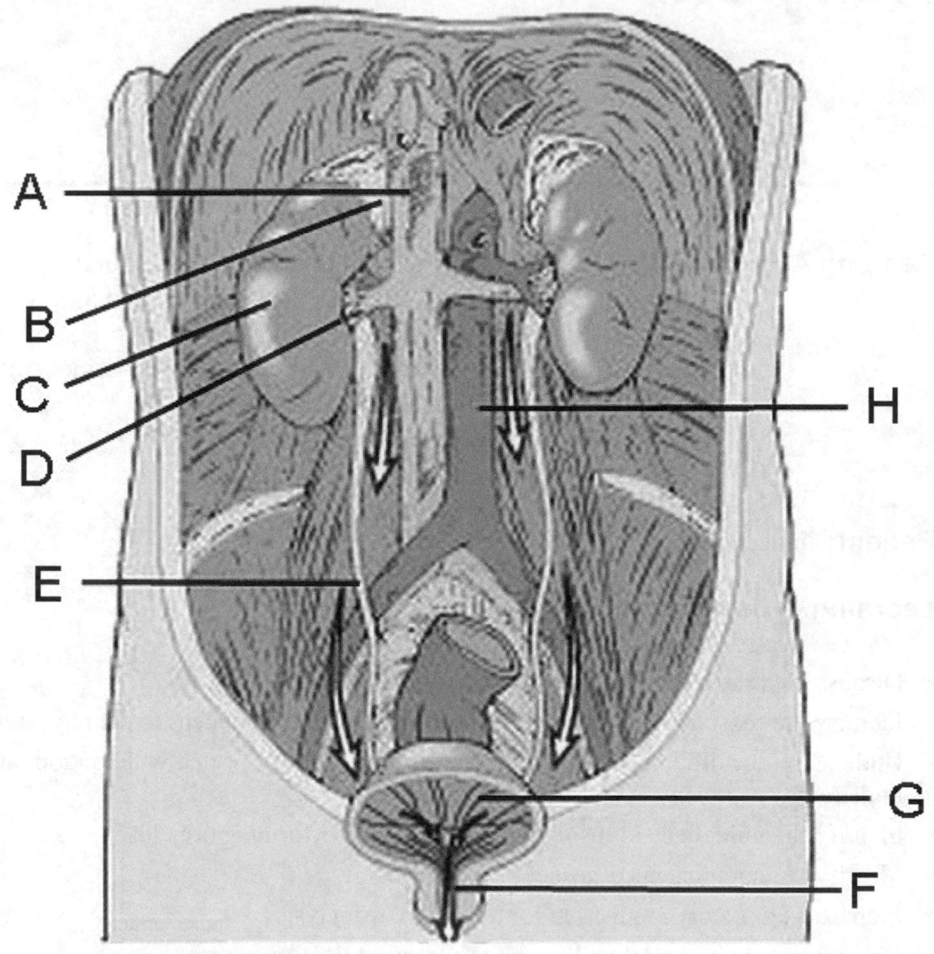

_____	Abdominal aorta	a. A
_____	Inferior vena cava	b. B
_____	Renal artery and vein	c. C
_____	Right adrenal gland	d. D
_____	Right kidney	e. E
_____	Ureter	f. F
_____	Urethra	g. G
_____	Urinary bladder	h. H

Copyright © 2014, 2011, 2007 by Saunders, an imprint of Elsevier Inc. All rights reserved.

2. Which are valid reasons for performing urinalyses?
   a. For assessment of pathologic conditions in body systems
   b. As a screening measure for the possibility of pathologic conditions
   c. To assist in evaluation of the effectiveness of medical treatment
   d. For detection of abused substances
   e. All of the above

3. Which urine collection methods may be used for testing specimens in the medical office? Select all that apply.

   _____ Random samples

   _____ Last-voided specimen of the day

   _____ 24-hour urine specimens

   _____ Clean-catch midstream specimen

   _____ Catheterized specimens

   _____ Early-morning voided specimens

   _____ First-voided morning specimens

   _____ Sterile specimens

4. Which guidelines are important in collecting a urine specimen? Select all that apply.

   _____ Obtain a full cup of urine.

   _____ Obtain 12-50 mL of urine, with 50 mL being the ideal volume.

   _____ Label the specimen with the patient's name only.

   _____ Label the specimen with the patient's name and the date and time of collection.

   _____ Label the specimen with the patient's name, the date and time of collection, and the type of specimen.

   _____ Label the specimen with the patient's name, the date and time of collection, and the initials of the person handling the specimen.

   _____ Medications should be recorded on the laboratory requisition.

   _____ Collection of urine should be avoided during menstruation.

   _____ The medical assistant should allow time for the patient to void and supply water for the patient to drink if necessary.

   _____ The medical assistant should not allow the patient to leave the office until the specimen has been collected.

Copyright © 2014, 2011, 2007 by Saunders, an imprint of Elsevier Inc. All rights reserved.

5. What instructions should be given to the patient for a 24-hour urine specimen?

Exercise 2

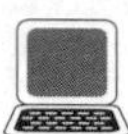

Online Activity—Performing a Urinalysis

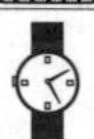

25 minutes

1. What differences in test results could be expected with random catch and clean-catch midstream urine specimens?

- Sign in to Mountain View Clinic.
- Select **Janet Jones** from the patient list.
- Click on **Exam Room**.
- Under the Watch heading, click on **Specimen Collection** and watch the video.

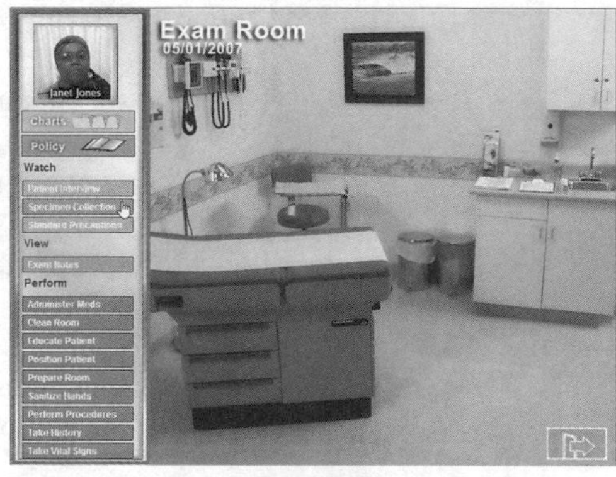

- Click the **X** on the video screen to close the video.
- Click the exit arrow.
- Click **Return to Map** and select **Yes** at the pop-up menu to return to the office map.
- Click on **Billing and Coding**.
- Click on **Charts**.
- Click on the **Workers' Comp** tab and select **2-Progress Notes**.
- Review Ms. Jones' Progress Notes, specifically watching for data regarding her previous medical history.

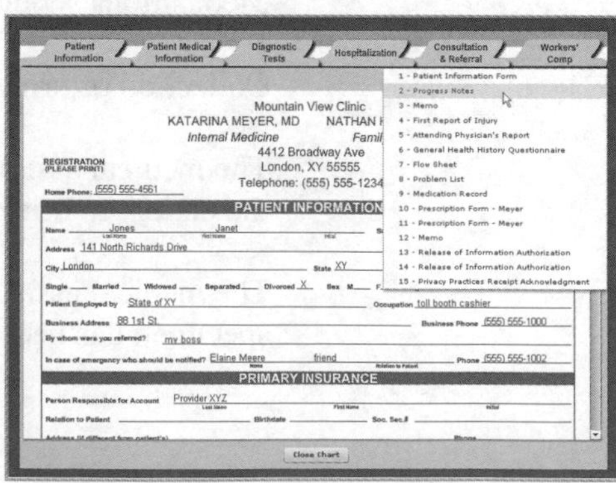

Copyright © 2014, 2011, 2007 by Saunders, an imprint of Elsevier Inc. All rights reserved.

Critical Thinking Question

2. Why do you think the medical assistant told Ms. Jones she would need for her to repeat the instructions given to her after listening to the directions for collecting a clean-catch mid-stream urine specimen?

3. Based on Ms. Jones' medical history, why would obtaining a urine specimen be important?

4. What is ureterolithiasis?

5. The three components of a urinalysis are ____________________,

____________________, and ____________________ analysis of the urine.

6. In a urinalysis, what four physical properties should be determined?

Copyright © 2014, 2011, 2007 by Saunders, an imprint of Elsevier Inc. All rights reserved.

7. Which terms are appropriate for describing the appearance of urine? Select all that apply.

_____ Clear

_____ Smokey

_____ Bright

_____ Cloudy

_____ Heavily cloudy

_____ Slightly cloudy

_____ Turbid (very cloudy)

_____ OK

_____ Hazy

8. What are some of the causes of odoriferous urine?

9. Urine should have a slightly ____________________ odor.

10. Indicate whether each of the following statements is true or false.

a. _________ Cloudiness of urine is always a sign that the urine contains bacteria.

b. _________ Urine should be tested as soon as possible after collection.

c. _________ The smell of ammonia may be an indication of a UTI due to bacterial action.

d. _________ The color of urine is caused by the concentration of urochrome from the breakdown of hemoglobin.

e. _________ The presence of myoglobin from a muscle crush injury cannot be distinguished from hemoglobinuria with dipstick testing.

f. _________ Blood is always visually apparent in urine when present.

g. _________ A fruity odor to urine may be a sign of diabetes.

h. _________ The longer urine stands after collection, the more likely bacteria are to grow.

i. _________ Morphine, methadone, PCP, tricyclics, marijuana, Ecstasy, and methamphetamines are toxins that may be identified in a patient's urine by performing a rapid drug screen.

Copyright © 2014, 2011, 2007 by Saunders, an imprint of Elsevier Inc. All rights reserved.

11. _______________ (**Reliability** or **Accuracy**) refers to the reproducibility of a test procedure.

12. Do you think that the medical assistant in the video was professional in providing information to Ms. Jones? Support your answer.

13. What procedure would you follow to perform the chemical analysis of Ms. Jones' urine specimen? (*Hint:* For this question, assume that you are opening a new bottle of reagent strips.)

14. _______________ (**Reliability** or **Accuracy**) refers to how close the obtained value of a test result is to the real true value.

15. Which of the following can be found on a dipstick urine test? Select all that apply.

_____ Protein

_____ Alcohol

_____ Blood

_____ Leukocyte esterase

_____ Glucose

_____ Ketones

_____ Urobilinogen

_____ Bile

_____ Bilirubin

_____ Nitrite

_____ pH

_____ Specific gravity

_____ Color

Copyright © 2014, 2011, 2007 by Saunders, an imprint of Elsevier Inc. All rights reserved.

16. Which statements are proper guidelines for using reagent strips for urine testing? Select all that apply.

_____ The specimen should be freshly voided.

_____ Reagent strips may be used only with a clean-catch midstream specimen.

_____ The specimen container should be clean and dry.

_____ The container should be free of detergent.

_____ The container must be sterile.

_____ First-voided morning specimens provide the best results for nitrite and protein determination, bacterial culture, pregnancy testing, and microscopic examination.

_____ Specimens should be read against the color card for the test.

_____ The amount of lighting available when reading the test is not important.

_____ Reagent strips may be stored under any conditions.

_____ Quality control ensures reliability of the test results.

_____ Reagent strips are best when stored in the refrigerator.

_____ Discoloration of the strips has no effect on testing.

_____ Quality control on the strips should be performed each day.

17. On the blank Progress Notes below, document the following urine specimen testing results for Janet Jones (using today's date and time). Include color (amber) and turbidity (cloudy). The dipstick urine results are as follows: albumin 1+; glucose 3+; leukocytes moderate.

PATIENT'S NAME ____________________ ☐FEMALE ☐MALE Date of Birth: __/__/__

DATE	PATIENT VISITS AND FINDINGS

Copyright © 2014, 2011, 2007 by Saunders, an imprint of Elsevier Inc. All rights reserved.

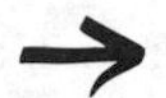

- Click **Close Chart** to return to the Billing and Coding area.
- Click the exit arrow.
- Click **Return to Map** and select **Yes** at the pop-up menu to return to the office map.
- Click on **Laboratory**.
- Click on the **Specimen Collection Tray**.
- Use the checkboxes to select the tests that need to be collected for the patient's visit. (*Hint:* If you wish to review the notes for this visit, click on Charts in the Exam Room sidebar menu, click on the **Workers' Comp** tab, and select **6-Progress Notes**.)

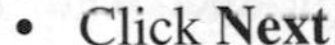

- Click **Next**.
- Answer all the questions related to each test using the checkboxes and radio buttons provided. (*Hint:* The Policy Manual can be opened at any time for reference as you answer the questions.)
- Click **Finish** to return to the Laboratory.

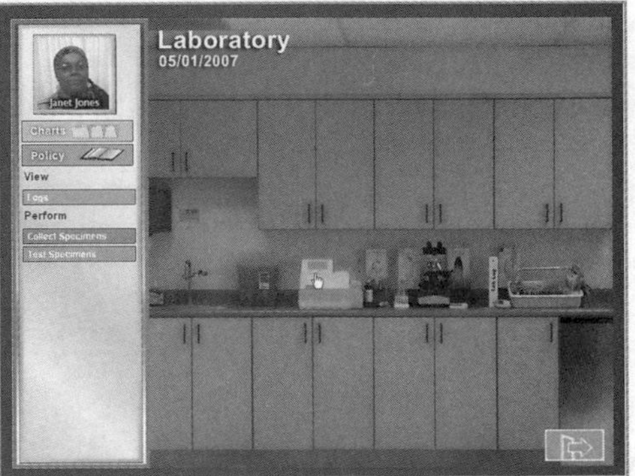

- Click on the **Specimen Analyzer**.
- Use the checkboxes to select the tests that need to be processed for the patient.
- Click **Next**.
- Answer all the questions related to each test using the checkboxes and radio buttons provided. (*Hint:* The Policy Manual can be opened at any time for reference as you answer the questions.)

18. On the following blank Progress Notes form, document the urine specimen testing results for Janet Jones (using today's date and time):

PATIENT'S NAME ____________________ ☐FEMALE ☐MALE Date of Birth: ___/___/___

DATE	PATIENT VISITS AND FINDINGS

Copyright © 2014, 2011, 2007 by Saunders, an imprint of Elsevier Inc. All rights reserved.

19. Indicate whether each of the following statements concerning microscopic examination of specimens is true or false.

a. _________ Microscopic examination of urine specimens is a CLIA-waived test.

b. _________ Red blood cells in urine are easily seen under a microscope.

c. _________ White blood cells are larger than red blood cells and are more easily seen.

d. _________ Epithelial cells in urine are the result of sloughing of the outer layer of skin.

e. _________ Squamous epithelial cells are not uncommon in urine specimens of females.

f. _________ Renal epithelial cells are considered normal in a urine specimen.

g. _________ Various crystals and casts may be found in urine.

h. _________ Drugs may produce crystals in urine.

i. _________ If urine is left to sit out or becomes cold, crystals may precipitate

Copyright © 2014, 2011, 2007 by Saunders, an imprint of Elsevier Inc. All rights reserved.

20. If Dr. Meyer believed it was necessary, she could have ordered a random urine specimen for Ms. Jones to be sent to the lab for routine urinalysis with a microscopic and quantitative analysis. Prepare the lab requisition form below to order this test for the patient (using today's date and the time of her appointment).

Lab Services

IMPORTANT
Patient instructions and map on back

PHYSICIAN ORDERS

Patient ______ (Last Name) ______ (First) ___ (M.I.) D.O.B. ______ M ☐ F ☐ Patient SS# ___ – ___ – ___

Address ______ City ______ Zip ______ Phone # ______

Physician ______

ATTACH COPY OF INSURANCE CARD

Date & Time of Collection: ______ ______

Drawing Facility: ______

Diagnosis/ICD-9 Code ______ (Additional codes on reverse)

☐ 789.00 Abdominal Pain
☐ 285.9 Anemia (NOS)
☐ 414.9 Coronary Artery Disease (CAD)
☐ 250.0 DM (diabetes mellitus)
☐ 780.7 Fatigue/Malaise
☐ 272.0 Hypercholesterolemia
☐ 244.9 Hypothyroidism
☐ 272.4 Hyperlipidemia
☐ 401.9 Hypertension
☐ 465.9 URI (upper respiratory infection)

☐ ROUTINE ☐ PHONE RESULTS TO: # ______
☐ ASAP ☐ FAX RESULTS TO: # ______
☐ STAT ☐ COPY TO: ______

HEMATOLOGY

☐ 1021 CBC, Automated Diff (incl. Platelet Ct.)
☐ 1023 Hemoglobin/Hematocrit
☐ 1020 Hemogram
☐ 1025 Platelet Count
☐ 1150 Pro Time Diagnostic
☐ 1151 Pro Time, Therapeutic
☐ 1155 PTT
☐ 1315 Reticulocyte Count
☐ 1310 Sed Rate/Westergren

URINE

☐ 1059 Urinalysis
☐ 1082 Urinalysis w/Culture if indicated
Urine-24 Hr ______ Spot ______
Ht. ______ Wt. ______
☐ 3033 Creatinine
☐ 3036 Creatinine Clearance (also requires blood)
☐ 3398 Protein
☐ 3096 Sodium/Potassium
☐ Microalbumin 24 Hr ____ Spot ____

SEROLOGY

☐ 8020 ANA (Antinuclear Antibody)
☐ 8040 Mono Spot
☐ 3494 Rheumatoid Factor
☐ 8010 RPR
☐ 5365 Rubella

CHEMISTRY

☐ 5550 Alpha Fetoprotein, Prenatal
☐ 3000 Amylase
☐ 3153 B12/Folate
☐ 3156 Beta HCG, Quantitative
☐ 3321 Bilirubin, Total
☐ 3324 Bilirubin, Total/Direct
☐ 3009 BUN
☐ 3159 CEA
☐ 3348 Cholesterol
☐ 3030 Creatinine, Serum
☐ 3509 Digoxin (recommend 12 hrs., after dose)
☐ 3515 Dilantin
☐ 3168 Ferritin
☐ 3193 FSH
☐ 3066 ▼ Glucose, Fasting
☐ 3061 Glucose, 1° Post 50 g Glucola
☐ 3075 ▼ Glucose, 2° Post Glucola
☐ 3060 Glucose, 2° Post Prandial (meal)
☐ 3049 ▼ Glucose Tolerance Oral GTT
☐ 3047 ▼Glucose Tolerance Gestational GTT
☐ 3650 Hemoglobin, A1C

CHEMISTRY

☐ 5232 HBsAg
☐ 3175 HIV (Consent required)
☐ 3581 Iron & Iron Binding Capacity
☐ 3195 LH
☐ 3590 Magnesium
☐ 3527 Phenobarbital
☐ 3095 Potassium
☐ 3689 Pregnancy Test, Serum (HCG, qual)
☐ 3653 Pregnancy Test, Urine
☐ 3197 Prolactin
☐ 3199 PSA
☐ 3339 SGOT/AST
☐ 3342 SGPT/ALT
☐ 3093 Sodium/Potassium, Serum
☐ 3510 Tegretol
☐ 3551 Theophylline
☐ 3333 Uric Acid

MICROBIOLOGY

Source ______
☐ 7240 Culture, AFB
☐ 7200 Culture, Blood x ______
☐ Draw Interval ______
☐ 7280 Culture, Fungus
☐ Culture, Routine
☐ 7005 Culture, Stool
☐ 7010 Culture, Throat
☐ 7000 Culture, Urine
☐ 7300 Gram Stain
☐ 7355 Occult Blood x ______
☐ 7365 Ova & Parasites x ______
☐ 7400 Smear & Suspension (includes Gram Stain/Wet Mount)
☐ 7060 Rapid Strep A Screen (Negs confir by cult)
☐ 7065 Rapid Strep A Screen only
☐ 7030 Beta Strep Culture
☐ 5207 GC by DNA Probe
☐ 5130 Chlamydia by DNA Probe
☐ 5555 Chlamydia/GC by DNA Probe
☐ 7375 Wright Stain, Stool

Additional Tests ______

PANELS & PROFILES

☐ ✗ 3309 CHEM 12 — Albumin, Alkaline Phosphatase, BUN, Calcium, Cholesterol, Glucose, LDH, Phosphorus, AST, Total Bilirubin, Total Protein, Uric Acid
☐ ▼ 3315 CHEM 20 — Chem 12, Electrolyte Panel, Creatinine, Iron, Gamma GT, ALT, Triglycerides
☐ ▼ 3357 CARDIAC RISK PANEL — Cholesterol, HDL, LDL, Risk Factors, VLDL Triglycerides
☐ ✗ 3042 CRITICAL CARE PANEL — BUN, Chloride, CO2, Glucose, Potassium, Sodium
☐ 3046 ELECTROLYTE PANEL — Chloride, CO2, Potassium, Sodium
☐ ▼ 3399 EXECUTIVE PANEL — Chem 20, Iron, Cardiac Risk Panel, CBC, RPR, Thyroid Cascade

☐ 5242 HEPATITIS PANEL, ACUTE — HAVIgMAb, HBsAg, HBsAb, HBcAb, HCVAb
☐ ▼ 3355 LIPID MONITORING PANEL — Cholesterol, Triglycerides, HDL, LDL, VLDL, ALT, AST
☐ 3312 LIVER PANEL — Alkaline Phospatase, AST, Total Bilirubin, Gamma GT, Total Protein, Albumin, ALT
☐ ✗ 3083 METABOLIC STATUS PANEL — BUN, Osmolality (calculated), Chloride, CO2 Creatinine, Glucose, Potassium, Sodium, BUN/Creatinine, Ratio, Anion Gap
☐ ✗ 3376 PANEL B — Chem 12, CBC, Electrolyte Panel
☐ ▼ 3382 PANEL D — Chem 20, CBC, Thyroid Cascade
☐ ✗ 3388 PANEL F — Chem 12, CBC, Electrolyte Panel, Thyroid Cascade

☐ ▼ 3391 PANEL G — Chem 20, Cardiac Risk Panel, CBC, Thyroid Cascade
☐ ▼ 3393 PANEL H — Chem 20, CBC, Cardiac Risk Panel Rheumatoid Factor, Thyroid Cascade
☐ ▼ 3397 PANEL J — Chem 20, Cardiac Risk Panel
☐ 5351 PRENATAL PANEL — Antibody Screen ABO/Rh, CBC Rubella, HBsAg, RPR
☐ 1059 with Urinalysis, Routine
☐ 1082 with Urinalysis w/Culture if Indicated
☐ ✗ 3102 RENAL PANEL — Metabolic Status Panel, Calcium, Phosphorus
☐ 3188 THYROID CASCADE — TSH, Reflex Testing

▼ - patient required to fast for 12-14 hours
✗ - patient recommended to fast 12-14 hours

LAB USE ONLY INIT ______

☐ SST ☐ PLASMA
☐ PURPLE ☐ SERUM
☐ YELLOW ☐ SWAB
☐ BLUE ☐ SLIDES
☐ GREEN ☐ DNA PROBE
☐ GREY ☐ B. CULT BTLS
☐ URINE
☐ BLACK
☐ OTHER ______

REC'V. SPECIMEN: ☐ FROZEN ☐ AMBIENT ☐ ON ICE

Special Instructions/Pertinent Clinical Information ______

Physician's Signature ______ **Date** ______

These orders may be FAXed to: 449-5288

7060-500 (7/96)

LAB

Copyright © 2014, 2011, 2007 by Saunders, an imprint of Elsevier Inc. All rights reserved.

Critical Thinking Question

21. If a patient is injured on the job, as Ms. Jones was, would you expect the employer to request a urine toxicology or drug screen on the employee after the injury occurred? Why or why not?

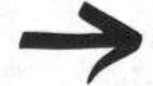

- Click **Finish** to return to the Laboratory.
- Click the exit arrow.
- On the Summary Menu, click **Look at Your Performance Summary**.
- Scroll down the Performance Summary to the Laboratory Collection and Lab Test sections and compare your answers with those chosen by the experts. Each test will have its own section. The summary can be printed or saved for your instructor.
- Click **Return to Map**, then click **Yes** at the pop-up menu to return to the office map or click **Exit the Program**.

Copyright © 2014, 2011, 2007 by Saunders, an imprint of Elsevier Inc. All rights reserved.

LESSON 27

Obtaining Specimens for Microbiological Testing

Reading Assignment: Chapter 37—Procedure 37-8
Chapter 55—Assisting in Microbiology and Immunology

Patient: Tristan Tsosie

Learning Objectives:

- Discuss the difference between pathogens and nonpathogens.
- Understand the proper procedure for obtaining wound exudate for microbiological testing.
- Identify the correct handling and transportation of a microbiological specimen.
- Discuss the reasons for using appropriate PPE when obtaining microbiological specimens.
- Document the transport of a microbiological specimen in the laboratory log.
- Apply critical thinking skills in answering questions regarding inconsistency in charting examples.

Overview:

In this lesson the information regarding obtaining a throat specimen and a specimen for microbiological testing is presented. Tristan Tsosie is an 8-year-old boy with a history of injury to his arm who is now visiting the clinic with a sore throat. You will determine the proper care of Tristan to fulfill the orders of the physician. The patient, who is to have suture removal and a cast check, is accompanied by his sister and another child. Some inconsistencies are present that you should note. These inconsistencies are addressed with Critical Thinking Questions in this lesson. Remember, when accessing the Progress Notes, that you have to be in the designated room to see the correct notes.

Copyright © 2014, 2011, 2007 by Saunders, an imprint of Elsevier Inc. All rights reserved.

Exercise 1

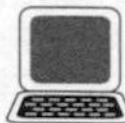

Online Activity—Obtaining a Wound Specimen for Microbiological Testing

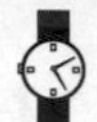

20 minutes

- Sign in to Mountain View Clinic.
- Select **Tristan Tsosie** from the patient list.
- If you need to refresh your memory from an earlier lesson, go to the Reception area and review Tristan's Check-In video.
- Click on **Exam Room**.
- Under the Watch heading, click on **Wound Care** and watch the video.

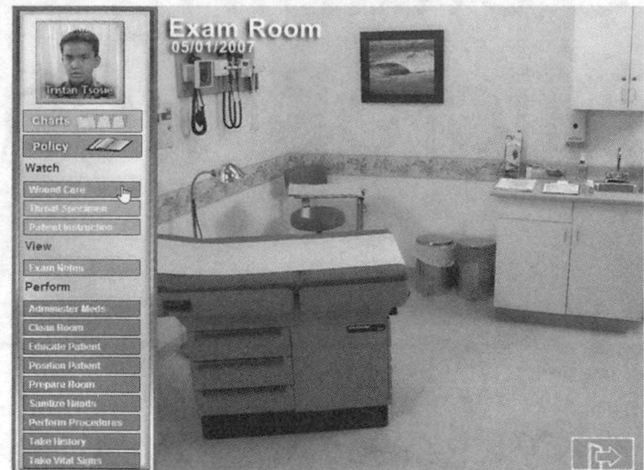

1. In the video, the medical assistant states that a wound specimen for testing will be obtained. Why is the wound specimen being taken from Tristan's arm?

2. Why should the specimen be taken before cleansing the wound?

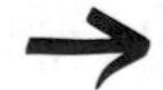

- Click the **X** on the video screen to close the video.
- Click on the **Exam Notes** file folder and read the documentation for Tristan Tsosie's visit.

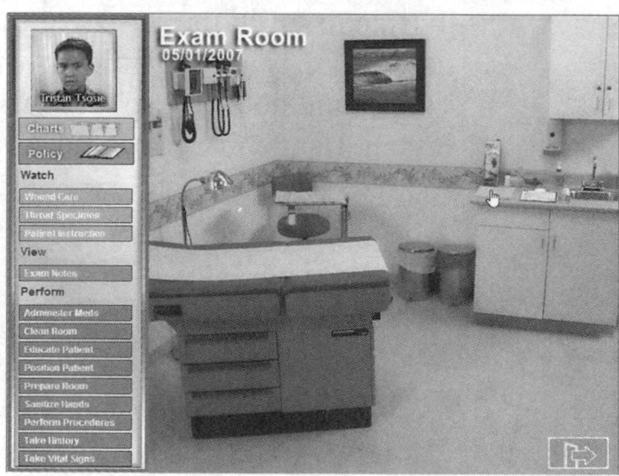

Copyright © 2014, 2011, 2007 by Saunders, an imprint of Elsevier Inc. All rights reserved.

3. What tests have been ordered for Tristan?

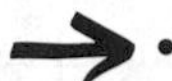

- Click **Finish** to return to the Exam Notes.
- Click on the **Supply Cabinet**.
- Add the supplies needed for the patient's exam by clicking on the supply from the Available Supplies list and clicking **Add Item** to confirm your choice.
- If you wish to remove a chosen supply, highlight the supply in the Selected Supplies box and click **Remove**.
- Repeat this step until you are satisfied you have everything you need from the list.
- Click **Finish** to return to the Exam Room.

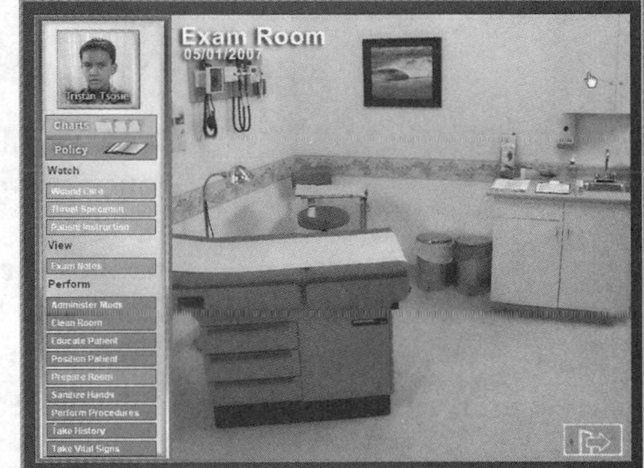

4. Describe the difference between pathogens and nonpathogens. Explain the importance of this difference in regard to wound care.

Copyright © 2014, 2011, 2007 by Saunders, an imprint of Elsevier Inc. All rights reserved.

5. Indicate whether each of the following statements is true or false.

   a. ________ The wound specimen should be taken from the cleanest area of the wound.

   b. ________ Wound specimens should be placed in the transport medium immediately after they are obtained.

   c. ________ Wound specimens should be dry for transport so that the chance of cross contamination is reduced.

   d. ________ Ideally, wound specimens should be obtained after antibiotic therapy has been initiated.

   e. ________ Hands should be sanitized before and after collecting the specimen, even though gloves have been worn.

   f. ________ Supplies used in the collection of the wound specimen should be disposed of in the biohazardous waste container.

   g. ________ Collection of all wound specimens requires the use of gowns and goggles.

   h. ________ Collection of the wound specimen is not complete until documentation has been completed.

   i. ________ The time between collecting the specimen and the laboratory processing of the specimen is not important.

6. Describe the means used by the medical assistant and the extern to place Tristan at ease during the procedure of collecting the wound specimen.

Critical Thinking Question

7. Would you have done anything differently if you were the medical assistant taking care of Tristan? (*Hint:* If you need to refresh your memory from an earlier lesson, such as when Tristan was checked in, you may go to the Reception area and review the check-in video.)

→ • Click on the **Exam Notes** file folder and reread the documentation concerning the wound.

Copyright © 2014, 2011, 2007 by Saunders, an imprint of Elsevier Inc. All rights reserved.

8. Below are the Progress Notes from Tristan's chart, showing how the wound specimen collection was documented. Compare this documentation against the Exam Notes. Is there any information that could be, or should be, added to this documentation?

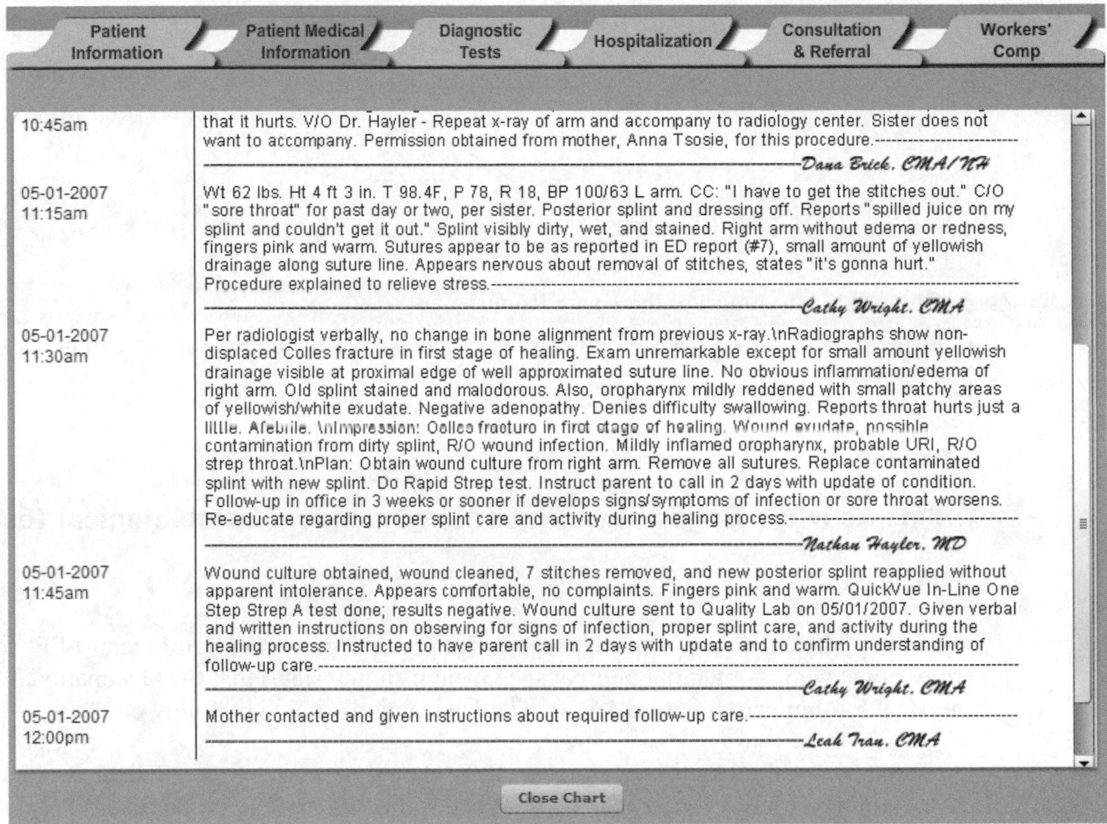

Critical Thinking Question

9. Assume the laboratory courier had already picked up the specimens on 5/1/07. What would be the appropriate measures to take to ensure specimen integrity?

Copyright © 2014, 2011, 2007 by Saunders, an imprint of Elsevier Inc. All rights reserved.

Critical Thinking Question

10. How will the medical assistant know the temperature in which to store the specimen until the laboratory courier arrives on the next day?

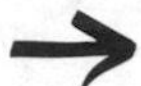

- Click **Finish** to return to the Exam Room.
- Remain in the Exam Room with Tristan Tsosie as your patient to continue to the next exercise.

Exercise 2

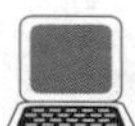

Online Activity—Collecting a Throat Specimen for Microbiological Testing

20 minutes

The Policy Manual does not specify the needed personal protective equipment (PPE) for a professional who is obtaining a throat specimen; it simply states that the Occupational Safety and Health Administration (OSHA) standard precautions should be followed.

1. What personal protective equipment (PPE) should be worn by the medical assistant while obtaining a routine throat specimen? When is it necessary to include other PPE, and what should these be?

- Under the Watch heading, click on **Throat Specimen** and watch the video.

2. What did the medical assistant do to be sure that she had Tristan's cooperation?

Copyright © 2014, 2011, 2007 by Saunders, an imprint of Elsevier Inc. All rights reserved.

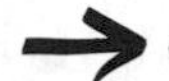

- Click the exit arrow.
- On the Summary Menu, click on **Look at Your Performance Summary**.
- Scroll down the Performance Summary to the Prepare Room section and compare your answers with those chosen by the experts. The summary can be printed or saved for your instructor.
- Click **Close** to return to the Summary Menu.
- Click **Return to Map** and select **Yes** at the pop-up menu to return to the office map.
- Click on **Laboratory**.
- Click on the **Specimen Collection Tray**.
- Use the checkboxes to select the tests that need to be collected for the patient's visit.
- Click **Next**.
- Answer all the questions related to each test using the checkboxes and radio buttons provided. (*Hint:* The Policy Manual can be opened at any time for reference as you answer the questions.)
- Click **Finish** to return to the Laboratory.
- Click on **Charts**.
- Click on the **Patient Medical Information** tab and select **1-Progress Notes**.
- Make a notation of the date documented in the Progress Notes for the transport of the specimen, and indicate that the specimen was sent to Quality Lab for analysis.

3. What are the results of the strep test that was processed using the specimen?

4. Was the documentation correct for the testing done? Explain your answer.

5. When you are obtaining a throat specimen for testing, what is the most appropriate site for collection?

Copyright © 2014, 2011, 2007 by Saunders, an imprint of Elsevier Inc. All rights reserved.

6. Why would it be advantageous to use two sterile swabs when collecting a specimen? In what situation(s) do you think a specimen would likely be sent to an outside laboratory?

7. Why is it important that the inside of the mouth not be touched while the throat specimen is being obtained?

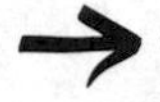

- Click on the **Diagnostic Tests** tab and select **3-Laboratory Requisition Form**.
- Review the Laboratory Requisition Form for accuracy and completeness.

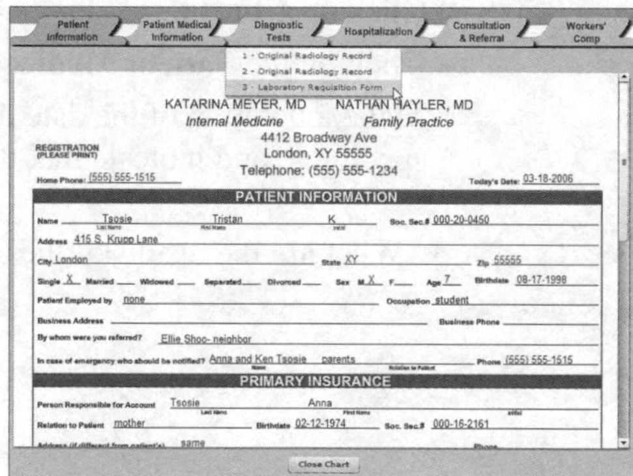

8. Is the Laboratory Requisition complete and correct? If not, describe any errors and explain what would need to be done to correct them.

9. What insurance information is to be provided with the requisition?

Copyright © 2014, 2011, 2007 by Saunders, an imprint of Elsevier Inc. All rights reserved.

- Click **Close Chart** to return to the Laboratory area.
- Click on the **Lab Log Binder**.

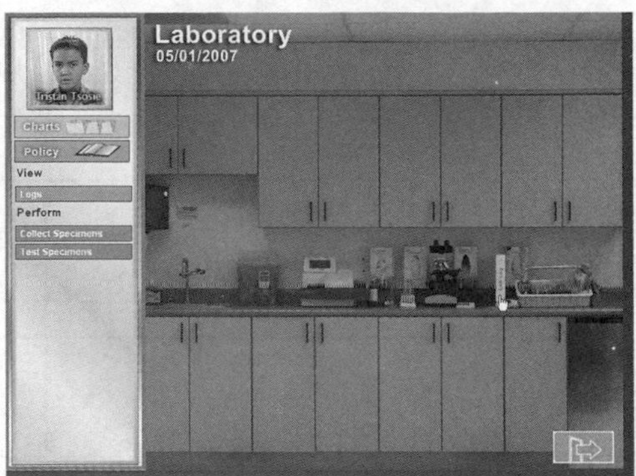

10. Are all of the tests properly logged for quality control and for following the results of the tests?

11. Earlier in the lesson, what did the Progress Notes say about the date of the transport of the culture to the reference laboratory? (*Hint:* See questions 8 and 9 in Exercise 1.)

Thought Question/Critical Thinking

12. Suppose the Progress Notes do not match the date on the laboratory log. Why would it be important to identify discrepancies when charting what happens in the medical office? Does it really matter which date is used?

Copyright © 2014, 2011, 2007 by Saunders, an imprint of Elsevier Inc. All rights reserved.

13. On the blank log below, document the transport of the wound specimen to the laboratory using the 05/01/07 date. Use the initials "CLW" as the person who collected the specimen.

Requisition Number	Date of Specimen Collected	Patient Name	Laboratory Test	Processing Laboratory	Initials: Specimen Collection	Date of Results Return	Initials: Results Return

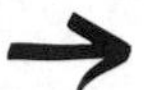

- Click **Finish** to return to the Laboratory.
- Click the exit arrow.
- On the Summary Menu, click on **Look at Your Performance Summary**.
- Scroll down the Performance Summary to the Collect Specimens and Logs section and compare your answers with those chosen by the experts. The summary can be printed or saved for your instructor.
- Click **Close** to return to the Summary Menu.
- Click the exit arrow.
- Click **Return to Map**, then click **Yes** at the pop-up menu to return to the office map or click **Exit the Program**.

Copyright © 2014, 2011, 2007 by Saunders, an imprint of Elsevier Inc. All rights reserved.

LESSON 28

Capillary and Venipuncture Procedures

Reading Assignment: Chapter 53—Assisting with Phlebotomy
- Venipuncture Equipment
- Routine Venipuncture
- Problems Associated with Venipuncture
- Specimen Recollection
- Chain of Custody

Patient: Kevin McKinzie

Learning Objectives:

- Identify the most commonly used venipuncture sites.
- Identify the types of specimens that can be obtained by venipuncture.
- Discuss the necessary preparation of the patient for a routine venipuncture.
- Determine what supplies are needed for a venipuncture.
- Review the need for standard precautions with venipuncture.
- Understand why proper positioning of the patient for venipuncture is necessary.
- Identify the process for safe capillary puncture on infants and older children or adults.
- Describe equipment and supplies needed for capillary puncture.
- Identify methods that can be used to increase blood flow when performing a capillary blood collection.
- Document the collection of blood specimens.
- Indicate how to properly label capillary specimens.

Overview:

In this lesson we will review phlebotomy procedures, including venipuncture and capillary puncture. The importance of standard precautions and risk management skills to prevent injury to the patient are also discussed. Using information obtained from the reading materials, you will analyze proper techniques for venipuncture and capillary puncture, including proper positioning and educating the patient before the procedure and the proper selection of blood collection tubes for certain types of blood samples. After completing this lesson, you will have an understanding of the different types of blood specimens, as well as the proper disposal of contaminated supplies. The importance of proper site selection for capillary puncture is also addressed to reduce discomfort and to ensure the safety of patients, especially infants.

Copyright © 2014, 2011, 2007 by Saunders, an imprint of Elsevier Inc. All rights reserved.

Exercise 1

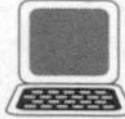

Online Activity—Identifying the Necessary Supplies for Venipuncture

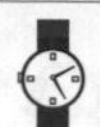

20 minutes

- Sign in to Mountain View Clinic.
- Select **Kevin McKinzie** from the patient list.
- Click on **Exam Room**.
- Click on the **Exam Notes** file folder to read the documentation for Kevin McKinzie's visit. Make note of any blood tests that will require phlebotomy during this visit.
- Click **Finish** to return to the Exam Room.
- Click on the **Supply Cabinet**.
- Add the supplies needed for the patient's examination by clicking on the supply from the Available Supplies list and clicking **Add Item** to confirm your choice.
- If you wish to remove a chosen supply, highlight the supply in the Selected Supplies box and click **Remove**.
- Repeat this step until you are satisfied you have everything you need from the list.
- Click **Finish** to return to the Exam Room.
- Click the exit arrow.
- On the Summary Menu, click on **Look at Your Performance Summary**.
- Scroll down the Performance Summary to the Prepare Room section and compare your answers with those chosen by the experts. The summary can be printed or saved for your instructor.
- Click **Close** to return to the Summary Menu.
- Click **Return to Map** and select **Yes** at the pop-up menu to return to the office map.

1. Which tests will require blood for completion of the physician's orders for the visit? Select all that apply.

_____ Urinalysis

_____ CBC with differential

_____ Hepatitis panel

_____ Liver panel

_____ EBV antibody

_____ MonoSpot test

Copyright © 2014, 2011, 2007 by Saunders, an imprint of Elsevier Inc. All rights reserved.

2. Which of the tests that you selected in question 1 would be sent to an outside laboratory for testing?

- Click on **Laboratory**.
- Click on the **Specimen Collection Tray**.
- Use the checkboxes to select the tests that need to be collected for the patient's visit.
- Click **Next**.
- Answer all the questions related to each test using the checkboxes and radio buttons provided. (*Hint:* The Policy Manual can be opened at any time for reference as you answer the questions.)
- Click **Finish** to return to the Laboratory.

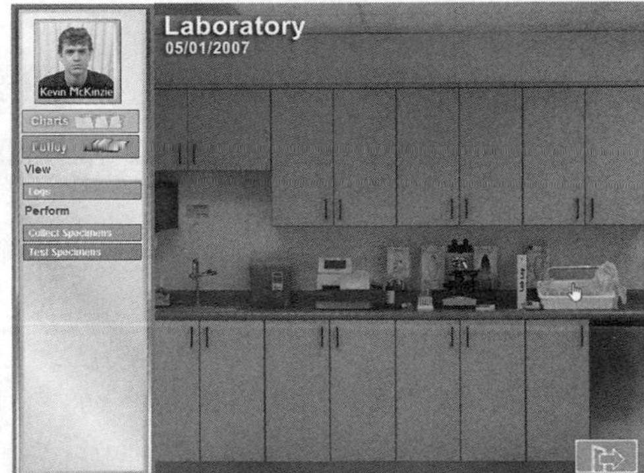

3. Indicate whether each of the following statements is true or false.

a. _________ Serum is obtained from whole blood that has an anticoagulant added to the test tube to prevent clotting.

b. _________ Plasma is obtained from whole blood that has an anticoagulant added to the test tube to prevent clotting.

c. _________ Whole blood is needed for a CBC with differential.

d. _________ Serum is needed for the hepatitis panel and the liver panel.

e. _________ Serum contains the chemicals found in the blood with the clotting factors removed.

f. _________ Plasma contains the chemicals found in the blood with the clotting factors removed.

g. _________ Evacuated tubes are available in only one size.

h. _________ Evacuated tubes have an expiration date and a label for writing the patient name.

i. _________ The evacuated tube may be pushed all the way into the Vacutainer adapter after the needle has entered the vein.

j. _________ If the top of the evacuated tube will need to be opened, a Hemoguard tube should be used.

k. _________ Before using an evacuated tube, you should check it for cracks and other breaches in quality control.

Copyright © 2014, 2011, 2007 by Saunders, an imprint of Elsevier Inc. All rights reserved.

l. _________ If a Vacutainer tube is dropped, it can still be used unless it is cracked or broken.

m. _________ The evacuated tube should be filled to the level of blood specified for the test, not to the size (volume capacity) of the tube.

n. _________ Tubes containing additives should be agitated or shaken 8 to 10 times to mix the blood with the additive.

4. Tubes with or without a clot activator and tubes with or without a gel barrier are used to collect ____________________ specimens.

5. List the parts of the Vacutainer system.

- Click the exit arrow.
- On the Summary Menu, click on **Look at Your Performance Summary**.
- Scroll down the Performance Summary to the Laboratory Collection section and compare your answers with those chosen by the experts. The summary can be printed or saved for your instructor.
- Click **Close** to return to the Summary Menu.
- Click **Return to Map** and select **Yes** at the pop-up menu to return to the office map.

Copyright © 2014, 2011, 2007 by Saunders, an imprint of Elsevier Inc. All rights reserved.

Exercise 2

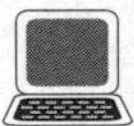

Online Activity—Choosing the Correct Position and Site for a Venipuncture

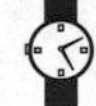

20 minutes

1. This diagram illustrates the most appropriate venipuncture sites for obtaining blood specimens. Match the columns below the diagram to identify each of the numbered sites.

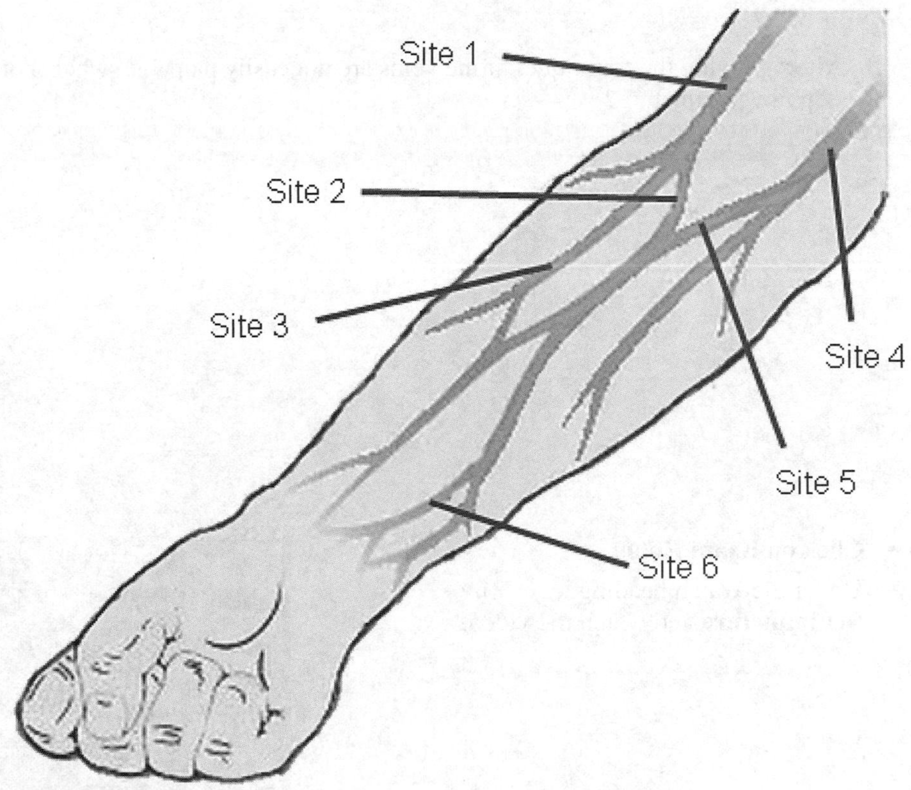

_____	Site 1	a. Basilic vein
_____	Site 2	b. Cephalic vein
_____	Site 3	c. Median antebrachial vein
_____	Site 4	d. Median basilic vein
_____	Site 5	e. Median cephalic vein
_____	Site 6	f. Supplementary cephalic vein

Copyright © 2014, 2011, 2007 by Saunders, an imprint of Elsevier Inc. All rights reserved.

2. What are the advantages of using the veins found in the antecubital area?

3. After applying the tourniquet, if the veins are not easily palpable, what should be the next step in venipuncture?

- Click on **Exam Room**.
- Under the Watch heading, click on **Venipuncture** and watch the video.

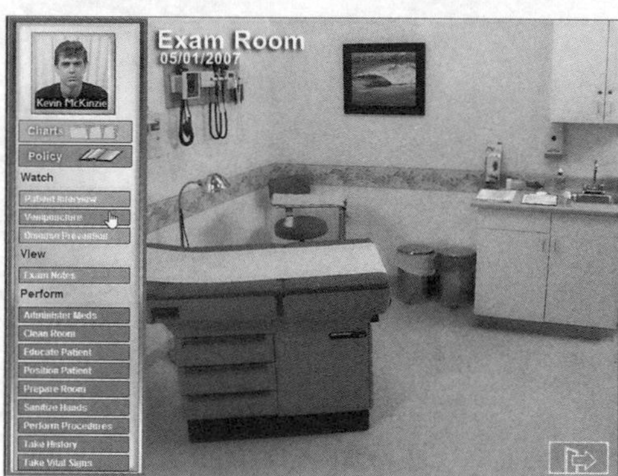

4. What additional steps should have been taken by the medical assistant to make the patient more at ease about the procedure?

Copyright © 2014, 2011, 2007 by Saunders, an imprint of Elsevier Inc. All rights reserved.

5. Why is it important for the patient to be in either a lying or sitting position during venipuncture?

6. Would it ever be appropriate to perform phlebotomy with the patient standing up? Explain your answer.

7. Indicate whether each of the following statements is true or false.

a. ________ Venipuncture may take place on the side of a mastectomy.

b. ________ Sclerosed veins feel hard and knotty and should not be used for venipuncture.

c. ________ Veins that are near the top of the skin are always the veins to use for venipuncture.

d. ________ The angle of the needle for venipuncture is 15 degrees.

e. ________ When blood is being drawn from the back of the hand, a butterfly needle or winged infusion set is more comfortable and more likely to provide a quality specimen.

f. ________ The tourniquet should be placed on the arm approximately 4 inches above the venipuncture site when finding the appropriate vein, and should remain in place until after the venipuncture is complete, no matter how long the time.

g. ________ The tourniquet should remain in place until after the needle is removed following venipuncture.

→ • Click the **X** on the video screen to close the video.
• Remain in the Exam Room with Kevin McKinzie as your patient to continue to the next exercise.

Copyright © 2014, 2011, 2007 by Saunders, an imprint of Elsevier Inc. All rights reserved.

Exercise 3

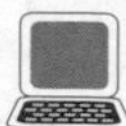

Online Activity—Disposal of Supplies and Handling of Specimen Following Venipuncture

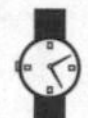

20 minutes

1. List some of the supplies that are used during a phlebotomy.

2. After venipuncture, what is the proper procedure for disposal of the venipuncture supplies?

- Click on the **Waste Receptacles**.
- Use the checkboxes to select the appropriate steps necessary to clean the Exam Room after the patient's exam.
- Click **Finish** to return to the Exam Room.
- Click the exit arrow.
- On the Summary Menu, click on **Look at Your Performance Summary**.
- Scroll down the Performance Summary to the Clean Room section and compare your answers with those chosen by the experts. The summary can be printed or saved for your instructor.
- Click **Close** to return to the Summary Menu.
- On the Summary Menu, click **Return to Map** and select **Yes** at the pop-up menu to return to the office map.

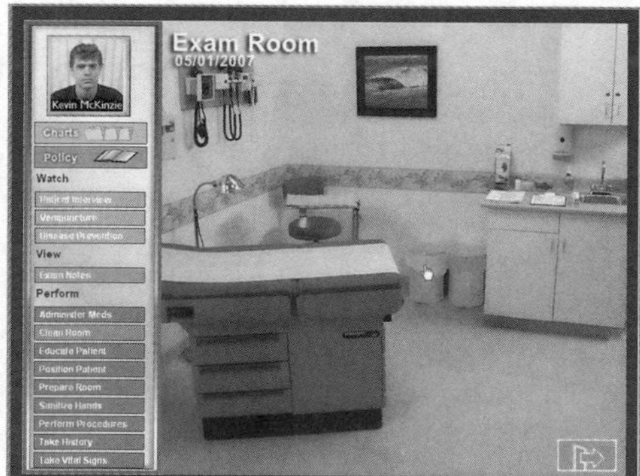

Copyright © 2014, 2011, 2007 by Saunders, an imprint of Elsevier Inc. All rights reserved.

3. Indicate whether each of the following statements is true or false.

   a. _________ OSHA has designated that safety-engineered devices on needles should be used to prevent needlestick injuries.

   b. _________ After venipuncture, all materials that have come in contact with the skin must be disposed of in biohazard waste.

   c. _________ OSHA requires that hands be sanitized following venipuncture.

   d. _________ The tourniquet used for the venipuncture should be made of latex and should be sanitized using alcohol so that it may be used for another patient.

   e. _________ Gloves may be removed immediately after the venipuncture, and the test tubes with no gross contamination may be handled without gloves.

   f. _________ Handwashing/hand sanitization should be done after removing gloves and before documentation in the medical record.

   g. _________ The length of time a specimen is held following venipuncture and before centrifuging has no significance.

   h. _________ Specimens that are not handled with care may have hemolysis.

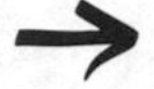

- Click on **Laboratory**.
- Click on **Charts**.
- Click on the **Diagnostic Tests** tab and select **1-Laboratory Requisition** from the drop-down menu.

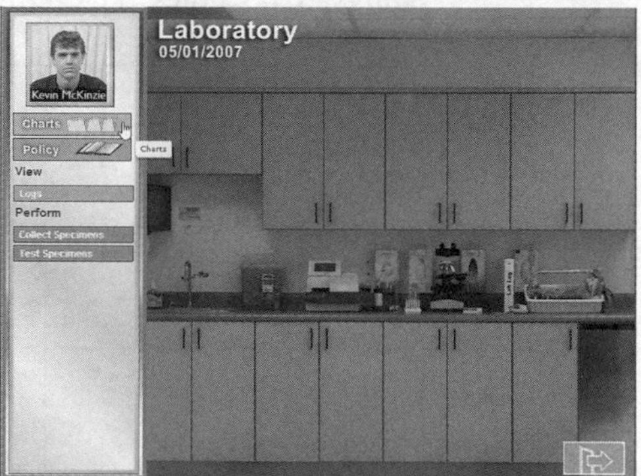

4. Review the Laboratory Requisition to ensure that all tests that are not Clinical Laboratories Improvement Act (CLIA)-waived have been ordered. Did you find that the tests were correctly ordered?

5. Should any of the tests have been done on the next day because of the need to fast?

Copyright © 2014, 2011, 2007 by Saunders, an imprint of Elsevier Inc. All rights reserved.

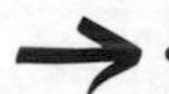

- Click **Close Chart** to return to the Laboratory area.
- Click on the **Lab Log Binder**.

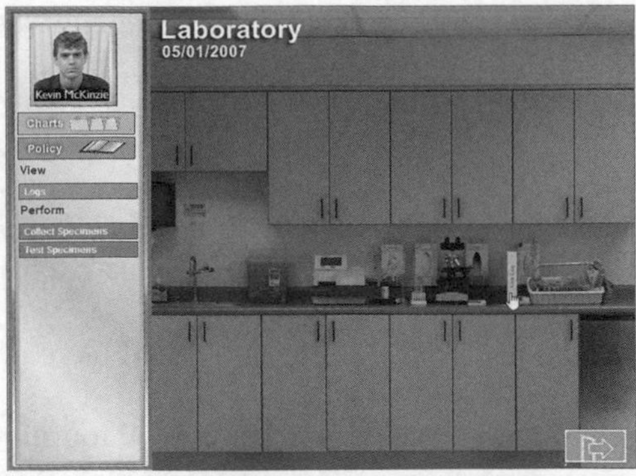

6. Are all of the tests properly logged for quality control and for following the results of the tests?

7. Using the following log, document the specimens for Kevin McKinzie as found in the physician's notes. The requisition number is 144756.

Requisition Number	Date of Specimen Collected	Patient Name	Laboratory Test	Processing Laboratory	Initials: Specimen Collection	Date of Results Return	Initials: Results Return

Copyright © 2014, 2011, 2007 by Saunders, an imprint of Elsevier Inc. All rights reserved.

Thought Question

8. Why is it unnecessary to include the patient's name and the date on each individual line if multiple tests are being ordered?

- Click **Finish** to close the log and return to the Laboratory.
- Click on the **Specimen Analyzer**.
- Use the checkboxes to select the tests that need to be processed for Kevin McKinzie.
- Click **Next**.
- Answer all the questions related to each test using the checkboxes and radio buttons provided. (*Hint:* The Policy Manual can be opened at any time for reference as you answer the questions.)

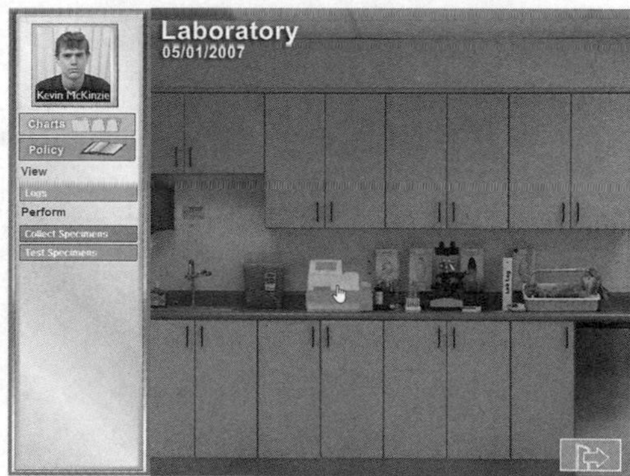

- Click **Finish** to return to the Laboratory.
- Remain in the Laboratory with Kevin McKinzie as your patient to continue to the next exercise.

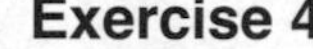

Exercise 4

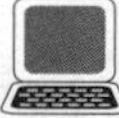

Online Activity—Documentation of the Specimens

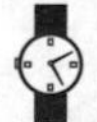

15 minutes

- Click on **Charts**.
- Click on the **Patient Medical Information** tab and select **1-Progress Notes**.

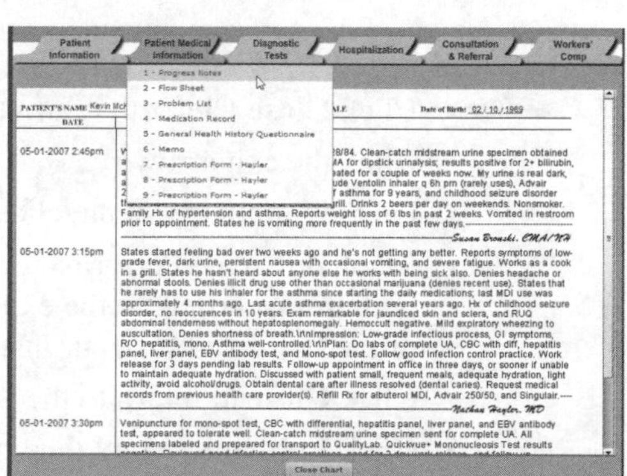

Copyright © 2014, 2011, 2007 by Saunders, an imprint of Elsevier Inc. All rights reserved.

1. Mr. McKinzie's appointment time was 2:45 p.m. Using this information and the tests ordered, document on the blank Progress Notes below the collection of the venipuncture specimens, including the laboratory to which the specimens were sent.

PATIENT'S NAME ______ ☐FEMALE ☐MALE Date of Birth: __/__/__

DATE	PATIENT VISITS AND FINDINGS

2. What information is lacking from the documentation of the venipuncture in the medical record?

3. What documentation should be placed on the tubes of blood before they are sent to the outside lab?

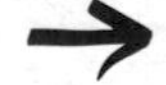

- Click **Close Chart** to return to the Laboratory area.
- Click the exit arrow.
- On the Summary Menu, click on **Look at Your Performance Summary**.
- Scroll down the Performance Summary to the Lab Test sections and compare your answers with those chosen by the experts. Each test will have its own section. The summary can be printed or saved for your instructor.
- Click **Close** to return to the Summary Menu.
- Click **Return to Map**, then click **Yes** at the pop-up menu to return to the office map or click **Exit the Program**.

Copyright © 2014, 2011, 2007 by Saunders, an imprint of Elsevier Inc. All rights reserved.

Exercise 5

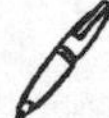

Writing Activity—Performing Capillary Puncture on Infants and Older Children or Adults

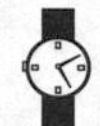

20 minutes

In this exercise you will determine the proper site for capillary puncture for infants and other patients. by showing the proper sites on the drawings below. This information will be obtained from your textbook readings.

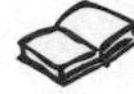

1. On the figure below, show the proper sites for adult capillary puncture. (*Hint:* Refer to your textbook for this information.)

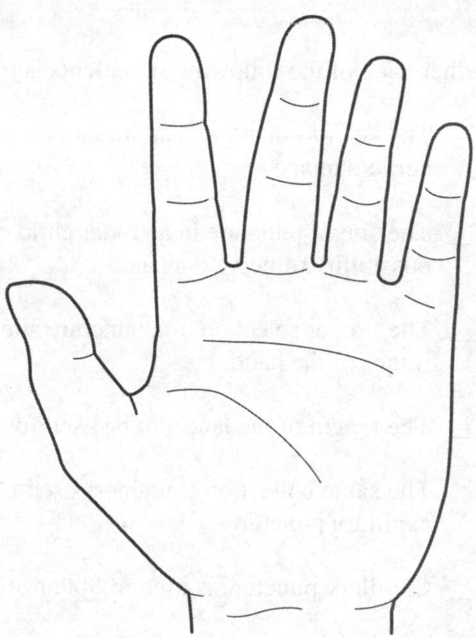

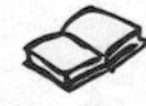

2. On the figure below, show the proper sites for infant capillary puncture. (*Hint:* Refer to your textbook for this information.)

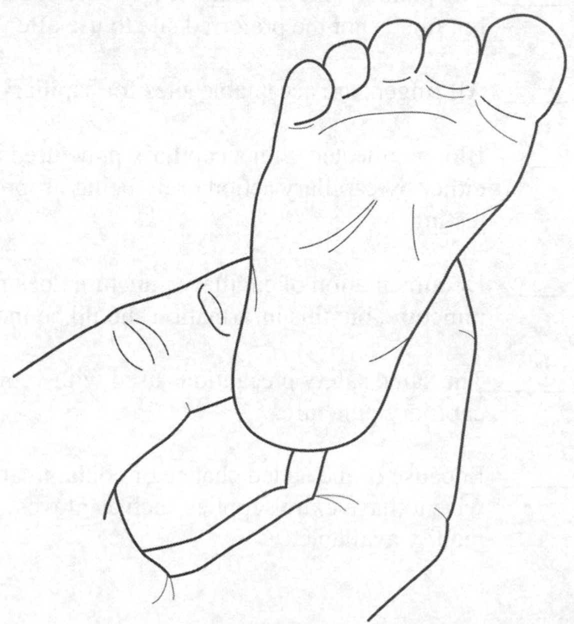

Copyright © 2014, 2011, 2007 by Saunders, an imprint of Elsevier Inc. All rights reserved.

3. List situations in which capillary puncture would be appropriate.

4. Indicate whether each of the following statements is true or false.

a. ________ The site of puncture in an infant is important to prevent the possibility of nerve damage.

b. ________ The site of puncture in an older child or an adult is important to prevent the possibility of nerve damage.

c. ________ The proper selection of a puncture site for an adult is the third or fourth finger of the hand.

d. ________ The length of the lancet to be used for adults and infants is the same.

e. ________ The same collection containers used for venipuncture may be used for capillary punctures.

f. ________ Capillary puncture is used to obtain small amounts of blood.

g. ________ Collection containers for capillary puncture have many of the same additives as those used for venipuncture.

h. ________ The plantar surface of the heel is used for infants who are not yet walking, but this is not the preferred site to use after a child begins walking.

i. ________ All fingers are acceptable sites for capillary puncture.

j. ________ Blood collected with a capillary puncture is pulled into the collection device either by capillary action or by being dropped onto a reagent strip for testing.

k. ________ Documentation of capillary puncture does not necessarily include the site of puncture, but this information should be included for infants.

l. ________ The same safety precautions used with venipuncture should be used with capillary puncture.

m. ________ Because of the added chance of contamination of surfaces by blood, it is wise to have extra supplies such as gloves, gauze pads, and disinfectant readily available.

Copyright © 2014, 2011, 2007 by Saunders, an imprint of Elsevier Inc. All rights reserved.

5. What is the most efficient way to transport capillary tubes?

6. What is one thing you can do to increase blood flow to the area in which you are collecting capillary blood?

Copyright © 2014, 2011, 2007 by Saunders, an imprint of Elsevier Inc. All rights reserved.

LESSON 29

Hematology Testing

Reading Assignment: Chapter 51—Assisting in the Clinical Laboratory
- Role of the Clinical Laboratory in Patient Care

Chapter 53—Assisting in Phlebotomy
- Capillary Puncture

Chapter 54—Assisting in the Analysis of Blood
- Hematology
- Collection of Blood Samples
- Hemoglobin
- Red Blood Cell Count
- White Blood Cell Count
- Red Cell Indices
- Differential Cell Count

Patient: Louise Parlet

Learning Objectives:

- Understand the three levels of laboratory testing as defined by CLIA.
- List the methods for obtaining specimens for CLIA-waived hematology testing.
- Read the Progress Notes correctly.
- List the normal reference range for components of blood that are tested in a complete blood count.
- Discuss the role of the hematology section of the laboratory.
- Describe the collection of blood in a hematocrit tube.
- Explain what is indicated by the MCH, MCV, and MCHC.
- Document laboratory test results on a laboratory flow sheet.

Overview:

In this lesson an understanding of CLIA-waived tests and hematology testing will be emphasized. You will use the Policy Manual to obtain the list of diagnostic tests for a patient, Louise Parlet, with a newly diagnosed pregnancy. Finally, you will be expected to add results of testing to a flow sheet for this patient.

Copyright © 2014, 2011, 2007 by Saunders, an imprint of Elsevier Inc. All rights reserved.

Exercise 1

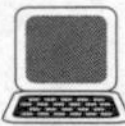

Online Activity—Performing Diagnostic Tests According to Office Policy

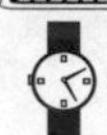

35 minutes

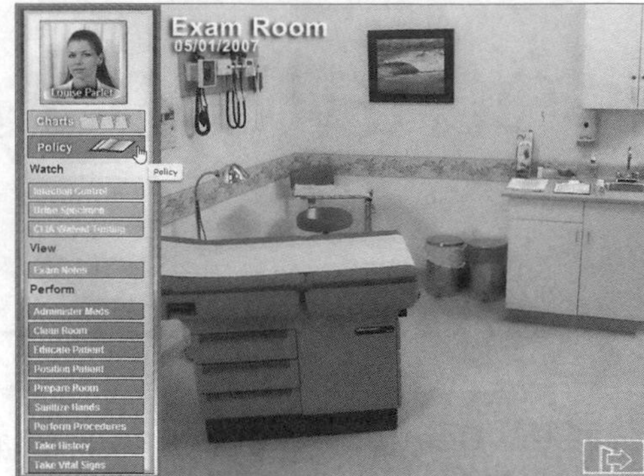

- Sign in to Mountain View Clinic.
- Select **Louise Parlet** from the patient list.
- Click on **Exam Room**.
- Click on the **Exam Notes** file folder and read the documentation for Ms. Parlet's visit. Make a notation of her primary diagnosis and the reason she is being seen in the office.
- Click **Finish** to return to the Exam Room.
- Click on **Policy** to open the office Policy Manual.
- Type "standing orders" in the search bar and click on the magnifying glass.
- Read the section of the Policy Manual on standing orders.

1. What is the primary diagnosis for Ms. Parlet?

2. According to office policy, what tests should be obtained from Ms. Parlet?

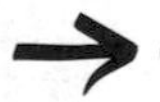

- From the menu on the left side of the screen, click on the arrow next to **Policy Manual** to expand the menu.
- Click on **Laboratory Policies** to read that section of the Policy Manual.

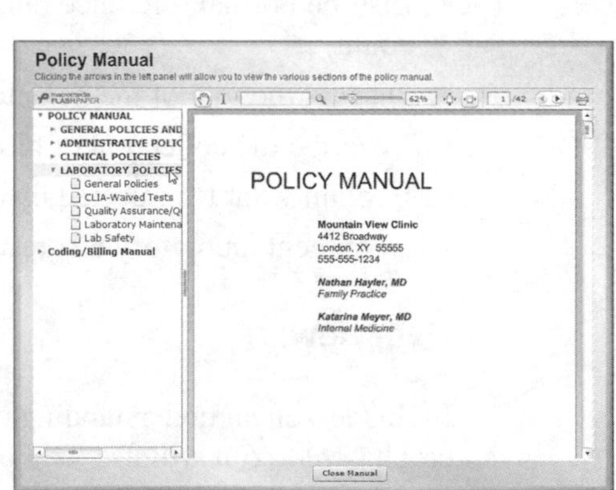

Copyright © 2014, 2011, 2007 by Saunders, an imprint of Elsevier Inc. All rights reserved.

3. What is meant by CLIA?

4. The three levels of CLIA testing are:
   a. simple, moderate, high complexity.
   b. waived, easy, high complexity.
   c. waived, moderate, high complexity.
   d. easy, medium, complex complexity.
   e. waived, medium, complex complexity.

5. Explain "waived tests" as defined by CLIA.

6. List at least four methods for obtaining CLIA-waived tests.

7. Which of the tests you identified in question 2 could be performed as CLIA-waived tests by the medical assistant before the physician sees Ms. Parlet?

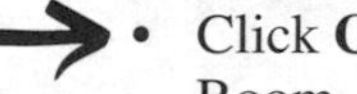

- Click **Close Manual** to return to the Exam Room.
- Click the exit arrow.
- Click **Return to Map** and select **Yes** at the pop-up menu to return to the office map.
- Click on **Billing and Coding**.

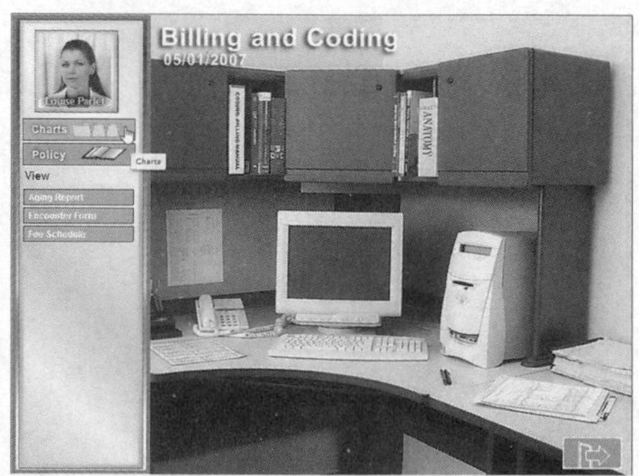

Copyright © 2014, 2011, 2007 by Saunders, an imprint of Elsevier Inc. All rights reserved.

- Click on **Charts**.
- Click on **Patient Medical Information** tab and select **3-Progress Notes** from the drop-down menu. Read the final Progress Notes for Ms. Parlet's visit.

8. According to the Progress Notes, what further blood tests were ordered for Ms. Parlet? Were any of these CLIA-waived?

9. Do the Progress Notes indicate that all the specimens were sent to Quality Lab?
   a. Yes
   b. No

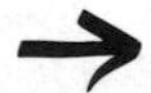

- Leave Louise Parlet's chart open since you will need it in Exercise 3.

Exercise 2

Writing Activity—Components of Hematology

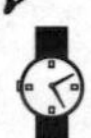

30 minutes

In this exercise, you will review hematology and its components, and the normal reference ranges for adult patients.

1. Explain the responsibilities of the hematology section of the laboratory.

2. What is the purpose of the "differential count" in the complete blood count (CBC)?

Copyright © 2014, 2011, 2007 by Saunders, an imprint of Elsevier Inc. All rights reserved.

3. Define *MCV*, *MCH*, and *MCHC*.

4. For each blood component listed below, identify the normal range for males and females.

Blood Component	Normal Range by Gender
Red blood cells (erythrocytes)	
White blood cells	
Hemoglobin (Hgb)	
Hematocrit (Hct)	
Platelets	
WBC differential	

5. Describe the collection of a capillary puncture specimen in a calibrated capillary tube for a spun hematocrit.

Copyright © 2014, 2011, 2007 by Saunders, an imprint of Elsevier Inc. All rights reserved.

6. What should the medical assistant do if air bubbles are present in the capillary tube?

7. Why is it important for no air bubbles to be in the capillary puncture specimen for a spun hematocrit?

8. On the diagram below, label the cellular elements found in a capillary tube following centrifuging.

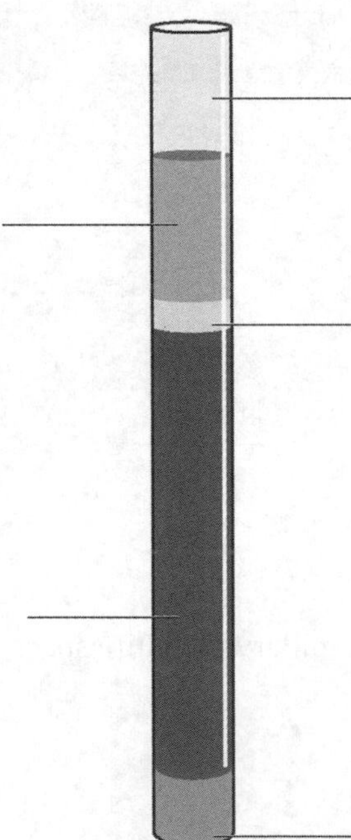

Copyright © 2014, 2011, 2007 by Saunders, an imprint of Elsevier Inc. All rights reserved.

9. When a capillary tube is being spun in a microhematocrit centrifuge, which of the following are necessary for safety? Select all that apply.

_____ PPE

_____ Placing the capillary tube anywhere in the centrifuge

_____ Placing the capillary tubes opposite each other for balance

_____ Placing the sealed edge of the capillary tube toward the exterior of the centrifuge

_____ Placing the capillary tube toward the center of the centrifuge

_____ Closing the lid of the centrifuge before spinning the capillary tube

_____ Opening the lid immediately after the centrifuge stops the cycle

_____ Opening the lid when the centrifuge stops spinning

Exercise 3

Writing Activity—Documenting Hematology Testing

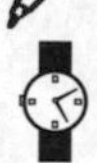

20 minutes

- Still working with Louise Parlet's chart, click on the **Patient Medical Information** tab and select **4-Flow Sheet**.

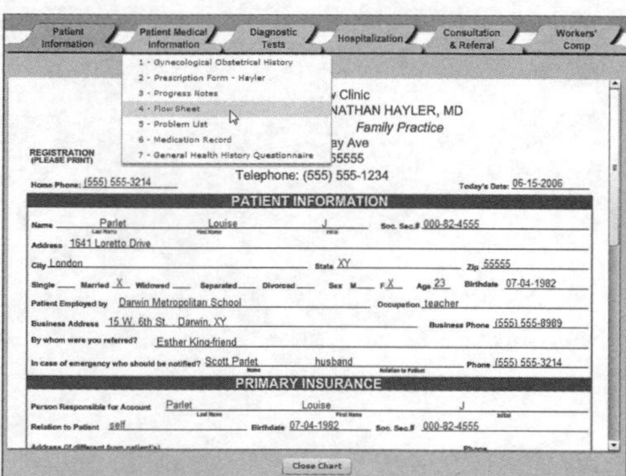

Copyright © 2014, 2011, 2007 by Saunders, an imprint of Elsevier Inc. All rights reserved.

1. The only CLIA-waived test documented for Ms. Parlet was her urine HCG. Her hemoglobin (Hgb), her glucose level, and a dipstick urine were also tested, but they were not documented until after the patient left the office at 9:45 a.m. On the blank Progress Notes below, document the following CLIA-waived test results for Ms. Parlet: Hgb 11.2 g/dL; BS 115, NF; dipstick urine negative for sugar, albumin (protein), leukocytes; pH 7; specific gravity 1.025. (*Note:* NF, nonfasting.)

PATIENT'S NAME ______________________ ☐FEMALE ☐MALE Date of Birth: ___/___/___

DATE	PATIENT VISITS AND FINDINGS

Copyright © 2014, 2011, 2007 by Saunders, an imprint of Elsevier Inc. All rights reserved.

2. Below, fill in the results from the CLIA-waived testing performed during her visit. (*Note:* To indicate that the glucose result was nonfasting, label as NF.)

FLOW SHEET

Name: Louise Parlet **Date of Birth:** 07/04/1982 **Age:** 23

Vital Signs Date:	05/01/07							
Weight	125 lbs							
Height	5 ft 5 in							
Temperature	98.2 F							
Pulse	72							
Respirations	16							
Blood Pressure	104/72							
Lab Tests Date:	05/01/07							
CBC								
RBC								
WBC								
HGB								
Hematocrit								
Alkaline Phosphatase								
Albumin								
Glucose								
Bilirubin total								
BUN								
Calcium								
Cholesterol								
Chloride								
CO2								
Creatinine								
Hb A1c								
LipidProfile								
LDL								
HDL								
Triglycerides								
SGGT								
SGOG/AST								
SGPT/ATL								
LDH								
T3								
T4								
T7								
TSH								
Triglycerides								
Total Protein								
Uric Acid								
Sodium								
Potassium								
Urinalysis								
Albumin								
Glucose								
PAPSmear								
PSA								
Other tests:								

Copyright © 2014, 2011, 2007 by Saunders, an imprint of Elsevier Inc. All rights reserved.

3. Dr. Hayler received a partial report on Ms. Parlet's laboratory results today. Document the results in the blank Progress Notes below, using 5/01/2007 as the collection date. Include the following results: Hgb 10.6 g/dL; Hct 38%; RBC 4.2; WBC 5,400; platelet count 200,000; rubella titer 1:1 (assumed immune); ABO O; Rh+; PAP negative; chlamydia negative.

PATIENT'S NAME ____________ ☐FEMALE ☐MALE Date of Birth: __/__/__

DATE	PATIENT VISITS AND FINDINGS

Copyright © 2014, 2011, 2007 by Saunders, an imprint of Elsevier Inc. All rights reserved.

4. Below, document the laboratory results from the Progress Notes onto the flow sheet.

FLOW SHEET

Name: Louise Parlet **Date of Birth:** 07/04/1982 **Age:** 23

Vital Signs Date:	05/01/07							
Weight	125 lbs							
Height	5 ft 5 in							
Temperature	98.2 F							
Pulse	72							
Respirations	16							
Blood Pressure	104/72							
Lab Tests Date:	05/01/07							
CBC								
RBC								
WBC								
HGB	11.2							
Hematocrit								
Alkaline Phosphatase								
Albumin								
Glucose	115							
Bilirubin total								
BUN								
Calcium								
Cholesterol								
Chloride								
CO2								
Creatinine								
Hb A1c								
LipidProfile								
LDL								
HDL								
Triglycerides								
SGGT								
SGOG/AST								
SGPT/ATL								
LDH								
T3								
T4								
T7								
TSH								
Triglycerides								
Total Protein								
Uric Acid								
Sodium								
Potassium								
Urinalysis								
Albumin	neg							
Glucose	neg							
PAPSmear								
PSA								
Other tests:								
urine HCG	pos							
urine leukocyte	neg							

Copyright © 2014, 2011, 2007 by Saunders, an imprint of Elsevier Inc. All rights reserved.

5. Should any of Ms. Parlet's laboratory test results be highlighted for the physician for special attention? If so, which one(s)? (*Hint:* Refer to your answers in Exercise 2, question 4.)

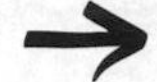

- Click **Close Chart** to return to the Billing and Coding area.
- Click the exit arrow.
- Click **Return to Map**, then click **Yes** at the pop-up menu to return to the office map or click **Exit the Program**.

Copyright © 2014, 2011, 2007 by Saunders, an imprint of Elsevier Inc. All rights reserved.

LESSON 30

Performing Blood Chemistry Testing

Reading Assignment: Chapter 51—Assisting in the Chemical Laboratory
- Quality Assurance and Quality Control

Chapter 54—Assisting in the Analysis of Blood
- Clinical Chemistry
- Blood Glucose Testing
- Cholesterol Testing

Patient: Rhea Davison

Learning Objectives:

- List the CLIA-waived chemistry tests commonly performed in a medical office.
- Name common blood chemistry tests performed in the medical office.
- Discuss the necessity of quality control for blood glucose tests in home and office testing.
- State the length of time to which fructosamine values correlate in regard to the patient's average glucose level.
- Identify the normal ranges of more commonly performed chemistry testing.
- Discuss the needed preparation for a fasting blood glucose or cholesterol test.
- Indicate which tests should be obtained as fasting chemistry tests when possible.
- State the patient teaching important in obtaining blood glucose tests using an Accu-Chek glucose meter.
- Describe the proper storage of blood glucose testing supplies.
- Complete the laboratory log for specimens being sent to an outside laboratory.
- Document the test results on a laboratory flow sheet and indicate those tests that need to be seen by the physician as soon as possible.

Overview:

In this lesson you will describe the collection and handling of some of the common CLIA-waived blood chemistry tests performed in the medical office. The normal range of blood chemistry results will be identified, and the ability to evaluate the test results will be emphasized. You will be expected to complete a laboratory log for specimens being sent to outside labs for testing. You will also document the return of the test results to the office. As the medical assistant, you will be asked to evaluate results that need immediate attention

Copyright © 2014, 2011, 2007 by Saunders, an imprint of Elsevier Inc. All rights reserved.

and those that can be seen by the physician at the end of the day. Rhea Davison is an established patient with a known history of diabetes mellitus. She has kept her diabetes well controlled until her last visit. The physician is concerned that the glucose meter (glucometer) she is using at home may be providing inaccurate results, so you are asked to assist Ms. Davison in learning how to perform routine maintenance on the glucose meter.

Exercise 1

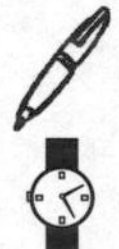

Writing Activity—Common Blood Chemistry Testing

25 minutes

1. What is measured through blood chemistry testing?

2. Into which classification (complexity) of CLIA tests do most chemistry analyzers fall?

3. Identify a few of the blood chemistry tests that are commonly performed in the medical office laboratory.

4. What patient preparation is preferred by physicians for cholesterol and other chemistry testing?

5. What is the best appointment time for the patient to have a blood chemistry test? Why?

Copyright © 2014, 2011, 2007 by Saunders, an imprint of Elsevier Inc. All rights reserved.

6. Express the blood glucose result that correlates with the glycosylated hemoglobin (HgbA1c) results.

7. What is the patient given to drink when having the glucose tolerance test?

8. If the physician orders a fructosamine test, how long will this correlate or "look back" at the results of the patient's glucose level?

Exercise 2

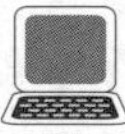

Online Activity—Patient Education for Quality Blood Glucose Tests

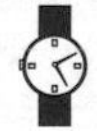

30 minutes

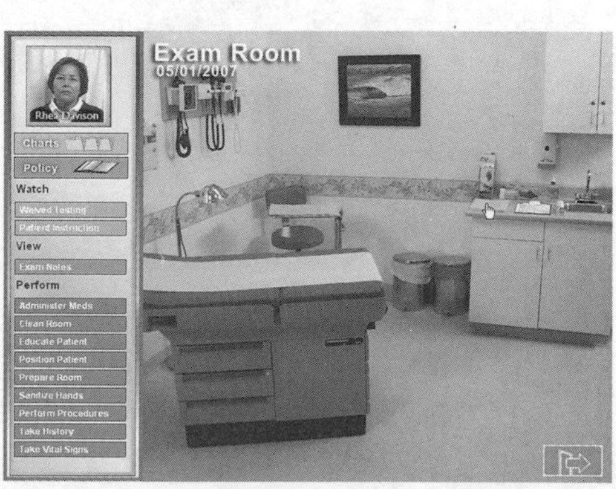

- Sign in to Mountain View Clinic.
- Select **Rhea Davison** from the patient list.
- Click on the **Exam Room**.
- Click on the **Exam Notes** file folder and read the documentation for Rhea Davison's visit.
- Click **Finish** to return to the Exam Room.
- Under the Watch heading, click on **Waived Testing** and watch the video.

Copyright © 2014, 2011, 2007 by Saunders, an imprint of Elsevier Inc. All rights reserved.

1. Now that you have read the Exam Notes and watched the video, why do you think that Dr. Meyer wants Ms. Davison to perform a glucose test using the equipment in the office?

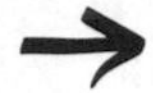

- Click the **X** on the video screen to close the video.
- Click on the **Supply Cabinet**.
- Add the supplies needed for the patient's exam by clicking on the supply from the Available Supplies list and clicking **Add Item** to confirm your choice.
- If you wish to remove a chosen supply, highlight the supply in the Selected Supplies box and click **Remove**.
- Repeat this step until you are satisfied you have everything you need from the list.

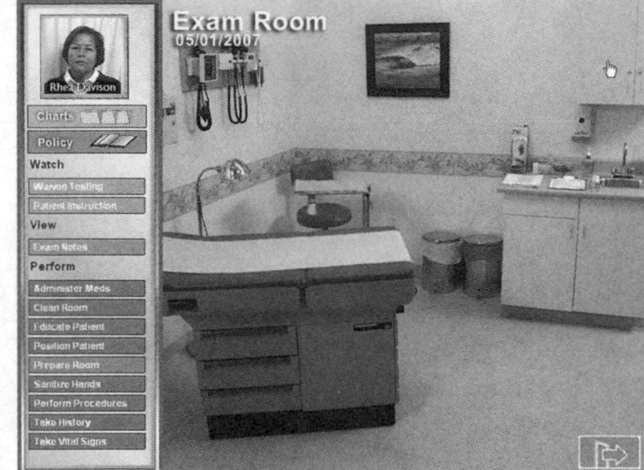

2. List the supplies needed by a medical assistant for blood glucose testing.

Copyright © 2014, 2011, 2007 by Saunders, an imprint of Elsevier Inc. All rights reserved.

3. Which supplies would be needed by Ms. Davison for performing quality control of the glucose testing equipment she currently uses at home? Select all that apply.

_____ Abnormal control sample

_____ Gloves

_____ Normal control

_____ Glucose meter

_____ Sterile wipes

_____ Container for sharps

_____ Glucose reagent strips

_____ Capillary lancet

4. Indicate whether each of the following statements is true or false.

a. _________ All chemistry tests results are confined to only a single number for normal readings.

b. _________ Cholesterol and blood glucose may be CLIA-waived tests.

c. _________ To perform cholesterol and blood glucose testing in the medical office, the equipment must be CLIA-waived unless highly qualified personnel are available for the testing.

d. _________ At home, a patient should store equipment away from light and heat sources.

e. _________ The fructose tests provide a record of the average of the patient's glucose level for 5 months.

f. _________ Quality control is necessary for ensuring that chemistry test equipment is working properly.

g. _________ Blood chemistry testing is used for differential diagnoses.

h. _________ The equipment used by patients at home is CLIA-waived.

i. _________ All types of blood glucose equipment have the same instructions for use.

5. What information needs to be supplied to Ms. Davison about the collection of the specimen immediately following the capillary puncture?

Copyright © 2014, 2011, 2007 by Saunders, an imprint of Elsevier Inc. All rights reserved.

6. What information should be supplied to Ms. Davison about the use of the glucose meter?

7. The medical assistant suggests that Ms. Davison ask the physician for a new glucose testing meter. Why do you think this is important?

8. In the Exam Notes, Ms. Davison reports having missed several doses of medication because of the inability to buy the medication. How would you expect this to affect the test results she obtained at home?

9. Would you expect Ms. Davison to have an increase in weight if she is following her prescribed diet? Explain your answer.

10. What information did Ms. Davison give about where she stores her glucose meter, and what affect may this have on the results of her tests?

Copyright © 2014, 2011, 2007 by Saunders, an imprint of Elsevier Inc. All rights reserved.

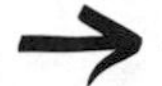

- Click **Finish** to return to the Exam Room.
- Click the exit arrow.
- On the Summary Menu, click on **Look at Your Performance Summary**.
- Scroll down the Performance Summary to the Prepare Room section and compare your answers with those chosen by the experts. The summary can be printed or saved for your instructor.
- Click **Close** to return to the Summary Menu.
- On the Summary Menu, click **Return to Map** and select **Yes** at the pop-up menu to return to the Office Map.

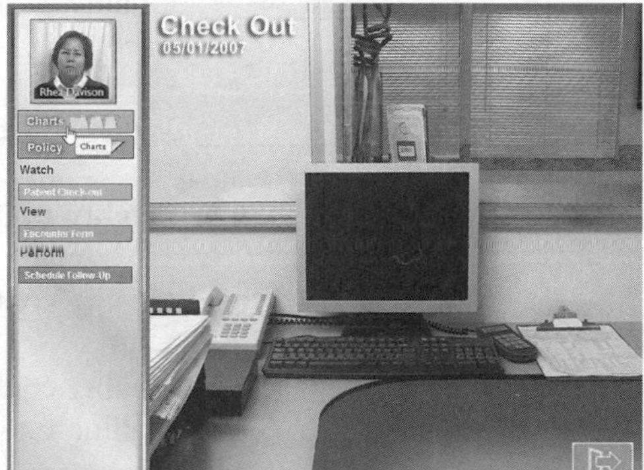

- Click on **Check Out**.
- Click on **Charts**.
- Click on the **Patient Medical Information** tab and select **1-Progress Notes**.
- Read the results of today's blood glucose test and the testing that is to be done on the next day.
- Click on the **Patient Medical Information** tab and select **6-Home Glucose Monitoring Record**.
- Review the results of Rhea Davison's home monitoring record.

11. Is the test result for Ms. Davison's blood glucose obtained in the office within the limits expected when compared with the results from her home testing? Explain your answer.

12. Dr. Meyer ordered an HgbA1c. What information does this test provide? Why is this an important test for Dr. Meyer to use in treating Ms. Davison?

Copyright © 2014, 2011, 2007 by Saunders, an imprint of Elsevier Inc. All rights reserved.

Exercise 3

Writing Activity—Quality Control with Blood Chemistry Testing

15 minutes

In this exercise you will use your knowledge to decide whether quality control has been accomplished.

1. Indicate whether each of the following statements is true or false.

   a. _________ Quality control for blood chemistry testing should be done no more than once a day.

   b. _________ When new reagent strips are opened, quality control sampling should occur.

   c. _________ Quality control samples have expiration dates.

   d. _________ Quality control samples may be used with any equipment.

   e. _________ Quality control is performed only so that the physician will have an accurate reading for comparison.

   f. _________ If the quality control samples are consistently inaccurate, the patient should try to repair the equipment used at home, because the patient is the person who best understands how that specific equipment works.

   g. _________ One method of checking for quality control of a machine in the medical office is to compare results obtained from a reference lab on a specific specimen with the results obtained on that same specimen in the office laboratory.

2. What is the significance if samples for quality control fall out of the control range?

3. If a patient questions the importance of performing quality control on a regular basis, what should you tell the patient?

Copyright © 2014, 2011, 2007 by Saunders, an imprint of Elsevier Inc. All rights reserved.

Exercise 4

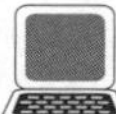

Online Activity—Preparing a Laboratory Log for Patient Specimens

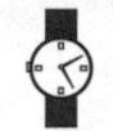

10 minutes

1. Rhea Davison's specimens were sent to an outside lab (Quality Lab) the day following her appointment. Using her Progress Notes, prepare the laboratory log below for these tests. (*Note:* The requisition number has been filled in for you.)

Requisition Number	Date of Specimen Collected	Patient Name	Laboratory Test	Processing Laboratory	Initials: Specimen Collection	Date of Results Return	Initials: Results Return
112417							

Copyright © 2014, 2011, 2007 by Saunders, an imprint of Elsevier Inc. All rights reserved.

Exercise 5

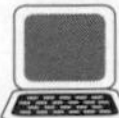

Online Activity—Adding Laboratory Results to the Flow Sheet

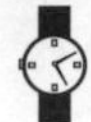

30 minutes

1. Using the flow sheet on the next page, transfer the test results recorded in Ms. Davison's Progress Notes for 5/1/07. In addition, add the following results, which were received by Dr. Meyer on 5/3/07:

   Blood chemistry

   - Alkaline phosphatase: 4
   - Bilirubin: 1.2
   - Serum glutamic oxaloacetic transaminase (SGOT): 14
   - Bicarbonate (CO2): 21
   - Calcium: 7.2
   - Chloride: 98
   - Creatinine: 0.6
   - Lactate dehydrogenase (LDH): 96
   - Glucose: 460
   - Potassium: 4.8
   - Total protein: 6.6
   - Sodium: 130
   - BUN: 18
   - Phosphorus: 3.2

   Thyroid profile

   - Thyroxine (T4): 10.8or
   - Triiodothyronine (T3): 185
   - Thyroid-stimulating hormone (TSH): 15.4 (normal values)
   - Cancer antigen (CA) 125: 3.6 (abnormal value)
   - Hemoglobin A1c: 10 (abnormal value)

   After you have charted all the results in the flow sheet, compare the results with the document entitled "Garrell's Common Chemistry Panels.pdf" located in the Simulations folder of your Evolve course. Place an asterisk (*) after any results that should be given prompt attention. Notations for normal and abnormal values have been included for tests that are not listed in the table.

Copyright © 2014, 2011, 2007 by Saunders, an imprint of Elsevier Inc. All rights reserved.

FLOW SHEET

Name: *Rhea Davison* **Date of Birth:** *08/16/1953* **Age:** *53*

Vital Signs Date:	05/01/07							
Weight	152 lbs							
Height	5 ft 1 in							
Temperature	98.6 F							
Pulse	86							
Respirations	24							
Blood Pressure	144/86							
Lab Tests Date:	05/01/07							
CBC								
RBC								
WBC								
HGB								
Hematocrit								
Alkaline Phosphatase								
Albumin								
Glucose								
Bilirubin total								
BUN								
Calcium								
Cholesterol								
Chloride								
CO2								
Creatinine								
HgbA1c								
LipidProfile								
LDL								
HDL								
Triglycerides								
SGGT								
SGOT/AST								
SGPT/ATL								
LDH								
T3								
T4								
T7								
TSH								
Triglycerides								
Total Protein								
Urea Nitrogen								
Sodium								
Potassium								
Urinalysis								
Albumin								
Glucose								
PAPSmear								
PSA								
Other tests:								

Copyright © 2014, 2011, 2007 by Saunders, an imprint of Elsevier Inc. All rights reserved.

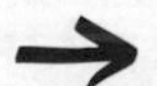

- Click **Close Chart** when finished to return to the Check Out area.
- Click the exit arrow in the lower right corner of the screen to exit the room.
- On the Summary Menu, click **Return to Map**, then click **Yes** at the pop-up menu to return to the Office Map or click **Exit the Program**.

Copyright © 2014, 2011, 2007 by Saunders, an imprint of Elsevier Inc. All rights reserved.

LESSON 31

Performing Immunology Testing

Reading Assignment: Chapter 41—Assisting in Obstetrics and Gynecology
- Diagnostic Testing

Chapter 52—Assisting in the Analysis of Urine
- Urine Pregnancy Testing

Chapter 55—Assisting in Microbiology
- Miscellaneous Microbiology Testing

Patients: Louise Parlet, Kevin McKinzie

Learning Objectives:

- Explain what information immunological tests can provide.
- Discuss what is meant by a false-negative result or false-positive result.
- Understand the importance of reading the package instructions before performing tests on a sample.
- Recognize when the antibody level is highest during an infection and when the antibody level starts to decline.
- Understand the importance of following directions for pregnancy testing.
- Describe the reaction that takes place in Mono testing.
- Document laboratory test results appropriately.

Overview:

In this lesson you will learn about the different types of immunology testing and the reasons this type of testing is used. A newly pregnant woman, Louise Parlet, provides urine for pregnancy testing and serology testing.

Copyright © 2014, 2011, 2007 by Saunders, an imprint of Elsevier Inc. All rights reserved.

Exercise 1

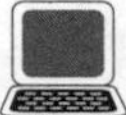

Online Activity—What Is Immunology Testing?

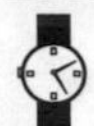

25 minutes

1. What information does immunological testing provide?

2. When does a person form antibodies?

3. Which antigens can cause the production of antibodies? Use your critical thinking skills while answering this question. Select all that apply.

_____ Viruses

_____ Bacteria

_____ Cat dander

_____ Electricity

_____ Pollen

_____ Water

_____ Earthworms

_____ Wheat

_____ Eggs

_____ Nuts (tree or ground)

Copyright © 2014, 2011, 2007 by Saunders, an imprint of Elsevier Inc. All rights reserved.

4. During which phase of a disease would the antibody level be the highest, and when does it start declining?

5. Which types of specimens can be used for immunology testing? Select all that apply.

_____ Feces

_____ Blood

_____ Urine

_____ Sputum

6. Which tests are based on immunology testing? Select all that apply.

_____ ABO blood typing

_____ QuickVue Mono test

_____ Hemoccult

_____ Sputum for acid-fast bacilla

_____ Syphilis titers

_____ VDRL

_____ Hepatitis titers

_____ CBC

_____ ASO test

7. Describe what is meant by a false-positive or false-negative test.

8. A false-negative result for immunology tests may be referred to as the ________________ ________________.

Copyright © 2014, 2011, 2007 by Saunders, an imprint of Elsevier Inc. All rights reserved.

9. What are the dangers of false-positive and false-negative test results? Apply critical thinking skills to answer this question.

10. Before performing any test, what should the medical assistant do once the test kit is opened?

11. Why is this step so important?

12. What is the name of the acute infectious disease that is also referred to as the "kissing disease"?

13. Patients of what age range are more frequently affected by mononucleosis?

Copyright © 2014, 2011, 2007 by Saunders, an imprint of Elsevier Inc. All rights reserved.

14. What virus causes mononucleosis?

15. Discuss the antigen-antibody reaction in the Mono tests.

- Sign in to Mountain View Clinic.
- Select **Kevin McKinzie** from the patient list.
- Click on **Check Out**.
- Click on **Charts**.
- Click on the **Patient Medical Information** tab and select **1-Progress Notes**.

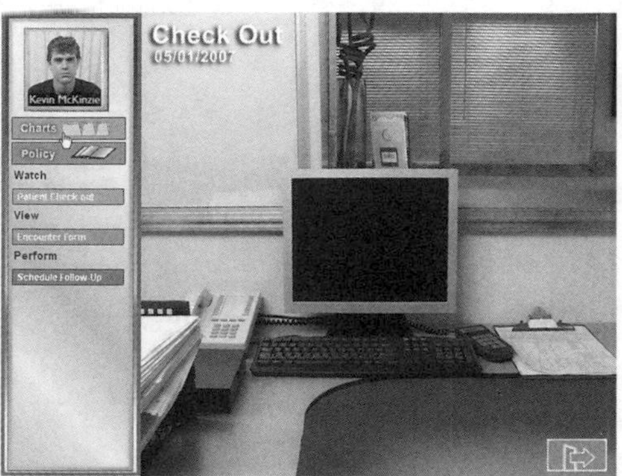

16. What was the result of Mr. McKinzie's QuickVue Mono test?

17. What type of specimen was used for this screening?

- Click **Close Chart** to return to the Check Out area.
- Click the exit arrow.
- Click **Return to Map**, then click **Yes** at the pop-up menu to return to the office map.

Copyright © 2014, 2011, 2007 by Saunders, an imprint of Elsevier Inc. All rights reserved.

Exercise 2

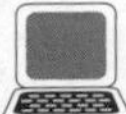

Online Activity—Immunology Testing with Urine Pregnancy Testing

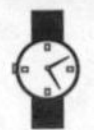

40 minutes

In this exercise you will work with Louise Parlet, a newly pregnant patient. She has performed a pregnancy test at home that was positive and has now come to the physician's office to verify the pregnancy.

1. The most common type of test used for pregnancy testing is the ____________________ ____________________ ____________________.

2. What substance in urine is present and produces a positive pregnancy test?

3. When is the substance you identified in question 2 at its highest peak in plasma?

4. Identify whether each of the following statements is true or false.

   a. _________ hCG is first apparent as early as 1 week after implantation or 4 to 5 days before a missed menstrual period.

   b. _________ The level of hCG remains the same throughout pregnancy.

   c. _________ Most pregnancy tests take 20 minutes to perform.

   d. _________ The best urine specimen to use for a pregnancy test is the first morning specimen.

   e. _________ When properly used, urine pregnancy tests are only 75% effective.

   f. _________ Pregnancy tests do not have built in "controls" to ensure that the test is performed correctly.

   g. _________ If a pregnancy test is performed early in the pregnancy, the test should be repeated later to confirm results.

Copyright © 2014, 2011, 2007 by Saunders, an imprint of Elsevier Inc. All rights reserved.

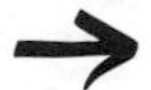

- Select Louise Parlet from the patient list.
- Click on **Exam Room**.
- Under the Watch heading, click on **Urine Specimen Collection** and watch the video.
- Click the **X** on the video screen to close the video.
- Under the Watch heading, click on **CLIA-Waived Testing** and watch the video.

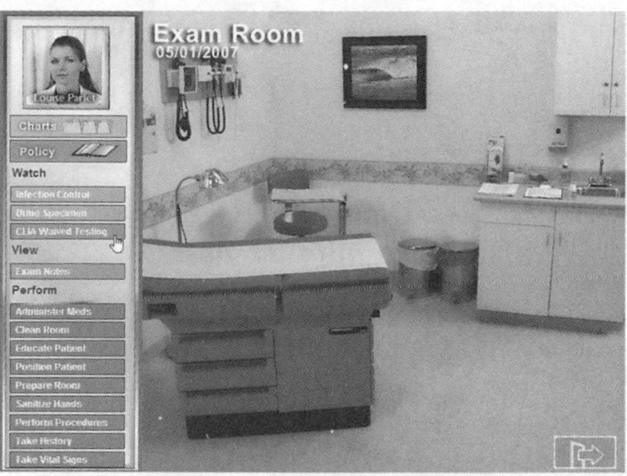

5. Ms. Parlet states that she has waited to void until her appointment. Why is the first-voided specimen more likely to provide accurate test results?

6. Why is it important for Ms. Parlet to collect a clean-catch midstream urine specimen?

7. The medical assistant who is training the student tells her that they do not keep a large inventory of pregnancy tests. What does she state as the reason for this?

8. How many drops of urine are supposed to be used in this particular test kit?

9. How long should the medical assistant wait before reading the results?

Copyright © 2014, 2011, 2007 by Saunders, an imprint of Elsevier Inc. All rights reserved.

- Click the **X** on the video screen to close the video.
- Click on **Policy** to open the office Policy Manual.
- Type "standing orders" and click on the magnifying glass.
- Read the policies on Pregnancy Testing that are part of the standing orders for this office.

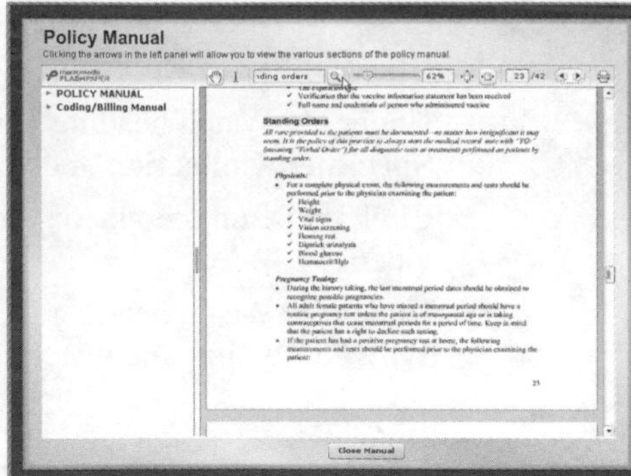

10. Why could the medical assistant perform a pregnancy test on Louise Parlet without a specific order from the physician?

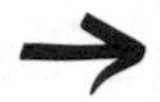

- Click **Close Manual** to return to the Exam Room.
- Click on the **Exam Notes** file folder and read the documentation for Louise Parlet's visit.

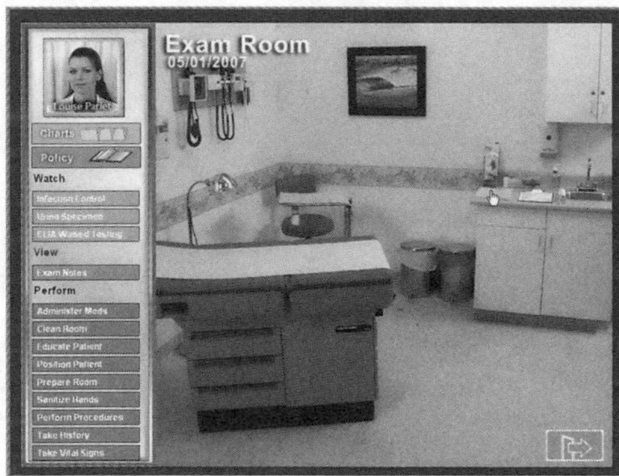

11. According to the Exam Notes, what other immunology tests were ordered for Ms. Parlet?

Copyright © 2014, 2011, 2007 by Saunders, an imprint of Elsevier Inc. All rights reserved.

12. Joan Smith, born 7/28/1982, has come to Mountain View Clinic for a pregnancy test. Below, accurately document this test and its result, which was negative. This is the second testing of Joan Smith's urine using a QuickVue test. Use today's date and time. Be sure to sign the entry.

PATIENT'S NAME ______________________ ☐FEMALE ☐MALE Date of Birth: ___/___/___

DATE	PATIENT VISITS AND FINDINGS

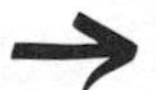

- Click **Finish** to return to the Exam Room.
- Click the exit arrow.
- Click **Return to Map**, then click **Yes** at the pop-up menu to return to the office map or click **Exit the Program**.

Copyright © 2014, 2011, 2007 by Saunders, an imprint of Elsevier Inc. All rights reserved.

LESSON 32

Wrapping Items for Sterilization

Reading Assignment: Chapter 56—Surgical Supplies and Instruments
- Care and Handling of Instruments

Chapter 57—Surgical Asepsis and Assisting with Surgical Procedures
- Sterilization
- Procedure 57-1
- Table 57-2

Patient: Jose Imero

Learning Objectives:

- Identify the things to check for proper working order when instruments are received in the medical office.
- Identify reasons for performing sanitization before sterilization.
- State the reason for using indicator strips in sterilization techniques and quality control.
- Identify the items needed for wrapping articles for sterilization.
- Sequence the steps required for wrapping items for sterilization.
- Match causes of improper sterilization with problems that will result if the proper technique is not followed.
- Discuss the storage requirements for items that have been autoclaved.

Overview:

In most cases, items that will come in contact with body tissues must be sterile. After a reusable item has been used for a patient, that item is sanitized and then prepared for sterilization. Preparation for sterilization of items that must remain sterile requires wrapping the item for storage after sterilization. A certain technique is necessary when wrapping items for the autoclave. We will review this technique in this lesson.

Copyright © 2014, 2011, 2007 by Saunders, an imprint of Elsevier Inc. All rights reserved.

Exercise 1

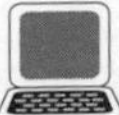

Online Activity—Sanitizing and Sterilizing Equipment

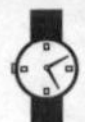

45 minutes

1. What are some of the things that you should check to ensure that new instruments are in good working order after you receive them from a supply company?

2. What does it mean to sanitize equipment?

3. When do instruments need to be sanitized?

4. If instruments cannot be sanitized immediately, what should you do?

5. What is the rationale for soaking instruments before sanitization?

Copyright © 2014, 2011, 2007 by Saunders, an imprint of Elsevier Inc. All rights reserved.

6. What should the medical assistant wear while sanitizing sharp instruments?

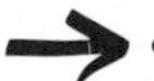

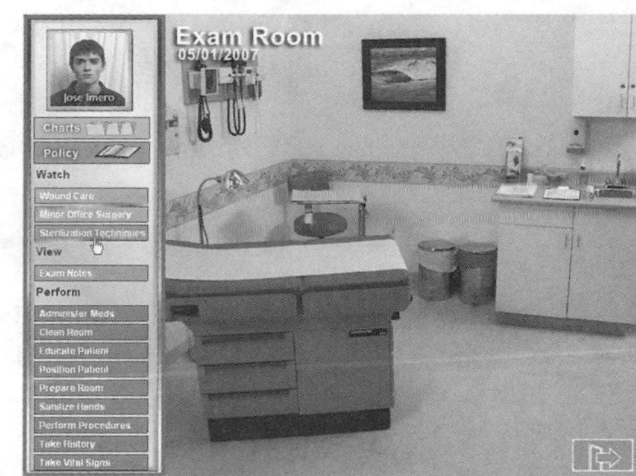

- Sign in to Mountain View Clinic.
- Select **Jose Imero** from the patient list.
- Click on **Exam Room**.
- Under the Watch heading, click on **Sterilization Techniques** and watch the video.
- Click the **X** on the video screen to close the video.
- Click on **Policy** to open the office Policy Manual.
- Type "instruments" in the search bar and click on the magnifying glass.
- Read about who is responsible for the sterilization of instruments.

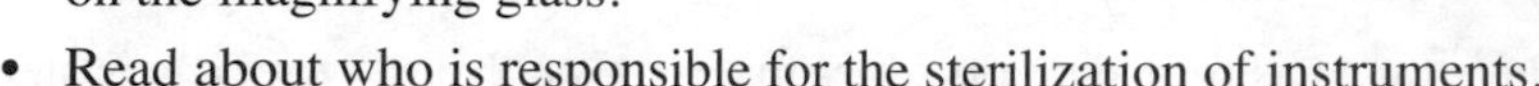

7. In the video, Charlie asks Danielle whether she has counted the instruments to see whether everything needed is on the tray. Why do you think he asked this question?

8. Why do you think Charlie asked whether the indicator strip was "in date"?

Copyright © 2014, 2011, 2007 by Saunders, an imprint of Elsevier Inc. All rights reserved.

9. What is the reason for the indicator strip?

10. Which supplies are needed when wrapping instruments and equipment for sterilization? Select all that apply.

_____ Wrapping paper or cloth/sterilization pouches

_____ Waterproof, felt-tipped pen

_____ Sterilization indicator

_____ Pencil

_____ Autoclave tape

11. If your autoclave tape has turned colors, does this indicate that the package is sterile? Support your answer.

12. Why is it important to make sure the wrapping material is an appropriate size for the item being wrapped? Use your critical thinking skills while answering this question.

13. Charlie told Danielle to begin with the wrapping material in a diamond shape. Why is this important when wrapping articles for sterilization?

Copyright © 2014, 2011, 2007 by Saunders, an imprint of Elsevier Inc. All rights reserved.

14. Indicate whether each of the following statements is true or false.

a. _________ When instruments with movable parts are being wrapped, the joint should be closed to prevent moisture from adhering to the instrument and causing rust.

b. _________ When instruments with sharp edges are being wrapped, the edges should first be wrapped in gauze.

c. _________ The sterilization strip shows that the package has been sterilized.

d. _________ Autoclave tape indicates that the package is sterile.

e. _________ Any ballpoint pen is acceptable for labeling a package for the autoclave.

f. _________ The first fold made in wrapping an instrument should be the fold closest to your body at the bottom of the package.

15. What information should appear on the label of a wrapped article for the autoclave? Select all that apply.

_____ Type of instrument or equipment found in the package

_____ Indicator strip inside

_____ Date of sterilization

_____ Initials of person preparing package

_____ Expiration date for the package

16. Match the columns below to show the correct sequence of steps in wrapping an instrument for autoclaving.

	Action	Step Number
_____	Fold the bottom corner of the wrap toward the center and fold a tab.	a. Step 1
_____	Open any hinged instruments	b. Step 2
_____	Place the autoclave tape across the outside corner.	c. Step 3
_____	Place the item(s) diagonally at the approximate center of the wrapping material.	d. Step 4
_____	Fold each side of the wrap into the center, leaving a tab on each side.	e. Step 5
_____	Place a sterilization indicator in the pack	f. Step 6

Copyright © 2014, 2011, 2007 by Saunders, an imprint of Elsevier Inc. All rights reserved.

17. Below are problems that may be experienced when autoclaving instruments. Match each problem with its possible cause.

	Problem	**Causes**
_____	Ebullition	a. Too rapid exhausting of the chamber
_____	Corroded instruments	b. Vacuum in the chamber
_____	Damp linens	c. Dirty chamber
_____	Steam leakage	d. Poor cleaning
_____	Stained linens	e. Corrosion or soil in the joint
_____	Spotted or stained instruments	f. Clogged chamber drain
_____	Chamber door not opening	g. Mineral deposits on instruments
_____	Instruments with soft hinges or joints	h. Worn gasket

18. Once the medical assistant has sterilized the instruments, how should they be stored?

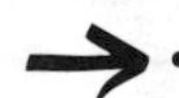

- Click the **X** in the upper right corner to close the video and return to the Exam Room.
- Click the exit arrow in the lower right corner of the screen to exit the room.
- On the Summary Menu, click **Return to Map** and select **Yes** at the pop-up menu to return to the Office Map or click **Exit the Program**.

Copyright © 2014, 2011, 2007 by Saunders, an imprint of Elsevier Inc. All rights reserved.

Exercise 2

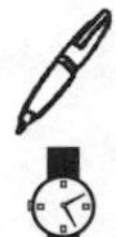

Writing Activity—Identifying Instruments Used in the Medical Office

15 minutes

Identify the following images of instruments by choosing the correct name.

1. Scissors

Images	Names
_____ 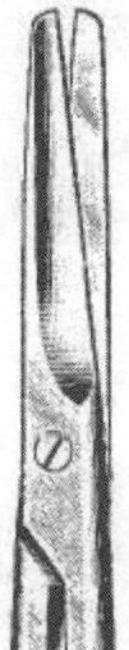	a. Lister bandage scissors
	b. Littauer suture scissors straight
	c. Mayo dissecting scissors curved
	d. Mayo dissecting scissors straight
	e. Operating scissors sharp-blunt
	f. Operating scissors sharp-sharp
_____ 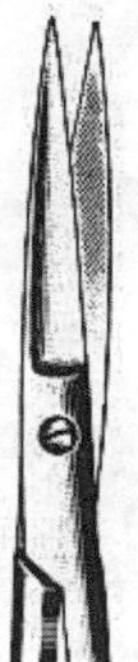	g. Operating scissors straight
_____ 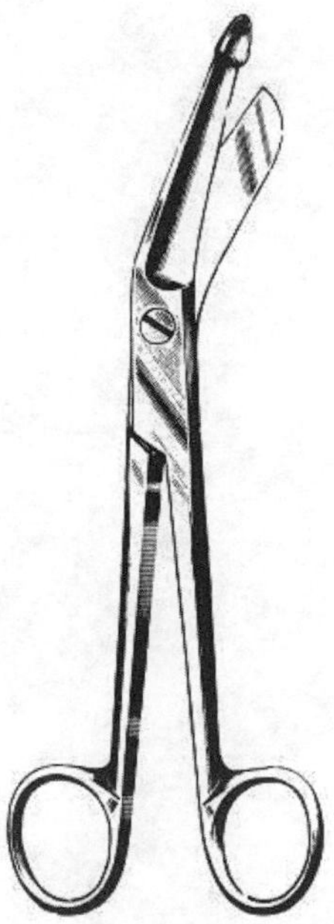	

Copyright © 2014, 2011, 2007 by Saunders, an imprint of Elsevier Inc. All rights reserved.

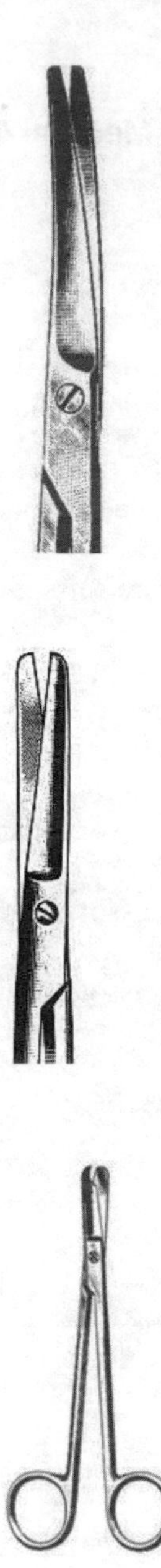

Copyright © 2014, 2011, 2007 by Saunders, an imprint of Elsevier Inc. All rights reserved.

2. Thumb Forceps

Images **Names**

_____ 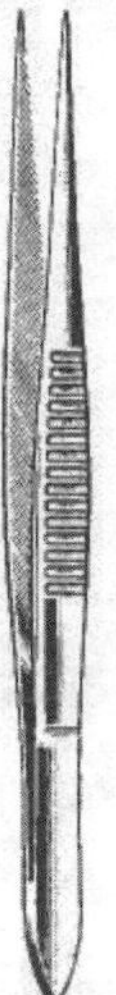

_____ 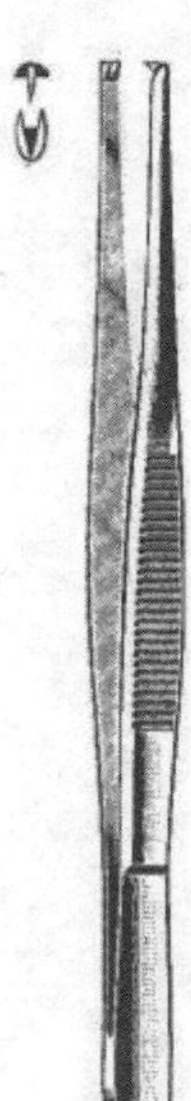

a. Adson dressing forceps

b. Plain splinter forceps

c. Standard tissue forceps

d. Straight thumb forceps

Copyright © 2014, 2011, 2007 by Saunders, an imprint of Elsevier Inc. All rights reserved.

_____ 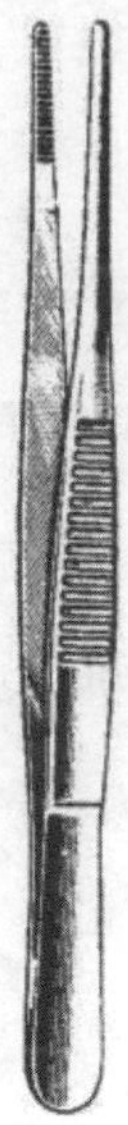

_____ 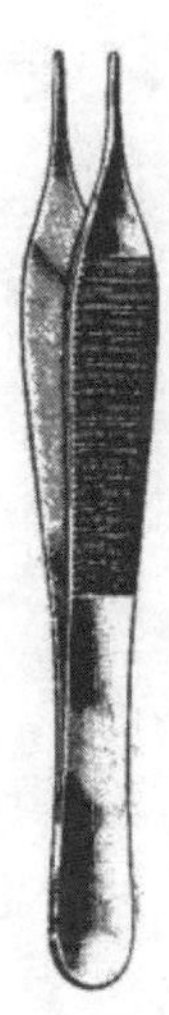

Copyright © 2014, 2011, 2007 by Saunders, an imprint of Elsevier Inc. All rights reserved.

3. Ring-Handled Forceps

Images	Names
____	a. Allis tissue forceps
	b. Foerster sponge forceps
	c. Halsted mosquito hemostatic forceps
	d. Kelly hemostatic forceps
	e. Ochsner-Kocher hemostatic forceps
	f. Rochester-Pean hemostatic forceps

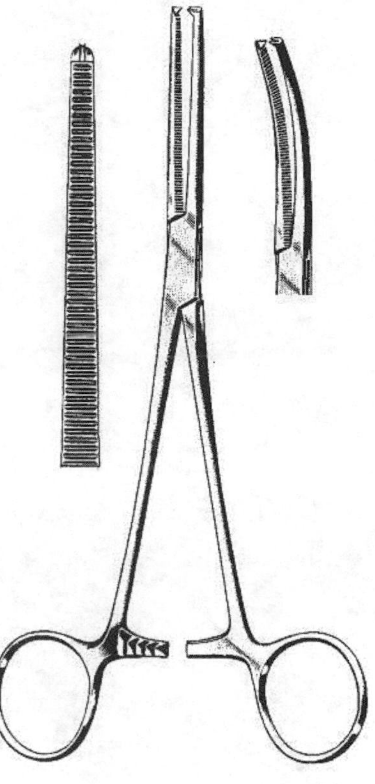

____

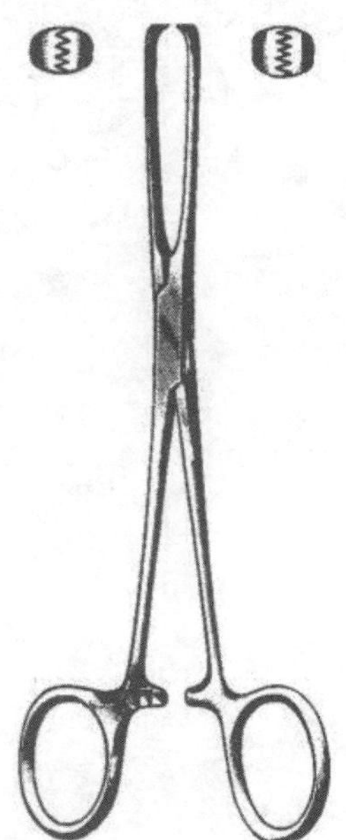

Copyright © 2014, 2011, 2007 by Saunders, an imprint of Elsevier Inc. All rights reserved.

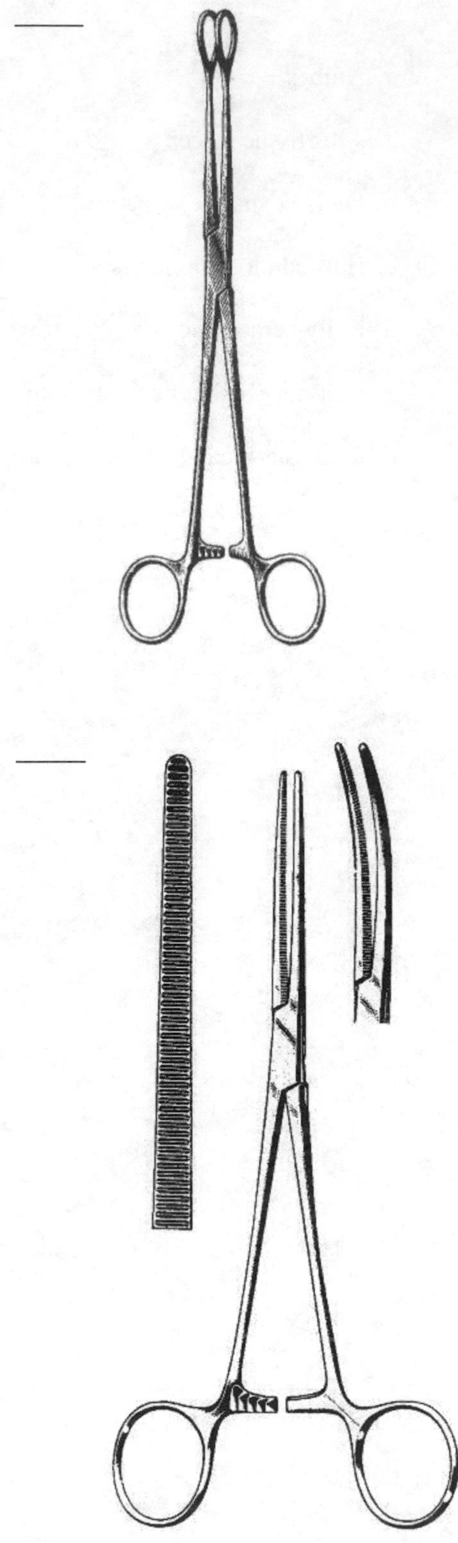

Copyright © 2014, 2011, 2007 by Saunders, an imprint of Elsevier Inc. All rights reserved.

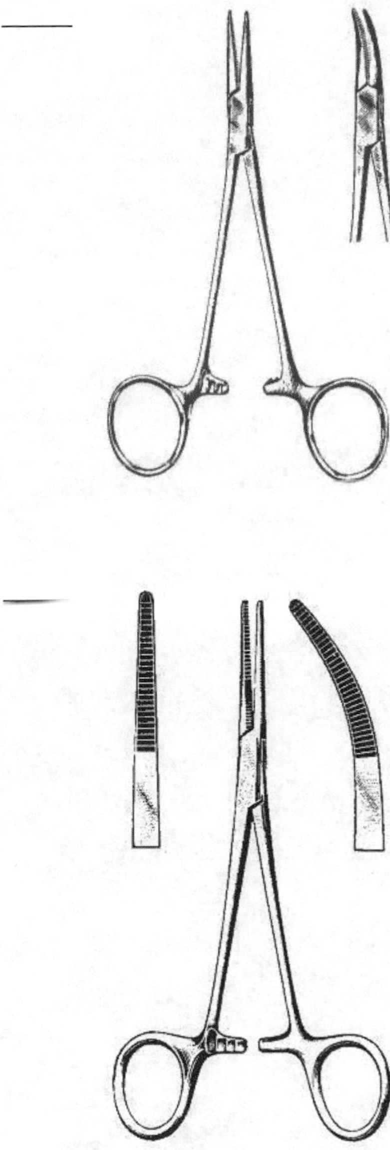

Copyright © 2014, 2011, 2007 by Saunders, an imprint of Elsevier Inc. All rights reserved.

LESSON 33

Assisting with Minor Office Surgery

Reading Assignment: Chapter 56—Surgical Supplies and Instruments
Chapter 57—Surgical Asepsis and Assisting with Surgical Procedures
- Surgical Procedures
- Assisting with Surgical Procedures
- Wound Care

Patients: Jose Imero, Tristan Tsosie

Learning Objectives:

- Identify instruments by their use or function.
- Understand the importance of good communication skills when preparing the patient for suture removal.
- Describe the importance of infection control and sterile aseptic technique with minor surgery.
- Understand appropriate disposal of biohazardous materials when performing wound care.
- Identify instructions given to the patient during minor office surgery regarding the care of the wound and returning for suture removal.
- Discuss the need for patient education after suturing a laceration and after removing sutures.
- Chart entries pertaining to minor office surgery and suture removal.
- Apply critical thinking skills in regard to patient education related to minor office surgery.

Overview:

This lesson focuses on the medical assistant's role in assisting the physician with minor office surgery. You will observe and evaluate the medical assistant's preparation of patient Jose Imero for suturing of lacerations. Another patient, Tristan Tsosie, has a laceration that needs suture removal. The necessary steps for this will be shown and evaluated.

Copyright © 2014, 2011, 2007 by Saunders, an imprint of Elsevier Inc. All rights reserved.

Exercise 1

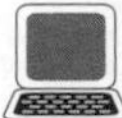

Online Activity—Assisting with Minor Office Surgery

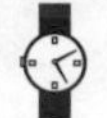

45 minutes

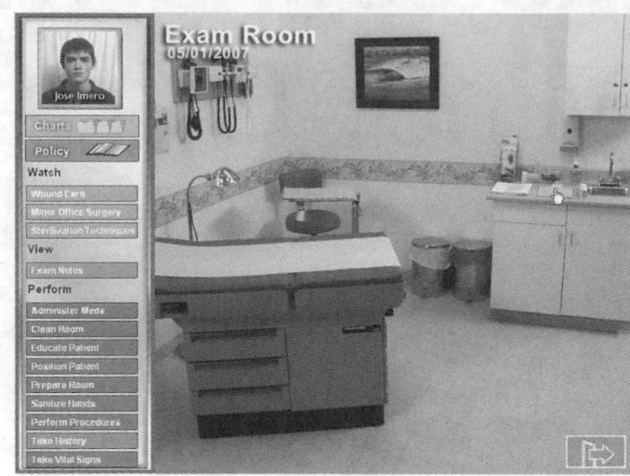

- Sign in to Mountain View Clinic.
- Select **Jose Imero** from the patient list.
- Click on **Exam Room**.
- Click on the **Medical Record** clipboard.
- Click on the **Ask** buttons to view the patient's answers to the questions regarding his medical history.
- Record the information into the patient's medical record in the box under "Document all findings below." Enter your name after your documentation as requested by your instructor.
- At the bottom of the page, click **Next** to view additional questions and responses related to the Jose Imero's history.
- Use the checkboxes to select any other information you would need to ask Jose Imero.
- If requested by your instructor, print the information by clicking on **Print** at the bottom of the screen.
- Click **Finish** to close the History Taking window and answer **Yes** at the pop-up window to return to the Exam Room.

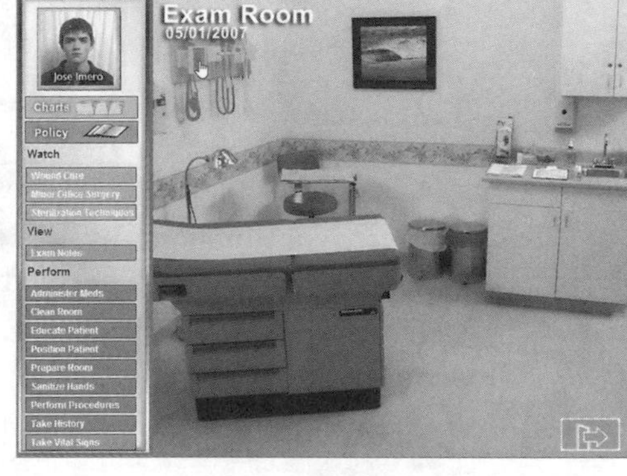

- Click on the **Vital Signs Wall Unit**.
- Click **Take Blood Pressure**.
- Record the readings in the appropriate box at the bottom of the screen.
- Repeat this for all vital signs.
- If any of the patient's results are abnormal, check the box next to "Check if Physician needs to be notified of abnormality."
- Click **Finish** to return to the Exam Room.
- Click on the **Exam Notes** file folder and read the documentation for Jose Imero's visit regarding the procedures he is to have performed during his examination and the patient instructions.
- Click **Finish** to return to the Exam Room.

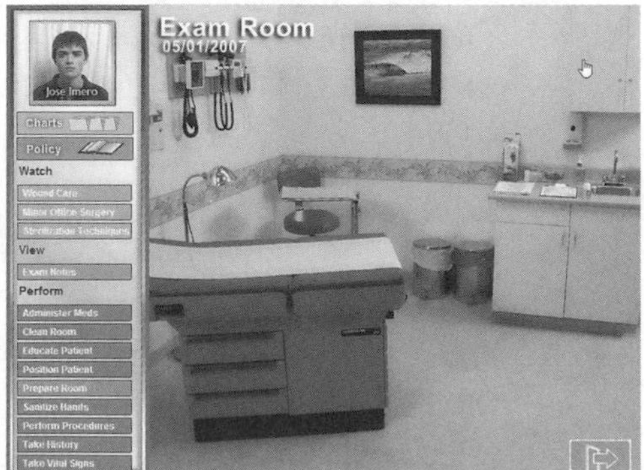

- Click on the **Supply Cabinet**.
- From the list of Available Supplies, click on **Wound Care** and review the contents on the tray as shown in the photograph.

Copyright © 2014, 2011, 2007 by Saunders, an imprint of Elsevier Inc. All rights reserved.

1. Listed below are the supplies provided for wound care as shown in the photograph from the Prepare Room wizard. Explain why you think each item is needed.

Sterile water or saline—

Surgical soap—

Gauze pads—

Gloves—

Antiseptic swabs—

→ • From the list of Available Supplies, click on **Surgical Supply Tray** and review the tray's contents as shown in the photograph.

2. What disposable supplies are found on the supply tray that will be needed for the suturing of Jose's foot? (*Note:* You can check your answers when you watch the video later in this exercise.)

(1)

(2)

(3)

(4)

(5)

(6)

(7)

→ • Next, click on **Surgical Instrument Tray** in the Available Supplies list. Again, review the tray's contents as shown in the photograph.

3. In the video that you will be watching, Dr. Hayler will specifically state that he is going to probe Jose's wound for possible foreign objects. With that information, what sterile materials necessary for preparing to suture a laceration are missing from the surgical instrument tray?

Copyright © 2014, 2011, 2007 by Saunders, an imprint of Elsevier Inc. All rights reserved.

4. Match each of the following surgical instruments with its use or description.

	Instrument	Use or Description
_____	Scalpel	a. Used to find foreign objects in a wound
_____	Forceps	b. Used for grasping and squeezing
_____	Operating scissors	c. Used to open or distend orifice or cavity
_____	Hemostats	d. Have straight sharp blades for cutting through tissue
_____	Needle holders	e. Small surgical knife used to cut through tissue
_____	Retractors	f. Used to pull back tissue and skin
_____	Speculum	g. Forceps-like instrument used to hold circular needles
_____	Suture scissors	h. Used to clamp blood vessels and to hold tissue
_____	Probe	i. Forceps with straight sharp points for removing foreign objects from wounds
_____	Splinter forceps	
		j. Scissors used to cut sutures

- Add the supplies needed for the patient's exam by clicking on the supply from the Available Supplies list and clicking **Add Item** to confirm your choice.
- If you wish to remove a chosen supply, highlight the supply in the Selected Supplies box and click **Remove**.
- Repeat this step until you are satisfied you have everything you need from the list.
- Click **Finish** to return to the Exam Room.
- Under the Watch heading, click on **Wound Care** and watch the video.

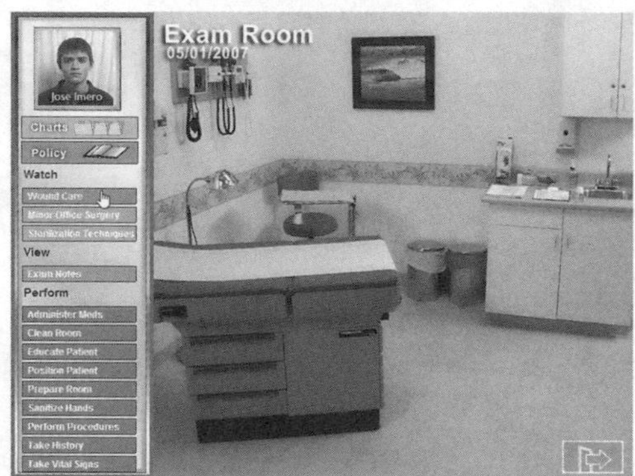

5. Why do you think the red bag was taped onto the Mayo stand?

6. Why did Charlie place a protective sheet under Jose's foot?

Copyright © 2014, 2011, 2007 by Saunders, an imprint of Elsevier Inc. All rights reserved.

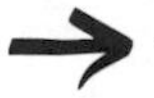

- Click the **X** on the video screen to close the video.
- Under the Watch heading, click on **Minor Office Surgery** and watch the video.
- While watching this video, look for a distinct break in sterile technique.

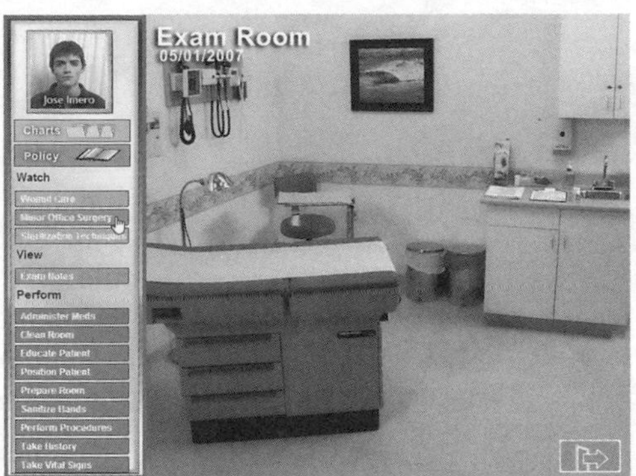

7. What is the break in sterile technique that Charlie allows to happen?

8. Why was it important that Charlie pass the suture material around the surgical tray?

9. Apply critical thinking skills and your knowledge from the chapter and chart to indicate whether each of the following statements is true or false.

   a. ________ The medical assistant is responsible for supplying a light source when assisting with minor surgery.

   b. ________ When setting a sterile field, the entire area is considered sterile.

   c. ________ When preparing a tray for suturing during minor surgery, it is most time efficient to place the instruments in the order of use.

   d. ________ The medical assistant should pay close attention as the surgery is being performed so he or she can anticipate anything with which the physician will need assistance.

   e. ________ Once a minor surgery suture tray has been set, the medical assistant cannot add instruments or supplies to the tray.

   f. ________ Surgical scissors may have sharp blades, blunt blades, or a combination of the two.

   g. ________ When assisting with minor surgery, the medical assistant must always use sterile gloves.

Copyright © 2014, 2011, 2007 by Saunders, an imprint of Elsevier Inc. All rights reserved.

h. _________ The application of sterile gloves requires a different technique from the application of nonsterile gloves.

i. _________ When pouring a solution onto a sterile field, the medical assistant should first pour the solution over the lip of the container into a waste receptacle container that is not on the sterile field and then discard it; the solution should then be poured into the sterile container on the sterile field (this applies to containers that do not have a double-cap system).

j. _________ When opening a sterile pack, the flap closest to you should be opened first.

k. _________ Suture material is always the same for each wound and each physician.

l. _________ Suture material comes in absorbable and nonabsorbable types.

m. _________ Absorbable suture is usually used for deep incisions or lacerations that require inner layers of sutures to close the wound.

n. _________ Nonabsorbable suture is usually used for deep tissue.

o. _________ Suture material comes in varying sizes, lengths, and absorbability.

p. _________ Skin may be closed with staples and adhesive skin closures.

q. _________ Selection of suture material depends on the site, length, and depth of the wound.

r. _________ According to the chart notes, Jose had 16 sutures placed in his foot.

10. What instructions did Dr. Hayler give Jose as he was suturing his laceration?

11. Why did Dr. Hayler tell Jose to use the crutches?

Copyright © 2014, 2011, 2007 by Saunders, an imprint of Elsevier Inc. All rights reserved.

Critical Thinking Question

12. Identify some of the other reasons patients must be given instructions to follow when they have had an area sutured.

13. What was one other measure Dr. Hayler took to prevent Jose from getting an infection? (*Hint:* You may wish to reopen the Exam Notes in the Exam Room.)

14. What other instructions were given to the patient according to the Exam Notes?

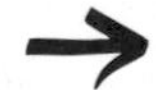

- Click the **X** on the video screen to close the video.
- Click the exit arrow.
- On the Summary Menu, click on **Look at Your Performance Summary**.
- Scroll down the Performance Summary to the Prepare Room, Take History, and Take Vital Signs sections and compare your answers with those chosen by the experts. The summary can be printed or saved for your instructor.
- Click **Close** to return to the Summary Menu.
- On the Summary Menu, click **Return to Map** and select **Yes** at the pop-up menu to return to the Office Map.

Copyright © 2014, 2011, 2007 by Saunders, an imprint of Elsevier Inc. All rights reserved.

Exercise 2

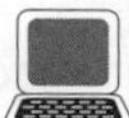

Online Activity—Assisting with Suture Removal

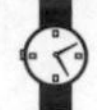

20 minutes

Your instructor may indicate that watching the video is an optional assignment. In an earlier lesson, we watched Tristan Tsosie's wound care video and prepared his room for wound care.

- Select **Tristan Tsosie** from the patient list.
- Click on **Exam Room**.
- Under the Watch heading, click on **Wound Care** and watch the video.

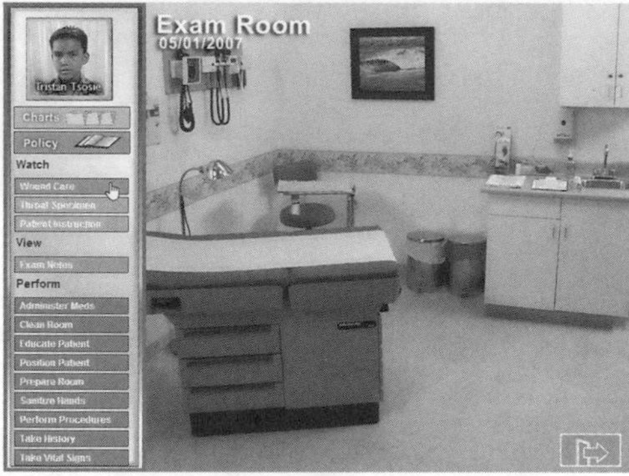

1. Tristan had a wound culture taken. When should the cleansing of the wound take place?

2. When the medical assistant was preparing Tristan for the removal of sutures, Tristan asked whether the procedure would hurt. Should the medical assistant have answered the question before continuing with the procedure, or was it effective communication to ignore the question at that point?

Critical Thinking Question

3. Why do you think Tristan asked if it was going to hurt?

Copyright © 2014, 2011, 2007 by Saunders, an imprint of Elsevier Inc. All rights reserved.

Critical Thinking Question

4. Would you expect most children to be as calm as Tristan was?

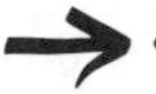

- Click the **X** on the video screen to close the video.
- Click on the **Supply Cabinet**.
- From the list of Available Supplies, click on **Suture Removal** and review the tray's contents as shown in the photo.
- The tray contains surgical soap, nonsterile gloves, sterile gloves, bandaging materials, gauze pads, suture-removing scissors, forceps, and a protective drape.

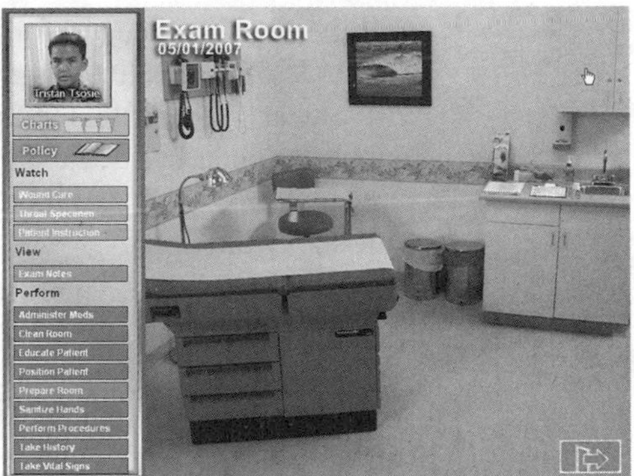

5. When removing sutures, what supplies should be sterile and what supplies can be aseptically clean?

6. Indicate whether each of the following statements is true or false. Remember to use critical thinking skills in addition to your knowledge from the reading assignment.

a. _________ Before removing sutures, the medical assistant should obtain the permission of the physician.

b. _________ If the wound appears to gape open during suture removal and the physician has stated that all sutures should be removed, the medical assistant should continue to remove the sutures.

c. _________ When sutures are being removed, the patient should be placed in a comfortable position to prevent injury or unnecessary discomfort.

d. _________ Following injury, all sutures will be ready to be removed at the same time.

Copyright © 2014, 2011, 2007 by Saunders, an imprint of Elsevier Inc. All rights reserved.

e. _________ The size and location of the wound are important factors that the physician will take into consideration when instructing the patient when to return to the office for suture removal.

f. _________ All sutures may be removed using the same size suture scissors and forceps, regardless of the location of the sutures.

g. _________ When cleansing the area before removing the sutures, the skin should be thoroughly cleansed and the dry exudate should be removed.

h. _________ When removing sutures, it is not important to count the sutures removed, since you need to remove only those you can see.

- Add the supplies needed for the patient's examination by clicking on the supply from the Available Supplies list and clicking **Add Item** to confirm your choice. The items you select will appear in the Selected Supplies box. When you click on an item, a photograph of that item will appear, which can be used for reference as you review your list of supplies. (*Note:* You can reopen the Exam Notes located in the lower left corner for reference as you make your selections.)
- If you wish to remove a chosen supply, highlight the supply in the Selected Supplies box and click **Remove**.
- Repeat these steps until you are satisfied you have everything you need from the list.
- Once you have made your selections, click **Finish** to return to the Exam Room.

- Click on the **Waste Receptacles**.
- Use the checkboxes to select the appropriate steps necessary to clean the Exam Room after Tristan's examination.
- Click **Finish** to return to the Exam Room.

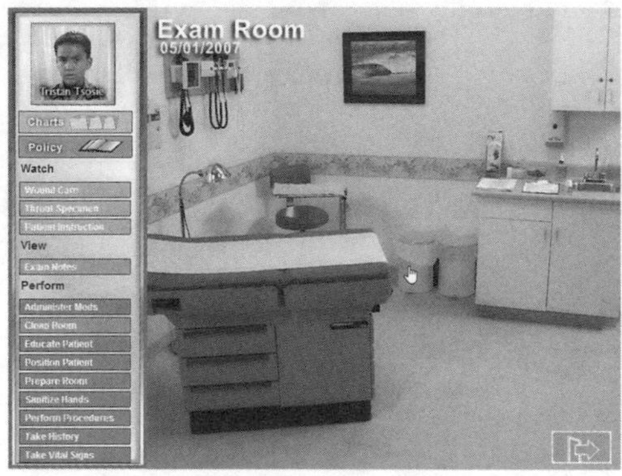

7. Why was it important for Tristan to keep his arm covered and splinted as the physician instructed?

Copyright © 2014, 2011, 2007 by Saunders, an imprint of Elsevier Inc. All rights reserved.

8. Below, document the removal of sutures from a clean wound on Tristan Tsosie's leg. The sutures were inserted 6 days earlier Be sure to document that the physician, Dr. Hayler, has observed the sutures and has told you to remove these seven sutures. Also document the dressing of the wound following removal and that the patient did not seem to have any problems. Use today's date for the documentation and your initials for the entry.

PATIENT'S NAME ______________________ ☐FEMALE ☐MALE Date of Birth: ___/___/___

DATE	PATIENT VISITS AND FINDINGS

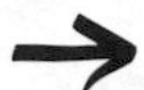

- Click the exit arrow.
- On the Summary Menu, click on **Look at Your Performance Summary**.
- Scroll down the Performance Summary to the Clean Room and Prepare Room sections and compare your answers with those chosen by the experts.
- You may save and print the Performance Summary for your records or turn it in to your instructor. The icons for saving and printing the Performance Summary are located at the top right corner of the screen.
- Click **Close** to return to the Summary Menu.
- On the Summary Menu, click **Return to Map**, then click **Yes** at the pop-up menu to return to the Office Map or click **Exit the Program**.

Copyright © 2014, 2011, 2007 by Saunders, an imprint of Elsevier Inc. All rights reserved.